THE RIGHT TEST

A Physician's Guide to Laboratory Medicine

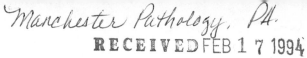

THE
RIGHT
TEST

A Physician's Guide
to Laboratory Medicine

2nd Edition

Carl E. Speicher, M.D.

Director, Clinical Laboratories,
The Ohio State University Hospitals
Professor and Vice-Chairman,
Department of Pathology
The Ohio State University
Columbus, Ohio

W.B. SAUNDERS COMPANY
A Division of Harcourt Brace & Company
Philadelphia   London   Toronto   Montreal   Sydney   Tokyo

W.B. Saunders Company
A Division of
Harcourt Brace & Company

The Curtis Center
Independence Square West
Philadelphia, Pennsylvania 19106

Library of Congress Cataloging-in-Publication Data

Speicher, Carl E.
   The right test: a physician's guide to laboratory medicine / Carl
E. Speicher.—2nd ed.
     p.   cm.
   Includes bibliographical references and index.
   ISBN 0-7216-3782-5
   1. Diagnosis, Laboratory—Handbooks, manuals, etc. I. Title.
   [DNLM: 1. Diagnosis, Laboratory—handbooks.   QY 39 S742r]
RB38.2.S64   1993
616.07′5—dc20
DNLM/DLC   92-49099

THE RIGHT TEST: A Physician's Guide to Laboratory Medicine   ISBN 0-7216-3782-5

Printed in the United States of America

Last digit is the print number: 9   8   7   6   5   4   3   2

To Our Patients

ACKNOWLEDGMENT

I am grateful to my colleagues and students at The Ohio State University as well as to my associates across the country for their help in formulating the ideas expressed in this book. Special thanks are extended to William Z. Borer, M.D., at the Thomas Jefferson University Hospital for his critical reading of the manuscript and his invaluable comments and suggestions; to Chris Anderson for her meticulous attention to committing these concepts to paper; and to John Dyson and Ray Kersey for their unhesitating, enthusiastic, and friendly support on behalf of the W. B. Saunders Company.

Carl E. Speicher, M.D.

PREFACE

In the context of ever-increasing health-care costs physicians are faced with the dilemma of providing optimal patient care at an affordable price. Since clinical laboratory tests are an important component of this care, a current guide to choosing and interpreting laboratory tests seems in order—hence, the second edition of *The Right Test*.

The warm reception of the first edition validates the Strunk and White format for presenting a short, user-friendly physician's guide to laboratory medicine.

In the second edition, I revised the original clinical problems and added a significant number of new problems with only a modest increase in the number of pages. The feedback from readers indicated that I should keep the book small. I accomplished this by eliminating the introductions to problems, using more tables, and restricting discussions to essential material. For additional information, readers are encouraged to consult the annotated bibliography at the end of each problem and the general bibliography at the end of the book.

Moreover, the second edition of *The Right Test* is in accordance with the national movement to develop practice parameters, which is being coordinated by the American Medical Association. The perception is that a significant percentage of all medical care is unnecessary and that practice parameters represent a way to improve the quality of health care and eliminate waste. In the area of laboratory medicine, the second edition of *The Right Test* provides parameters—authoritative whenever possible—to help achieve the best patient care at the lowest cost. Although hundreds of practice parameters are available, not many have received widespread endorsement. National medical societies are actively working with the American Medical Association to develop better parameters. In the absence of practice parameters for many patient-care problems, I have turned to the most authoritative sources available for laboratory medicine recommendations. Thus, I have tried to provide at least one good way to approach each patient-care problem that relies on laboratory medicine for its solution.

BIBLIOGRAPHY

Speicher CE: The Right Test, 1st ed. Philadelphia, WB Saunders Co, 1990, p vii.
Strunk W, White EB: The Elements of Style, 3rd ed. New York, Macmillan Publishing Co, 1979.

CONTENTS

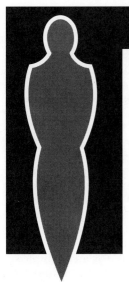

INTRODUCTION

Practice Parameters
Need for a Better Way for Physicians to Use
    Laboratory Tests
Decision-Making Model as a Framework for
    Laboratory Testing
Problem-Solving, Clinical Decision-Making
    Approach to Laboratory Testing
Useful Techniques for Interpreting Laboratory
    Data
Format for Discussing Medical Problems in This
    Book
Additional Considerations

In the United States a national effort is underway to improve the quality of patient care while eliminating waste. Examples of this effort include the development of practice parameters by the American Medical Association and national medical societies and the quality improvement and utilization review program of the Joint Commission on the Accreditation of Healthcare Organizations. In the context of this effort, there is a need to improve the quality and use of laboratory tests.

An aggravating factor is the escalating cost of health care. In 1990 spending on United States health care grew to $666 billion, an amount equal to 12.2% of the gross national product and representing a 10.5% increase over the previous year. In 1992, the annual cost of health care exceeded $800 billion. It has been estimated that laboratory tests are responsible for up to 10% of the total health care dollars.

Practice Parameters

Although widely used, the term *practice parameters* sometimes is not clearly understood. Practice parameters are simply recommendations to help physicians take care of their patients. The intent is to improve patient care and eliminate waste. Conceptually, there are several different kinds of parameters:

- **Standards:** should be followed exactly; strictly speaking, there are hardly any real standards.

1

- **Guidelines:** give limits that allow some freedom of choice.
- **Options:** provide a wider spectrum of choice than guidelines.
- **Nonoptions:** describe choices that are inappropriate or obsolete.

Practice parameters are the foundation for the recommendations in this book. If specific practice parameters are unavailable for particular patient-care problems, the most authoritative recommendations that can be found in the literature are used.

In the discussions of various problems in this book, the strongest type of recommendation is indicated by a simple imperative verb (e.g., **Use** the Pap smear to screen for cervical cancer in all women 18 years and older and in those women who have been sexually active regardless of age). A recommendation that allows more freedom of choice will often use the term *consider* (e.g., **Consider** testing for human papillomavirus [HPV] in cervical smear and biopsy specimens as tests become available). A nonoption is designated as follows: **Do not screen** for high serum cholesterol in patients who are acutely ill or pregnant, and **do not use** serum lipoprotein electrophoresis for general screening. The lupus erythematosus (LE) test is an example of an obsolete test. It should be replaced with a test for serum antinuclear antibody (ANA).

Need for a Better Way for Physicians to Use Laboratory Tests

More than 1000 individual tests are available to physicians each time they face a clinical decision that depends on laboratory tests, and it has been estimated that the number of new tests is growing at the rate of nearly one per week. The physician's task of learning about tests is often frustrating and time-consuming. It makes sense to organize the approach to laboratory testing in terms of a limited number of common and important clinical problems rather than an almost endless list of individual laboratory tests. These problems encompass a wide variety of test-dependent clinical decisions.

In applying a clinical decision-making approach to the use of laboratory tests, sound, scientifically based protocols for test ordering in common patient-care situations, although urgently needed, are not always available. Testing standards, guidelines, options, and nonoptions must be developed. The goal of appropriate laboratory testing can be conceptualized as follows:

AMOUNT AND KIND OF TESTING	OUTCOMES			
	POOR	AVERAGE	GOOD	EXCELLENT
Too little	A			
About right			C	X
Too much		B		(the ideal result)

Source: Adapted from Robert H. Brook, M.D., Director, Health Sciences Program, Rand Corporation, Santa Monica, Calif.

The goal is not *A*, *B*, or even *C*. It is *X*. To achieve the ideal result, physicians must not only choose the right tests, but they also must have the tests performed in an accredited laboratory. Moreover, the test results must be properly interpreted, and the appropriate therapy must be implemented.

Decision-Making Model as a Framework for Laboratory Testing

The decision-making model is a useful framework for characterizing the role of laboratory tests in clinical problem solving:

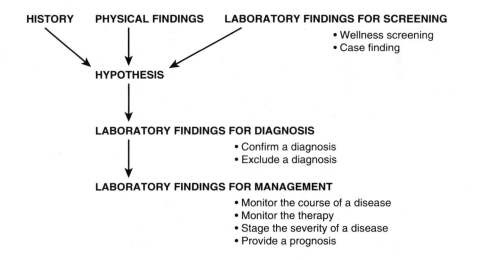

HISTORY   PHYSICAL FINDINGS   LABORATORY FINDINGS FOR SCREENING

• Wellness screening
• Case finding

HYPOTHESIS

LABORATORY FINDINGS FOR DIAGNOSIS

• Confirm a diagnosis
• Exclude a diagnosis

LABORATORY FINDINGS FOR MANAGEMENT

• Monitor the course of a disease
• Monitor the therapy
• Stage the severity of a disease
• Provide a prognosis

In addition to their use for diagnosis and management, laboratory tests are used for screening, of which there are two different types: (1) wellness screening, in which the individuals are asymptomatic and basically healthy; and (2) case finding, in which the individuals are symptomatic or have a disease (i.e., they are patients).

Test strategies for diagnosis, management, or screening may consist of single tests or combinations of tests. Test combinations in turn can be formulated in parallel, in series, or both. These test combinations are called *batteries*, *panels*, or *profiles* (the terms are used interchangeably). Serial serum creatine kinase–MB (CK-MB) determinations for the diagnosis of acute myocardial infarction (AMI) exemplify tests in series; the classic 12-test serum biochemical profile is an example of tests in parallel.

Test panels or profiles should be developed according to clinical decision-making requirements rather than according to which tests are more common or which tests a given instrument can perform. Although the serial CK-MB test panel was determined on the basis of clinical decision-making needs, the 12-test biochemical profile was determined on the basis of which tests could be done on a given instrument. In fact, testing panels should transcend laboratory instruments and laboratory disciplines alike. A good testing profile for the diagnosis of meningitis using cerebrospinal fluid transcends laboratory instruments and the combined laboratory disciplines of hematology, chemistry, and microbiology; a good testing profile for risk assessment for coronary heart disease (CHD) includes not just total serum cholesterol, but also high-density lipoprotein (HDL) cholesterol, low-density lipoprotein (LDL) cholesterol, and triglycerides.

Problem-Solving, Clinical Decision-Making Approach to Laboratory Testing

The effective use of laboratory data can be understood only in the context of the clinical decisions they influence. In addition to a requirement for generic problem-solving strategies, specific clinical decision-making approaches to using laboratory tests also are needed. The physician's task of managing a particular patient's problem comprises a series of clinical decisions. Some decisions rely heavily on laboratory tests for their solution; some decisions use test results as ancillary information to clinical, radiographic, or electrocardiographic data; and other decisions do not depend on laboratory tests at all.

The clinical, decision-oriented view of laboratory testing is a powerful one. For example, when caring for a patient with an AMI, physicians are confronted with a number of clinical decisions, some of which depend mainly, some only partially, and some not at all on laboratory tests:

DISCRETE CLINICAL DECISIONS WITHIN THE PROBLEM OF ACUTE MYOCARDIAL INFARCTION

CLINICAL DECISION	DEPENDENCE ON LABORATORY TESTS
Deciding to admit the emergency department patient with chest pain	NO—although a positive CK/CK-MB test result could detect an unexpected AMI
Diagnosing AMI in the coronary care unit	YES—serial CK/CK-MB tests are the gold standard for diagnosis
Estimating the size of an AMI	PARTIALLY—although the prognostic information may not be reliable
Diagnosing AMI in the post-noncardiac surgery patient	YES—similar to diagnosing AMI in the coronary care unit
Deciding to use thrombolytic therapy in a patient with AMI	NO—therapy should be initiated prior to CK/CK-MB elevations
Evaluating the effectiveness of thrombolytic therapy for AMI	PARTIALLY—an early rise in serum CK/CK-MB can signal reperfusion of ischemic muscle

Source: Speicher CE: Decision-oriented test request forms: A system for implementing practice parameters in laboratory medicine. Clin Lab Med 11:259, 1991.

Certain decisions presently cannot be made by using laboratory tests. For example, the decision to use thrombolytic therapy in a patient with probable AMI must be made clinically—not by laboratory tests. A test for the even earlier diagnosis of AMI needs development (perhaps a CK isoform analysis). Thrombolytic therapy has significant risks, and if an earlier diagnosis of AMI could be made, the clinical decision about whether or not this therapy is appropriate for a particular patient could be improved. Similarly, in the emergency department the diagnosis of probable AMI must be made clinically—not by laboratory tests. In the hospital coronary unit serial measurements of CK-MB have high diagnostic sensitivity and specificity for diagnosing AMI; whereas in the emergency department setting the diagnostic sensitivity and specificity of a single measurement of CK-MB for diagnosing AMI are much lower because there is usually time for only one measurement of CK-MB. This emergency department dilemma can be approached by either developing a better test for AMI or holding the patient for serial CK-MB determinations.

In a recent study it was possible to decrease inappropriate serum triiodothyronine (T_3) testing by 38% and thyrotropin (thyroid-stimulating hormone [TSH]) testing by 61% through an educational program plus implementation of a decision-oriented test request form for hyperthyroidism and hypothyroidism in place of a menu of individual thyroid tests as follows:

	T_3 uptake
	T_4 (RIA)
	T_3 (RIA)
A	TSH

☐ Thyroid function screen (T_4 [RIA], T_3 uptake, plus index)
☐ Hyperthyroid panel (T_4 [RIA], T_3 uptake, plus indexes)
☐ Hypothyroid panel (T_4 [RIA], T_3 uptake, TSH, plus index)
☐ Other thyroid tests
B   Specify

A, Thyroid function tests as listed on previous comprehensive laboratory test request form. **B,** Problem-oriented format for thyroid function tests on new request form. T_3 = triiodothyronine; T_4 = thyroxine; RIA = radioimmunoassay; TSH = thyrotropin.

Wong ET, McCarron MM, Shaw ST, Jr: Ordering of laboratory tests in a teaching hospital. JAMA 249:3076-3080, 1983. Copyright 1983, American Medical Association.

This new form accomplished the reduction by eliminating inappropriate testing (e.g., requesting a TSH test for hyperthyroidism and a T_3 test when it was unnecessary). Moreover, the physicians were assured of obtaining the correct tests for the diagnosis they had in mind. A similar effort to improve the use of serum creatine kinase and lactate dehydrogenase isoenzyme tests for the diagnosis of AMI failed when the educational program was conducted but the decision-oriented test request form was omitted.

The use of decision-oriented test request forms represents an effective way to encourage physicians to use the right tests and eliminate unnecessary ones. Historically, efforts to modify physicians' behavior using various techniques, including education, have not been very successful. Interestingly, when house officers were reminded about the charges for tests, they ordered 14% fewer tests—apparently, without adverse effects on patient outcomes.

Useful Techniques for Interpreting Laboratory Data

It is important to understand how the information obtained from the performance of a laboratory test changes the pretest probability of disease to the posttest probability (predictive value) of disease. This can be illustrated using Bayes' theorem, likelihood ratios, and odds. Using a receiver operating curve (ROC) is a way to analyze the overall performance of a test. One of the problems with calculating posttest probability (predictive value) is the requirement for an estimate of pretest probability. This estimate may be obtained by using prevalence data available in the literature for various clinical settings and estimates based on clinicians' experience.

PREDICTIVE VALUE

Several definitions are needed:

- Predictive value (posttest probability) of a positive test: probability of a disease being present if the test is positive
- Predictive value (posttest probability) of a negative test: probability of a disease being absent if the test is negative
- Prevalence (pretest probability): the frequency of patients with a certain disease in the group being tested with the measurement
- Diagnostic sensitivity: the percentage of true-positive results in patients with the disease
- Diagnostic specificity: the percentage of true-negative results in healthy patients

The relationships of these statistical concepts can be summarized in this table:

PREDICTIVE VALUE TABLE

	No. With Positive Test Result	No. With Negative Test Result	Totals
No. with disease	TP	FN	TP + FN
No. without disease	FP	TN	FP + TN
TOTAL	TP + FP	FN + TN	TP + FP + TN + FN

TP = True positives; the number of sick subjects correctly classified by the test.

FP = False positives; the number of subjects free of the disease who are misclassified by the test.

TN = True negatives; the number of subjects free of the disease who are correctly classified by the test.

FN = False negatives; the number of sick subjects misclassified by the test.

Prevalence = Percent of total subjects examined who are diseased.

Sensitivity = Positivity in disease

$$= \frac{TP}{TP + FN} \times 100 = \frac{TP}{\text{No. diseased}} \times 100$$

Specificity = Negativity in health $= \frac{TN}{TN + FP} \times 100$

$$= \frac{TN}{\text{No. without disease}} \times 100$$

Predictive value of a positive test $= \frac{TP}{TP + FP} \times 100$

$$= \frac{TP}{\text{No. positive}} \times 100$$

Predictive value of a negative test $= \frac{TN}{TN + FN} \times 100$

$$= \frac{TN}{\text{No. negative}} \times 100$$

Source: Galen RS, Gambino SR: Beyond Normality: The Predictive Value and Efficiency of Medical Diagnoses. New York, John Wiley & Sons, Inc, 1975, p 124. By permission of Churchill Livingstone, New York.

It is important to appreciate the effects of prevalence (pretest probability) on predictive value as follows:

EFFECT OF PREVALENCE ON PREDICTIVE VALUE

| **EFFECT OF PREVALENCE*** | | **EFFECT OF PREVALENCE†** | |
PREVALENCE (%)	PREDICTIVE VALUE OF A POSITIVE TEST (%)	PREVALENCE (%)	PREDICTIVE VALUE OF A POSITIVE TEST (%)
0.1	1.9	0.1	9.0
1.0	16.1	1.0	50.0
2.0	27.9	2.0	66.9
5.0	50.0	5.0	83.9
50.0	95.0	50.0	99.0

*Sensitivity = 95%; specificity = 95%.
†Sensitivity = 99%; specificity = 99%.
Source: Adapted from Galen RS, Gambino SR: Beyond Normality: The Predictive Value and Efficiency of Medical Diagnoses. New York, John Wiley & Sons, Inc, 1975, p 16. By permission of Churchill Livingstone, New York.

The predictive value (posttest probability) of a test is simply the a posteriori probability as computed using a mathematical expression, Bayes' theorem. It allows quantification of how the performance of a test changes the pretest probability of a disease to the posttest probability of a disease.

An example of these relationships is illustrated in the following table for which a pregnancy test of a given sensitivity and specificity was performed on a group of women with a certain prevalence (pretest probability or a priori probability) of pregnancy.

PREVALENCE OF PREGNANCY, SENSITIVITY OF PREGNANCY TEST, AND SPECIFICITY OF PREGNANCY TEST PLUS PREDICTIVE VALUE OF PREGNANCY TEST RESULT

	No. WITH POSITIVE RESULT	No. WITH NEGATIVE RESULT	TOTAL
No. pregnant	90	10	100
No. not pregnant	180	720	900
TOTAL	270	730	1000

Prevalence: 10.0%
Sensitivity: 90.0%
Specificity: 80.0%
Predictive value of a positive: 33.3%
Predictive value of a negative: 98.6%

Source: Speicher CE, Smith JS: Choosing Effective Laboratory Tests. Philadelphia, WB Saunders, 1983, p 49.

In practice, today's pregnancy tests have higher positive predictive values (posttest probabilities) than the one depicted in the table for two reasons. First, the prevalence (pretest probability) of pregnancy is usually higher than 10% because women who have pregnancy tests have a very high prevalence of pregnancy (i.e., they preselect themselves from nonpregnant women because they have findings of pregnancy such as a missed menstrual period). Second, modern pregnancy tests have higher diagnostic sensitivities and specificities than the one depicted in the table.

LIKELIHOOD RATIOS AND ODDS

Likelihood ratios (LR) and odds are other methods that may be used to interpret quantitative test results. These methods are helpful when interpreting sequential tests or single tests with multiple cutoffs. See the discussion of early detection of alcohol abuse in Chapter 1 for the use of LR to interpret the results of the CAGE questionnaire.

The greater posttest probability for disease of markedly abnormal test results than minimally abnormal test results is an important concept that has general applicability, not just for the CAGE questions but for other tests as well (e.g., a markedly high serum cholesterol concentration has a greater positive predictive value for risk of coronary heart disease than a minimally high cholesterol concentration; a markedly high serum glucose concentration has a greater positive predictive value for diabetes mellitus than a minimally high glucose concentration; a markedly high serum human immunodeficiency virus [HIV] antibody titer has a greater positive predictive value for HIV infection than a minimally high HIV antibody titer; and a markedly high serum prostate-specific antigen [PSA] concentration has a greater positive predictive value for prostate cancer than a minimally high PSA concentration).

Format for Discussing Medical Problems in This Book
PROBLEM ORGANIZATION

In this book each medical problem is discussed in terms of individual clinical decisions: when to choose certain tests and which tests to choose, how to evaluate the tests and the results, what to do if test results are positive, what to do if test results are negative, and how to use tests to monitor the patient if the diagnosis is confirmed. The format is to state the decision recommendation in bold type, followed by a justification of the recommendation in regular type.

WHICH TESTS TO CHOOSE

In this section are clues that affect the pretest probability of the clinical condition under consideration. Information is provided about appropriate tests to request in a given screening or diagnostic decision-making situation. In addition, there is a brief explanation of the reasons for obtaining these tests. Sometimes tests that should not be obtained are also mentioned. Unfortunately, in practice the use of a new test does not usually replace the other tests for which it provides an alternative. Rather, the new test often is done in addition to the old tests.

If patient preparation or specimen collection and handling issues are important, instructions are provided on how to perform these tasks properly. For example, accurate measurement of the plasma activated partial thromboplastin time depends on filling the citrated collection tube completely with blood, thoroughly mixing it, and promptly delivering it to the laboratory.

HOW TO EVALUATE THE TESTS AND THE RESULTS

Physicians should learn more about laboratory tests. The clinical laboratory is not simply a "black box" from which tests are requested and equivalent results are always received. There are pitfalls related to specimen collection and handling, methodologies, and the skills of the individuals performing the tests. All laboratory tests are not created equal, and test differences can affect results, which in turn can affect clinical decisions. Greater knowledge about laboratory tests not only will enable physicians to use tests more effectively but also will help them to understand better the nuances of office laboratory testing and home (self) testing. In some situations it occasionally is helpful for physicians actually to know how to perform the tests themselves: (1) preparation and examination of a Gram-stained smear of the sputum for pneumonia, of the urine for urinary tract infection, and of wound drainage for an infected wound; (2) performance of a macroscopic reagent strip (dipstick) urinalysis and microscopic examination of the urinary sediment for urinary tract disorders; and (3) preparation and examination of a Wright-stained peripheral blood smear for red cell, white cell, and platelet disorders. For certain clinical decisions it is imperative to know not only which test or tests to request but also which method or methods to use and how the methods should be standardized and controlled. For example, the National Cholesterol Education Program recommendations for desirable, borderline-high, or high levels of serum cholesterol cannot be used unless a method for measuring cholesterol is used that is equivalent to the Program method. It is also important to know the diagnostic utility of tests (i.e., how effective they are in confirming or excluding a diagnosis).

Physicians should use the reference ranges of the laboratory that performs their tests, because reference ranges vary based on the methodology. Common reference ranges are provided inside the front and back covers of this book, and special reference ranges are included in the test evaluation section of each problem. Reference ranges and other laboratory values are given in conventional units followed by international units in parentheses. Reference ranges should address important variables (analytic; biologic, genetic, and ethnic; environmental; and life-style).

Clinical decision levels are also included in this section. The term *decision level* refers to a threshold value above which or below which a particular management action is recommended. The use of decision levels recognizes the importance of additional information content in knowing not only whether a test result is high or low, but also how high or low. For example, the reference range for serum calcium is 8.4 to 10.2 mg/dL (2.10 to 2.55 mmol/L). The decision level above which hypercalcemic coma can occur is 13.5 mg/dL (3.37 mmol/L), and the decision level below which tetany can occur is 7 mg/dL (1.75 mmol/L). It would be inappropriate to assign the cause of a patient's coma to hypercalcemia if the level were 11.5 mg/dL (2.87 mmol/L); even though 11.5 mg/dL (2.87 mmol/L) is above the upper limit of the reference range for serum calcium, it is below the decision level for hypercalcemic coma. Moreover, decision levels can help in deciding whether an unexpected or unexplained abnormal test result is true positive or false positive—with markedly abnormal test results more likely to be true positive than slightly abnormal test results.

HOW TO INTERPRET POSITIVE AND NEGATIVE TEST RESULTS

In this section is information on the posttest probability of the disease or disorder under consideration. For example, consider thyroid function tests for the diagnosis of hyperthyroidism or hypothyroidism. Serum thyroxine (T_4), a triiodothyronine resin uptake (T_3RU), and a calculated free thyroxine index (FT_4I) are only approximately 95% sensitive for hyperthyroidism, and if the T_4 and FT_4I test results are normal in the presence of clinical findings suggestive of hyperthyroidism, a serum triiodothyronine (T_3) test or the new highly sensitive immunoradiometric assay for thyrotropin, S-TSH, is indicated to confirm the diagnosis. On the other hand, a serum T_4 or FT_4I test is even less sensitive to detect hypothyroidism, and if the T_4 and FT_4I are normal in the presence of clinical features of hypothyroidism, a serum S-TSH assay is indicated to confirm the diagnosis. Alternatively, the decision-making strategy for diagnosing thyroid dysfunction could be simplified by ordering one test—an S-TSH assay.

If a test result does not make sense or is indeterminate, a useful tactic is to repeat it. For example, when testing for HIV infection, if the enzyme-linked immunosorbent assay (ELISA) is positive and the Western blot analysis is indeterminate, repeat the Western blot test monthly. Another useful technique is to use a second test to confirm the significance of the indeterminate test (e.g., using a serum gamma-glutamyl transferase test to confirm the significance of an isolated high serum alkaline phosphatase value for diagnosing liver disease).

HOW TO MONITOR THE PATIENT'S DISORDER

If a diagnosis is confirmed and the patient is treated, this section gives information on which tests are useful to monitor the patient's condition and how often these tests should be ordered. For example, in patients with acute hepatitis B who are e antigen positive, it is appropriate to test for anti-hepatitis B e antibody monthly since development of the antibody indicates when the patient is less infectious to others.

ADDITIONAL ABNORMAL TEST RESULTS

Sometimes test results are available that are not really necessary for the diagnostic strategy, but they have been ordered as part of a profile or for some other reason. It is important to know whether or not these test results can occur in the condition under consideration and whether or not another disease process must be hypothesized to explain them. If available, information on the pathophysiological derangements responsible for these abnormal test results is included.

Instead of an alphabetical listing of tests and their abnormal values, the abnormal test results are organized conceptually according to the way the results are usually grouped and considered. This same organization is used for common reference ranges located inside the front and back covers of this book.

Additional Considerations

Data in the medical literature support the approach used in this book, that is, a series of recommendations followed by an explanation of the underlying reasons. Individuals often have difficulty with rote memorization of recommendations unless the underlying reasons are understood. Further, physicians will not use rules for clinical decision making unless they have confidence that the rules are correct. This confidence comes from an understanding of the underlying reasons and the credibility of the source of the rules.

Material for this book comes from several sources: the author's experience, general references at the end of the book, annotated references at the end of each problem, and occasional references included within the problem discussion. The annotated references and occasional references were chosen mainly, but not entirely, to highlight important information that has surfaced between the publication of the general references and the present time. Sometimes an older reference is included to emphasize information that has not found its way into standard texts.

Finally, it is hoped that a more scientific approach to clinical decision making using laboratory tests will help assure the quality of patient care. This quality assurance through appropriate laboratory testing is not only good for patients but also is economical (i.e., good medicine is cost-effective). Moreover, physicians' anxiety about medicolegal risk should be lessened because, to the extent possible, the recommendations in this book are based on the best information currently available; by following these recommendations, physicians are practicing the best clinical medicine they can.

BIBLIOGRAPHY

Brook RH: Quality of care: Do we care? Ann Intern Med 115:486, 1991.
  Believes that physicians should become involved with guideline development and outcome analysis.
Burke MD: Clinical decision making and laboratory use. In Fenoglio-Preiser C (ed): Advances in Pathology, vol 3. St. Louis, Mosby–Year Book, 1990, p 207.
  Reviews the use of laboratory studies in clinical decision making.
Elstein AS, Shulman LS, Sprafka SA: Medical Problem Solving: An Analysis of Clinical Reasoning. Cambridge, Mass, Harvard University Press, 1978, p 199.
    Schwartz S, Griffin T: Medical Thinking: The Psychology of Medical Judgement and Decision Making. New York, Springer-Verlag, 1986, p 169.
  Literature that supports the approach used in this book.

Findlay S: Medicine by the book: A gusher of guidelines for doctors can educate patients, too. U.S. News and World Report, July 6, 1992, p 68.
Lay magazine encourages patients to read guidelines and gives information on where to obtain guidelines.

Fine MJ, Orloff JJ, Rihs JD, et al: Evaluation of housestaff physicians' preparation and interpretation of sputum Gram stains for community-acquired pneumonia. J Gen Intern Med 6:189, 1991.
Hirschmann JV: The sputum Gram stain. J Gen Intern Med 6:261, 1991.
Housestaff physicians should receive formal training in the preparation and interpretation of Gram stains.

Galen RS, Gambino SR: Beyond Normality: The Predictive Value and Efficiency of Medical Diagnoses. New York, John Wiley & Sons, 1975.
A key text that highlights the importance of Bayes theorem in clinical decision making.

Garnick DW, Hendricks AM, Brennan TA: Can practice guidelines reduce the number and costs of malpractice claims? JAMA 266:2856, 1991.
Discusses the potential effect of practice guidelines on malpractice claims.

Kassirer JP, Kopelman RI: Learning Clinical Reasoning. Baltimore, Md, Williams & Wilkins, 1991.
Excellent new text that describes the process of clinical reasoning using 63 cases. The role of laboratory tests is clearly described.

Lee TH, Goldman L: Serum enzyme assays in the diagnosis of acute myocardial infarction: Recommendations based on a quantitative analysis. In Sox HC Jr (ed): Common Diagnostic Tests: Use and Interpretation, 2nd ed. Philadelphia, American College of Physicians, 1990, p 35.
Good review of the use of serum enzymes for the diagnosis of AMI.

Panzer RJ, Black ER, Griner PF (eds): Diagnostic Strategies for Common Medical Problems. Philadelphia, American College of Physicians, 1991.
Good discussion of Bayes' theorem, likelihood ratios, and odds.

Speicher CE: All laboratory tests are not created equal. Arch Pathol Lab Med 109:709, 1985.
Discusses the differences in test results caused by methodology and other miscellaneous factors.

Speicher CE: Decision-oriented test request forms: A system for implementing practice parameters in laboratory medicine. Clin Lab Med 11:255, 1991.
Suggests a way to implement practice parameters in laboratory medicine.

Speicher CE: Practice parameters: An opportunity for pathologists to take a leadership role in patient care. Arch Pathol Lab Med 114:823, 1990.
Describes the development of practice parameters for laboratory medicine.

Swartwout JE (ed): Directory of Practice Parameters: 1992 edition. Chicago, American Medical Association, 1991.
Summarizes available practice parameters as of 1992.

Tierney WM, Miller ME, McDonald CJ: The effect on test ordering of informing physicians of the charges for outpatient diagnostic tests. N Engl J Med 322:1499, 1990.
When informed of test charges, house officers ordered 14% fewer tests.

U.S. health-care spending increased 10.5% in 1990. *Wall Street Journal*, October 3, 1991, p B4.
Spells out the escalating cost of health care in the United States.

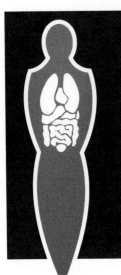

CHAPTER 1

SCREENING

Wellness Screening and Case Finding
Unexplained Abnormal Test Result
Pregnancy Testing
Pap Smear and Cervical Cancer
Serum Cholesterol and Coronary Heart Disease
Occult Fecal Blood Testing and Colorectal Cancer
Digital Rectal Examination, Prostate-Specific
    Antigen, and Prostate Cancer
Detection of Alcohol Abuse
Urine Screening for Drug Abuse
Hemochromatosis

Wellness Screening and Case Finding

1.   In wellness screening request a complete blood count (CBC), biochemical tests, urinalysis, and other studies when the individual examined belongs to a clinical class that is at risk for significant conditions that can be detected by abnormalities in these tests. Otherwise, do not routinely request tests without a good reason. For an example of wellness screening guidelines, see the schedule that follows this discussion for testing asymptomatic men and women, which was developed for the Ohio State University Health Plan (OSUHP).

Wellness screening is the testing of asymptomatic individuals who are basically healthy. General screening of everyone for every disorder may lead to false-positive test results and fruitless follow-up testing with little gain and potential for real harm. Selective screening refers to testing of asymptomatic persons who are at risk for the target condition. Baseline information against which to compare future test results, data that make other studies unnecessary, and reassurance that the patient is free of disease are legitimate reasons for requesting screening tests. One should screen for diseases that are relatively common, that can be detected before clinical findings develop, that are easy to treat, and that have harmful consequences if left untreated.

Although it generally is more cost-effective to perform wellness screening only on individuals who are at risk (i.e., only screen those with a high pretest probability for the disease), for some diseases clinical findings are not reliable for determining who is at risk, or the cost of determining who is at risk may be more than the cost of performing the tests. Using modern analyzers, screening for certain diseases with laboratory tests may actually be the most cost-effective strategy.

The use of test batteries, panels, or profiles for screening is controversial. Some argue that no data demonstrate the usefulness of profiles, whereas others argue that long medical tradition and experience support the use and benefits of profiles.

Several decades ago the advent of multitest chemistry analyzers introduced a wave of enthusiasm for screening patients with multiple laboratory tests. During the last decade there has been a swing back to a restrictive view of screening by laboratory tests, based on studies that failed to reveal significant benefits. Many of these studies were flawed. They emphasized the generation of test data and not the use of test data for patient care. Usually they did not address the selection of the right tests. The true role of screening by laboratory tests remains undetermined. Clearly there are situations in which laboratory tests and test profiles can detect disease better than the history and physical examination. The use of profiles has been criticized as inappropriate and sometimes wasteful; however, it is the content of the profile—not the concept of the profile—that has been problematic.

HEMATOLOGY

Examples of individuals who are at risk for anemia and who may benefit from a CBC include infants in the first year of life; institutionalized, elderly persons; pregnant women; and recent immigrants from Third World countries. Mild iron deficiency anemia may provide the first clue to colorectal cancer in an otherwise healthy older individual. The CBC often is performed on an automated instrument that usually gives values for hemoglobin, hematocrit, red blood cell indices, and white blood cells—and often platelets and an electronic white cell differential as well. If only the detection of anemia is of interest and a discrete hemoglobin or hematocrit measurement is available, one or both of these tests may be requested.

CHEMISTRY

Screening for gestational diabetes is clearly beneficial, and screening for diabetes might be helpful for particular patients (e.g., obese persons who would be spurred to lose weight by a demonstration of glucose intolerance). Measurements of serum cholesterol in adults 20 years of age and over are worthwhile because of the high prevalence of hypercholesterolemia as a risk factor for coronary heart disease (CHD). Although some experts believe that screening serum calcium or uric acid determinations are valuable, others argue that since there is no advantage in treating asymptomatic hyperparathyroidism or hyperuricemia, screening for abnormal calcium and uric acid values should be omitted. Screening for abnormal iron metabolism (iron deficiency and iron overload) using fasting serum iron, transferrin saturation, and ferritin determinations may be worthwhile. Thyroid function testing in older patients may be worthwhile because of the increased prevalence of thyroid dysfunction with increasing age. Because many of these tests are performed on an automated instrument that may include other tests as well (a biochemical profile), it may be cost-effective simply to request the profile. The cost and trouble of collecting and processing a specimen are significant and not something that should be repeated frequently. With a biochemical profile, transaminase, alkaline phosphatase, and bilirubin measurements can be used to screen for liver disease, and serum proteins can be used to detect dysproteinemia. New instruments are emerging that allow performance of only the individual tests desired.

URINALYSIS

Examples of individuals with a high prevalence of urinary tract disorders who may benefit from a urinalysis include pregnant women; older men with prostatic hypertrophy, obstruction, and possible infection; and anyone known to have a history of recurrent urinary tract disease. Because a urine reagent strip (dipstick) test (including nitrite and leukocyte esterase) is such an effective and economical way to detect urinary tract disease, it may be appropriate to incorporate it into wellness screening to detect occult pyuria, hematuria, and proteinuria.

MISCELLANEOUS

Since the prevalence of sexually transmitted diseases is increasing, consider testing for *Chlamydia* and gonorrhea in sexually active patients with multiple partners. Screening for drug abuse, alcohol abuse, syphilis, and the human immunodeficiency virus (HIV) may be appropriate for groups at high risk.

The American Cancer Society recommendations for cancer screening are as follows:

CANCER	TEST	WHO SHOULD BE SCREENED AND HOW OFTEN
Cervical	Pap smear	Women 18 yr and older, annually
		Sexually active girls, annually
Prostate	Rectal examination	Men 40 and older, annually
	Ultrasound and blood test*	Not recommended for general screening
Breast	Professional examination	Women 20 to 40, every 3 yr
		Women over 40, annually
	Mammogram	Women 35 to 39, once
		Women 40 to 49, every 1 or 2 yr
		Women 50 and older, annually
Ovarian	Ultrasound and blood test	Not recommended for general screening

*Recently, the American Cancer Society issued this new guideline: annual digital rectal examination and prostate-specific antigen should be performed on men 50 years and older. If either is abnormal, further evaluation should be considered.

CANCER	TEST	WHO SHOULD BE SCREENED AND HOW OFTEN
Colon	Rectal examination	Men and women 40 and older, annually
	Stool blood test	Men and women 50 and older, annually
	Sigmoidoscopy	Men and women 50 and older, every 3 to 5 yr
Lung	X-ray	Not recommended for general screening

Source: Screening the tests that detect cancer. *The New York Times Magazine,* April 28, 1991, p 9. Copyright © 1991 by The New York Times Company. Reprinted by permission.

2.   In case finding request tests that are appropriate for the clinical situation.

Case finding is the testing of patients seen for unrelated symptoms or diseases. In contrast to wellness screening in which the individuals are asymptomatic, these persons have a medical problem. In case finding, appropriate testing depends on the good judgment of the attending physician. Testing may range from a few tests to a wide variety of routine and special laboratory studies. A recent study concluded that the usefulness of a CBC as a case-finding tool in middle-aged outpatients is limited. If an otherwise healthy patient is seen with a minor injury or for an elective minor surgical procedure, little testing may be necessary. Minimal preoperative test recommendations developed in the Mayo Clinic from a study of 3782 otherwise healthy patients undergoing elective surgery are as follows:

AGE (YR)	TESTS REQUIRED*
<40	None
40–59	Electrocardiography, creatinine, and glucose
≥60	Electrocardiography, chest radiograph, CBC, glucose, and creatinine

*In addition, the following guidelines apply:

- A CBC is indicated in all patients who undergo blood typing and who are screened or crossmatched.
- Measurement of potassium is indicated in patients taking diuretics or undergoing bowel preparation.
- A chest radiograph is indicated in patients with a history of cardiac or pulmonary disease or with recent respiratory symptoms.
- A history of cigarette smoking in patients older than 40 years of age who are scheduled for an upper abdominal or thoracic surgical procedure is an indication for spirometry (forced vital capacity).

Source: Narr BJ, Hansen TR, Warner MA: Preoperative laboratory screening in healthy Mayo patients: Cost-effective elimination of tests and unchanged outcomes. Mayo Clin Proc 66:158, 1991.

Based on a study of 520 patients undergoing elective surgery, similar recommendations from Letterman Army Medical Center suggest performing electrocardiography for patients age 30 to 60 and electrocardiography, chest radiograph, hematocrit, glucose, urea nitrogen, creatinine, and nutritional studies (total protein, albumin, and lymphocyte count) for patients older than 60.*

---

*Velanovich V: The value of routine preoperative laboratory testing in predicting postoperative complications. Surgery 109:236, 1991.

Although the Mayo Clinic and Letterman Army Medical Center recommendations may be adequate for addressing operative and postoperative complications, the number of other significant diseases (e.g., thyroid dysfunction, dyslipidemia) that may have been overlooked is unknown.

On the other hand, if there are specific indications for laboratory testing, appropriate tests should be done. A diabetic patient with ketoacidosis requires a large number of tests to diagnose and manage the immediate problem and to look for coexisting conditions and complications such as urinary tract infection. As in wellness screening, baseline information, reassurance of normality, and data that make other studies unnecessary are appropriate reasons for testing.

3.   Interpret test results in the context of the complete health examination.

Clinical laboratory test results are valuable, but they are only one part of the assessment of patients and are best used in the context of information from other sources such as (1) the general history and physical examination, (2) blood pressure, (3) weight, (4) hearing and vision, (5) oral examination, (6) breast examination, (7) electrocardiography, (8) mammography, (9) sigmoidoscopy, and (10) radiography.

Follow significantly abnormal test results with additional testing. Sometimes an abnormal test result (just outside the reference range) makes no sense in the context of the clinical findings, and it is questioned. This constitutes the problem of the unexplained abnormal test result, which should be approached as outlined in the next discussion.

BIBLIOGRAPHY

Bates SE: Clinical applications of serum tumor markers. Ann Intern Med 115:623, 1991.
   Points out that thus far every tumor marker has failed as a screening test for cancer in asymptomatic persons.
Eddy DM (ed): Common Screening Tests. Philadelphia, American College of Physicians, 1991.
   Collection of position papers from the Annals of Internal Medicine *on screening for hypertension, coronary artery disease, cardiac risk factors, diabetes mellitus, thyroid disease, osteoporosis, breast cancer, cervical cancer, colorectal cancer, and lung cancer.*
Gambino R: The American College of Physicians and Blue Cross/Blue Shield Guidelines. Lab Report for Physicians 10:44, 1988.
   Content, not the concept, of the profile has been problematic.
Glenn GC (ed): A Critique of Blue Cross/Blue Shield Guidelines Based on Common

Diagnostic Tests: Use and Interpretation. Skokie, Ill, College of American Pathologists, 1988.
Critique of The Blue Cross/Blue Shield Guidelines for the use of common laboratory tests.

Guidelines for electrocardiography: A report of the American College of Cardiology/ American Heart Association Task Force on Assessment of Diagnostic and Therapeutic Cardiovascular Procedures (Committee on Electrocardiography). J Am Coll Cardiol 19:473, 1992.
Guidelines for reducing the number of baseline and preoperative ECGs performed in persons less than age 40 and the number of routine follow-up ECGs.

Hayward RSA, Steinberg EP, Ford DE, et al: Preventive care guidelines: 1991. Ann Intern Med 114:758, 1991.
Compares wellness screening guidelines from the American College of Physicians, the Canadian Task Force on the Periodic Health Examination, the United States Preventive Services Task Force, and other authorities.

Ohio State Faculty: Wellness screening and case finding. Columbus, Ohio, The Ohio State University Health Plan Clinical Notes, vol 1, no 1, Summer 1990.
Medical practice guidelines for screening.

Rüttimann S, Clémençon D, Dubach UC: Usefulness of complete blood counts as a case-finding tool in medical outpatients. Ann Intern Med 116:44, 1992.
Concludes from a study of 595 middle-aged medical outpatients that CBCs have limited use.

Sox HC Jr (ed): Common Diagnostic Tests: Use and Interpretation, 2nd ed. Philadelphia, American College of Physicians, 1990.
Reviews the CBC, biochemical profiles, and other common laboratory tests with American College of Physicians' guidelines for their appropriate use.

Sox HC Jr: The baseline electrocardiogram. Am J Med 91:573, 1991.
Suggests that baseline testing constitutes a different reason for testing than screening to detect disease and thus requires a different rationale.

Witte DL, Angstadt DS, Schweitzer JK: Chemistry profiles in "Wellness Programs": Test selection and participant outcomes. Clin Chem 34:1447, 1988.
Discusses the selection and interpretation of chemistry tests in wellness screening programs.

OSUHP HEALTH MAINTENANCE "PHYSICAL EXAM" GUIDELINES, FOR THE ASYMPTOMATIC ADULT FEMALE AT LOW MEDICAL RISK

Age: 20 21 22 23 24 25 26 27 28 29 30 31 32 33 34 35 36 37 38 39 40 41 42 43 44 45 46 47 48 49 50 51 52 53 54 55 56 57 58 59 60 61 62 63 64 65

Elements of the exam

History, physical and counselling regarding risk factors, every 5 years to age 40, then every year.

Gyn Exam: Begin age 18, yearly thereafter; or every 2 years after 3 negative Pap smears, until age 40. After age 40 every year or every other year.

Clinical Breast Exam, Same frequency as Gyn exam. Teach monthly self exam.

Pap smear, Same frequency as Gyn exam.

Blood Pressure Check, each visit.

Vision, dilated eye exam, age 20-39: every 3-5 years; age 40-64 every 2-4 years. (Covered under Vision Plan.)

Hearing, pure tone audiometry if exposed chronically to excessively loud noises, every 1-3 years, begin age 40.

Diagnostic/Screening Tests:

Mammogram, 35-39 baseline. 40-49 every 1-2 years. Age 50 yearly.

Stool for occult blood. Yearly after age 40, 3 consecutive stools, using Hemoccult II cards. Follow recommended diet and sampling procedure.

Urinalysis, multi-combination dipstick, same frequency as Gyn exam.

Sigmoidoscopy, with 60 cm flexible scope; age 50 or older, for individuals with first degree relatives with colorectal cancer, or other high risk conditions. Repeat every 5 years after 2 negative exams.

Blood Work: FBS, Cholesterol, CBC, BUN, Cr., Electrolytes. Every 5-10 yrs.

EKG, Baseline before age 40, every 5 years thereafter, or at the physician's discretion. [ONE EKG]

☐ **Recommended age to be performed.**
± **Can be performed at the discretion of physician or patient.**

Source: OSU Health Plan: Clinical Notes, vol 1, no 1, Summer 1990.

OSUHP HEALTH MAINTENANCE "PHYSICAL EXAM" GUIDELINES, FOR THE ASYMPTOMATIC ADULT MALE AT LOW MEDICAL RISK

Age: 20 21 22 23 24 25 26 27 28 29 30 31 32 33 34 35 36 37 38 39 40 41 42 43 44 45 46 47 48 49 50 51 52 53 54 55 56 57 58 59 60 61 62 63 64 65

Elements of the exam

History, physical and counselling regarding risk factors, every 5 years to age 40, then every year.

Blood Pressure Check, each visit.

Rectal/Prostate exam included with physical exam.

Vision, dilated eye exam, age 20-39; every 3-5 years; age 40-64 every 2-4 years. (Covered under Vision Plan.)

Hearing, pure tone audiometry if exposed chronically to excessively loud noises, every 1-3 years, begin age 40.

Diagnostic/Screening Tests:

Stool for Occult Blood. Yearly after age 40, 3 consecutive stools, using Hemoccult II cards. Follow recommended diet and sampling procedure.

Urinalysis, multi-combination dipstick, every 5-10 years.

Sigmoidoscopy, with 60 cm flexible scope; age 50 or older, for individuals with first degree relatives with colorectal cancer, or other high risk conditions. Repeat every 5 years after 2 negative exams.

Blood Work: FBS, Cholesterol, CBC, BUN, Cr., Electrolytes. Every 5-10 yrs.*

EKG, Baseline before age 40, every 5 years thereafter, or at the physician's discretion. — ONE EKG

□ Recommended age to be performed.
*PSA every year after age 50.
± Can be performed at the discretion of physician or patient.

Source: OSU Health Plan: Clinical Notes, vol 1, no 1, Summer 1990.

Unexplained Abnormal Test Result

1.   If a slightly abnormal test result (just outside the reference range) does not fit with the patient's clinical and other laboratory findings, consider that it may represent a statistical outlier that may be ignored.

Minor test result abnormalities are common during wellness screening and case finding. These results are statistical outliers that often may be ignored if they lie just outside the reference range (>2 but <3 standard deviations) and the patient has no other abnormal clinical, radiographic, or laboratory findings. The probability of occurrence for these statistical outliers increases with the number of different tests performed as follows:

NUMBER OF TESTS PERFORMED	PROBABILITY (%) OF FINDING RESULTS OUTSIDE REFERENCE RANGE*
1	5
6	24
12	43

*Using the mean ±2 standard deviations (95% confidence limits) for the reference range.

During wellness screening consider using the mean ±3 standard deviations (99.7% confidence limits) to define normal. This would considerably decrease false-positive test results.

The condition of a healthy person with a false-positive test result has been called the *Ulysses syndrome* because, like Ulysses, the patient must pass through a long journey of investigative procedures before returning to the previous state of health.

2.   If, however, an abnormal test result might be more than a minor statistical outlier and could have real clinical significance (e.g., increased serum calcium), verify the result rather than ignoring it. Pay attention to abnormal test results for critical analytes.

It is important to distinguish test results that are markedly abnormal from those that are minimally abnormal (possible statistical outliers). HIV testing illustrates this important point. In a low-risk group a weak HIV antibody titer is almost always a false-positive result since the probability of disease is very low. On the other hand, a strong HIV antibody titer is predictive of disease most of the time. Another way to clarify the significance of an unexplained abnormal test result is to follow it with a confirmatory test (e.g., clarifying the meaning of a positive Venereal Disease Research Laboratory [VDRL] test for syphilis by performing a fluorescent treponemal antibody absorption [FTA-ABS] test). Still another way is to wait awhile and repeat the test to determine whether it becomes normal, stays the same, or becomes more abnormal.

A general approach for verifying an unexplained test result abnormality follows:

- Repeat the measurement (only repeat tests that are abnormal; i.e., if a 12-test biochemical profile reveals an abnormal serum calcium result, only repeat the serum calcium measurement, not the entire 12-test biochemical profile).
  —Prepare the patient properly.
  —Obtain a proper sample.
  —Ensure appropriate specimen handling.
  —Use the best laboratory method available (e.g., for serum calcium, use the atomic absorption method, if available).
- Use the proper reference range for the age and sex of the patient.

3.   If the abnormal test result has been verified, consider a drug effect or a life-style effect, and if this does not explain the abnormality, consider the significance of the abnormal test result in the context of the individual's clinical and other laboratory findings.

A common example of an unexplained abnormal test result is increased serum alkaline phosphatase (ALP). Sometimes the increase can be explained by a specimen collection and handling problem, or a laboratory error, or the patient is a growing child or a pregnant woman, which explains the increased result. Occasionally the increase is due to a drug effect that can occur with agents such as chlorpromazine or methyltestosterone. The increase can also be caused by ALP's forming a macroenzyme complex with immunoglobulin, and the increase can persist for years and have no clinical significance. This macroenzyme phenomenon can also occur with amylase, creatine kinase, lactate dehydrogenase, aspartate aminotransferase, and glucose-6-phosphate dehydrogenase. Benign increase of ALP may be familial.

Life-style effects can be due to exercise, alcohol intake, and smoking. For example, vigorous exercise in an unconditioned person can increase serum creatine kinase; excessive alcohol intake can cause anemia, increased lipids, and numerous other test abnormalities; and smoking can increase serum carcinoembryonic antigen. Marathon runners, after the completion of a race, may have hematuria and a positive test for fecal occult blood; if enough blood is lost, anemia can occur.

Only if an unexplained abnormal test result such as a high level of serum ALP cannot be accounted for by factors such as those previously discussed should one consider obtaining a differential diagnosis and follow-up studies. Unrecognized disease may be the cause for an unexplained abnormality (e.g., Paget's disease) for an unexpected high ALP level. In the United States, osteoporosis is the only bone disease that is more prevalent than Paget's disease. Paget's disease affects an estimated 3% to 4% of people over the age of 45 and up to 8% of those over 80. The ALP of sons, daughters, and siblings of people with Paget's disease should be measured every 2 or 3 years after they reach age 40.

The significance of an unexplained test result may be clarified by considering it in the context of the patient's clinical and other laboratory findings. For example, an unexplained high ALP level in an elderly man with a history of prostate cancer takes on a special significance because the patient is at risk for metastatic bone disease, which may be manifested by an increased serum ALP. Similarly, if an unexplained high ALP level occurs in a middle-aged, overweight woman who has a slightly high serum bilirubin level, the possibility of cholelithiasis comes to mind, and additional studies are appropriate. When an initial test result such as an ALP is abnormal, the presence of another related abnormal test result such as increased gamma-glutamyl transferase helps to confirm that the initial abnormal test result is significant.

4.   In a patient with an unexplained high serum ALP level, perform a careful history and physical evaluation and obtain a CBC, chemistry profile, and gamma-glutamyl transferase (GGT) test. Repeat the ALP test in 1 to 3 months if there is no obvious diagnosis.

This workup is designed to detect the cause of the increased ALP, which includes the following diseases: malignancy, drug (e.g., phenytoin sodium [Dilantin]) therapy, congestive heart failure, bone disease, and hepatobiliary disease. Increased GGT testing is especially sensitive in detecting hepatobiliary disease. In the final analysis, none of these diseases may be present, and the isolated high ALP level may be due to a condition called *benign familial hyperphosphatasemia*.

BIBLIOGRAPHY

Brody JE: A fairly common bone disease that many sufferers may not recognize. *New York Times*, October 2, 1991, p B9.
  Points out the significant prevalence of Paget's disease and the role of increased ALP in its diagnosis.
Gambino R: The misuse of predictive value: Or why you must consider the odds. Lab Report for Physicians 11:65, 1989.
  Describes different techniques for clarifying an unexplained abnormal test result. The likelihood of disease varies with the strength of the signal.
Lieberman D, Phillips D: "Isolated" elevation of alkaline phosphatase: Significance in hospitalized patients. J Clin Gastroenterol 12:415, 1990.
  Recommends a workup for an isolated high serum alkaline phosphatase test result and discusses possible causes.
Litin SC, O'Brien JF, Pruett S, et al: Macroenzyme as a cause of unexplained elevation of aspartate aminotransferase. Mayo Clin Proc 62:681, 1987.
  Describes the benign elevation of many enzymes that can occur because of the macroenzyme phenomenon.
Rang M: The Ulysses syndrome. Can Med Assoc J 106:122, 1972.
  Coined the term Ulysses syndrome *to describe the state of a healthy person with a false-positive test result.*
Shulkin DJ, DeTore AW: When laboratory tests are abnormal and the patient feels fine. Hosp Pract 25:85, 1990.
  Points out that slightly abnormal results on routine biochemical screens often indicate a problem with the test results, not with the patient.
Siraganian PA, Mulvihill JJ, Mulivor RA, et al: Benign familial hyperphosphatasemia. JAMA 261:1310, 1989.
  Describes the increased serum ALP in benign familial hyperphosphatasemia.

Pregnancy Testing

1.   Perform a urine or serum pregnancy test to screen for or to confirm the diagnosis of pregnancy. Perform a serum pregnancy test if the earliest possible detection of pregnancy is important, if an ectopic pregnancy is suspected, or if there is any question about the validity of a previous urine pregnancy test. Serial quantitative serum human chorionic gonadotropin (hCG) determinations are useful to diagnose ectopic pregnancy.

Selective wellness screening for pregnancy is appropriate when a woman is contemplating the performance of a procedure that is potentially harmful to the fetus (e.g., having a radiographic study or ingesting a potentially teratogenic drug).

Modern pregnancy tests for serum or urinary hCG are very sensitive and specific. Keep several points in mind: (1) use serum or a concentrated first-morning urinary specimen collected in a clean, dry container; (2) carefully label the specimen; and (3) promptly deliver the specimen to the laboratory.

To perform the test yourself: (1) choose a kit that uses a monoclonal antibody to hCG; (2) make certain the test kit has been stored properly and is not outdated; (3) choose a kit that incorporates controls; (4) meticulously follow the directions; and (5) perform the test promptly.

2.   Evaluate the tests.

There are important differences between urine and serum tests for hCG. Obtaining accurate and precise serum hCG assays is necessary for the diagnosis of ectopic pregnancy.

URINE PREGNANCY TEST

Methods that use monoclonal antibody to hCG are preferable. Urine pregnancy tests are qualitative—the results are either positive or negative. The most sensitive methods give positive results at the time of the first missed menstrual period (hCG level, 20 to 50 mU/mL [20 to 50 U/L]), and most methods give positive results within 2 to 3 weeks after the first missed period. Blood, protein, or detergents in the urine can interfere with the test.

SERUM PREGNANCY TEST

Methods using antibody to beta-hCG or monoclonal antibody to hCG are best. Serum pregnancy tests may be either qualitative or quantitative. Serum hCG becomes detectable within 24 hours after implantation (5 mU/mL [5 U/L]), increases progressively, and reaches levels of 100 to 5000 mU/mL (100 to 5000 U/L) at 30 days, 50,000 to 140,000 mU/mL (50,000 to 140,000 U/L) at 10 weeks, and 10,000 to 50,000 mU/mL (10,000 to 50,000 U/L) after 16 weeks. Higher-than-expected levels are found with multiple pregnancies, polyhydramnios, eclampsia, and erythroblastosis fetalis.

Serum hCG can be increased in the following conditions:

- Normal pregnancy
- Ectopic pregnancy
- Abortion
- Gestational trophoblastic tumors: hydatidiform mole and choriocarcinoma
- Testicular tumors, germinal cell origin: choriocarcinoma, embryonal carcinoma with syncytiotrophoblastic giant cells, and seminoma with syncytiotrophoblastic giant cells
- Other tumors: breast, ovarian, pancreatic, cervical, gastric, and hepatic cancers

ECTOPIC PREGNANCY

Between 1970 and 1980 the rate of diagnosis of ectopic pregnancies increased from 4.5 to 16.8 ectopic pregnancies per 1000 pregnancies. Three diagnostic techniques have helped in the diagnosis: high-resolution ultrasonography, laparoscopy, and serum quantitative hCG assays. Currently available assays are more than 99% sensitive for detecting the presence of a pregnancy. Suspect ectopic pregnancy if serum hCG fails to increase to values seen in a normal pregnancy and if the rate of increase is less than that of a normal pregnancy. A normal intrauterine pregnancy should have at least a 66% increase of serum hCG over a 48-hour observation period. A lower rate of increase indicates an ectopic pregnancy or an intrauterine pregnancy destined to abort in approximately 85% of cases, whereas a significantly higher rate of increase might indicate a multiple pregnancy. Accurate and precise quantitative measurements of serum hCG are essential to assess the rate of increase.

3.   Remember that either false-positive or false-negative results can occur.

Modern pregnancy tests have pitfalls that may cause false-positive or false-negative results. They include mislabeled specimens, using dilute urine, dirty containers, deterioration of specimens kept at room temperature, outdated reagents, not following directions, and subjective bias when a woman performs a test on her own urine. See the Introduction of this book for a table that gives the relationships for predictive value, sensitivity, specificity, and prevalence for pregnancy testing.

4.   In pregnant women the following abnormal blood test results may occur:

↓ **Hemoglobin and hematocrit** related to increased plasma volume that can be aggravated by iron deficiency anemia.

↑ **Leukocytes** during late pregnancy and labor. Myelocytes occasionally can be found in the peripheral blood in pregnancy.

↑ **Chloride** caused by decreased bicarbonate secondary to respiratory alkalosis, which is especially prominent during labor.

↓ **Bicarbonate** caused by respiratory alkalosis.

↓ **Calcium** related to insufficient ingestion of calcium, phosphorus, and vitamin D.

↑ **Erythrocyte sedimentation rate** from third month to 3 weeks postpartum because of increased fibrinogen.

↓ **Partial pressure of carbon dioxide (PCO_2)** from respiratory alkalosis caused by increasing enlargement of the uterus and a stimulating effect on respiration by pregnancy hormones.

↑ **Glucose** from glucose intolerance caused by ovarian and placental hormones.

↓ **Urea nitrogen** because of expanded intravascular space and increased glomerular filtration rate: a decreased urea nitrogen-creatinine ratio (<10:1).

↓ **Creatinine.** A creatinine level of 1.2 mg/dL (106 μmol/L) or greater in pregnancy represents an increased level.

↓ **Sodium** caused by expanded intravascular space.

↓ **Phosphorus,** slight, with no significant implications.

↑ **Creatine kinase** during last few weeks that remains high during parturition and becomes normal 5 days postpartum.

↓ **Creatine kinase** during eighth to twentieth week, with minimal value at twelfth week.

↓ **Aspartate aminotransferase (SGOT)** caused by decreased pyridoxine levels during pregnancy.

↑ **Lactate dehydrogenase.**

↑ **Alkaline phosphatase** from the placenta. First appears in second trimester, increases in third trimester, and disappears 4 weeks postpartum.

↓ **Albumin** caused by expanded intravascular space.

↑ **Cholesterol** probably related to increased hepatic synthesis.

BIBLIOGRAPHY

Bakerman S: ABC's of Interpretive Laboratory Data, 2nd ed. Greenville, NC, Interpretive Laboratory Data, 1984, p 239.
Summarizes conditions in which hCG is increased.
Bluestein D: Monoclonal antibody pregnancy tests. Am Fam Physician 38:197, 1988.
Discusses the advantages of using a monoclonal antibody to hCG.
Fields SA, Toffler WL: Pregnancy testing: Home and office. West J Med 154:327, 1991.
Highlights the advantages and pitfalls of modern pregnancy tests.
Ory SJ: New options for diagnosis and treatment of ectopic pregnancy. JAMA 267:534, 1992.
Mayo Clinic recommendations for the diagnosis of ectopic pregnancy using serum hCG concentrations and other techniques.

Pap Smear and Cervical Cancer

1.   Use the Papanicolaou (Pap) smear to screen for cervical cancer in all women 18 years of age and older and in those women who have been sexually active regardless of age. Good technique is important.

Wellness screening for cervical cancer using the Pap smear has widespread endorsement by numerous authorities. Approximately 13,000 women develop cervical cancer in the United States each year, and approximately 7000 die from the disease. Worldwide, cervical cancer kills more than half a million women each year. Cervical cancer screening can reduce the incidence and mortality rate by up to 90%.

Poor technique is a significant cause of false-negative Pap smears. Common causes of poor smears are (1) using a thick smear from an abundance of red blood cells or inflammatory cells; (2) poor fixation, often caused by air drying the smear before fixation; (3) a scarcity of cells, caused by wiping the cervix before obtaining the smear; and (4) an absence of endocervical cells, which results from failure to obtain an endocervical sample.

2.   Consider testing for human papillomavirus (HPV) in cervical smear and biopsy specimens as tests become available. On the basis of currently available information, women with cervical abnormalities should receive evaluation, treatment, and follow-up using current Pap smear and biopsy technology for these abnormalities, regardless of the presence or absence of HPV. HPV typing may be appropriate when Pap smear results are equivocal or indicate the presence of low-grade disease and you wish to exclude the presence of high-risk (oncogenic) HPV.

HPV is the fastest rising sexually transmitted disease in the United States—up to one in three Americans are affected. It is a DNA virus that has been implicated as a cause of cervical cancer. There are more than 60 different types, and 20 types infect the anogenital tract. A simple classification differentiates HPVs into high-risk (oncogenic) and low-risk (nononcogenic) sets. Seven HPVs (types 6, 11, 16, 18, 31, 33, and 35) account for most clinically important infections, and five types (16, 18, 31, 33, and 35) are associated with the majority of cervical cancers. HPVs 6 and 11 are responsible for approximately 90% of exophytic condylomas of the external genitalia but only 10% of low-grade squamous intraepithelial lesions (SILs) of the cervix. Type 16, 18, 31, 33, and 35 are associated with all grades of SIL and invasive cancers of the cervix. The potential for false-negative Pap smears in the presence of an oncogenic HPV infection is a stimulus for developing HPV tests. The reported sensitivity of the Pap smear for cervical cancer and precursor lesions is as low as 70% and may never be much above 95%, even under the most ideal conditions. An HPV test or an HPV test and a Pap smear may eventually prove to have a higher sensitivity for cancerous or potentially malignant cervical lesions than a Pap smear alone so that fewer false-negative results would occur and women who should be closely monitored can be better identified. PCR-based assays for HPV have been positive for HPV infection in up to 46% of female university students.

3.   Request cervical cytologic reports that evaluate the Pap smear in terms of diagnostic implications rather than arcane numerical systems.

The "Bethesda System," developed in 1988 at a National Cancer Institute–sponsored workshop in Bethesda, Maryland, is the recommended format for reporting cervical and vaginal cytologic diagnoses. The report includes three elements: (1) a statement of the adequacy of the specimen; (2) a general categorization of whether the findings are normal or not; and (3) a descriptive diagnosis of the infection and/or neoplastic process.

4.   Evaluate every significantly abnormal result. A single negative report on a repeat smear does not eliminate the need for a thorough diagnostic evaluation.

A significantly abnormal result means atypia or worse, including inflammatory atypia. The diagnostic evaluation may include treatment of an inflammatory condition, visual inspection, colposcopically directed biopsy, endocervical curettage, and, when indicated, cervical conization. Inflammatory change may be a clue to important disorders, including sexually transmitted diseases, especially in women less than 25 years of age.

5.   If the cervical cytologic report is normal, repeat cervical cytologic screening annually. After therapy for preinvasive and invasive cancer, repeat screening every 3 months for 2 years and then every 6 months.

If results from three successive annual Pap smears are negative, starting when the individual reaches age 18 years or becomes sexually active, at the discretion of the physician the woman may have the tests less frequently.

6.   In patients who have had a hysterectomy for benign conditions and for whom there is adequate pathological documentation that the cervical epithelium has been totally removed and who have known previously normal smears, further screening is unnecessary.

This recommendation comes from the revised Canadian Task Force guidelines. In the United States recommendations for this particular situation have not been addressed.

7.   In patients with cervical cancer the following abnormal blood test results may occur:

↑ **Lactate dehydrogenase** from the cancer.

↑ **Carcinoembryonic antigen** from the cancer.

↑ **Alkaline phosphatase.** As a group, cancers of the ovary, endometrium, cervix, and breast exhibit the highest frequency of the Regan isoenzyme.

BIBLIOGRAPHY

American College of Obstetricians and Gynecologists: Cervical Cytology: Evaluation and Management of Abnormalities. Washington, DC, ACOG Technical Bulletin 81, October 1984.
   Recommendations by the American College of Obstetricians and Gynecologists for using the Pap smear to diagnose cervical cancer.
Bauer HM, Ting Y, Greer CE, et al: Genital human papillomavirus infection in female university students as determined by a PCR-based method. JAMA 265:472, 1991.
   HPV infection is very common in university students as determined by PCR-based assays.
Cates W Jr, Hinman AR: Sexually transmitted disease in the 1990's. N Engl J Med 325:1368, 1991.
   Centers for Disease Control (CDC) experts estimate that up to one in three Americans have HPV.
Cuzick J, Terry G, Ho L, et al: Human papillomavirus type 16 DNA in cervical smears as predictor of high-grade cervical cancer. Lancet 339:959, 1992.
   Suggests clinical indications for the use of HPV testing.

Eddy DM: Screening for cervical cancer. Ann Intern Med 113:214, 1990.
Excellent review of the data that support the use of Pap smears to diagnose cervical cancer.

Gambino R, Krieger P: False-negative fractions in cytology screening. Lab Report for Physicians 10:61, 1988.
Estimates the sensitivity of a Pap smear at 70% to 95%.

Hayward RSA, Steinberg EP, Ford DE, et al: Preventive care guidelines: 1991. Ann Intern Med 114:758, 1991.
Authoritative recommendations for the use of the Pap smear to screen for cervical cancer.

King A, Clay K, Felmar E, et al: The Papanicolaou smear. West J Med 156:202, 1992.
Good summary of recommendations by the American Cancer Society California Division's Ad Hoc Committee on Cervical Cancer.

Mandelblatt J: Papanicolaou testing following hysterectomy. JAMA 266:1289, 1991.
Recommendation for the Pap smear in a not uncommon situation.

Miller KE, Losh DP, Folley A: Evaluation and follow-up of abnormal Pap smears. Am Fam Physician 45:143, 1992.
Practical discussion of the management of patients with abnormal Pap smears.

Solomon D: The Bethesda System and Its Consequences. New Orleans, LA, American Society Clinical Pathologists/College of American Pathologists Symposium, September 24, 1991.

  Koss LG: The new Bethesda System for reporting results of smears of the uterine cervix. J Natl Cancer Inst 82:988, 1990.

  National Cancer Institute Workshop: The 1988 Bethesda System for reporting cervical/ vaginal cytologic diagnoses. JAMA 262:931, 1989.

  Key articles on the Bethesda System. As late as 1987, 72% of laboratories in one metropolitan area were using an outmoded numerical system for cytology reports.

Wilson JD, Robinson AJ, Kinghorn SA, et al: Implications of inflammatory changes on cervical cytology. BMJ 300:638, 1990.
Inflammatory changes are an important clue to sexually transmitted diseases or other colposcopic abnormalities, especially in women under 25.

Serum Cholesterol and Coronary Heart Disease

1.   Measure serum total cholesterol in every adult 20 years of age and over—whether the patient is fasting or nonfasting—at the time of the first visit. Consider also measuring high-density lipoprotein (HDL) cholesterol to calculate the total cholesterol:HDL cholesterol ratio (a 12- to 14-hour fast is desirable). Measure serum total cholesterol in children who have a strong family history of high cholesterol or coronary heart disease (CHD). Do not screen patients who are acutely ill or pregnant, and do not use serum apolipoprotein studies or lipoprotein electrophoresis for general screening.

Most authorities recommend wellness screening for hypercholesterolemia using serum total cholesterol values. CHD causes more than 500,000 deaths in the United States each year, and since up to 80% of the population may have high serum total cholesterol levels, screening is worthwhile. Each 1% reduction in serum total cholesterol reduces the CHD rate by approximately 2%. Many authorities believe that the serum total cholesterol:HDL cholesterol ratio is better than total cholesterol to estimate risk of CHD. The risk of CHD decreases by 2% to 3% for each increase of 1 mg/dL (0.026 mmol/L) of HDL cholesterol. This risk may prompt measurement of the total cholesterol and the HDL cholesterol during the first visit. If this is the case, a 12- to 14-hour fast is desirable.

Use either serum or plasma; plasma values are slightly lower. Draw blood without venous stasis since stasis can increase cholesterol concentration (e.g., after a tourniquet is applied for 5 minutes, the cholesterol level can increase 5% to 10%). Use good technique when collecting blood by skin puncture (e.g., excessive milking of the skin can significantly lower the cholesterol concentration because of dilution with tissue fluids). Serum cholesterol is quite stable at room temperature, but if delays in testing are anticipated, the specimen should be refrigerated.

The serum total cholesterol concentration is not significantly increased after a meal; therefore the screening specimen may be drawn any time the patient is seen. Since cholesterol values may be affected by an acute medical or surgical illness, do not screen acutely ill patients; evaluate only individuals who are ambulatory, in their usual state of health, on their normal diet, and not pregnant. In the first 24 hours after myocardial infarction the serum cholesterol concentration reflects preinfarction levels; therefore draw the blood specimen immediately after the patient is first seen—patients with increased values should be effectively managed.

Childhood cholesterol screening is controversial. Some propose that all children be screened for high cholesterol values, whereas others suggest that the risk-benefit ratio of childhood cholesterol screening is unfavorable and that children should not be screened. At this time it seems prudent to screen selectively, based on a family history of high cholesterol or premature CHD.

Do not use serum apolipoproteins as screening tests. Serum apolipoprotein A-I and the ratio of apolipoprotein A-I to apolipoprotein B may be better markers for CHD than serum lipids, but until these measurements are better standardized with better reference ranges and clinically relevant information, they are inappropriate for screening.

Do not use lipoprotein electrophoresis as a screening test. However, it can be useful in the diagnosis of certain lipid disorders such as abetalipoproteinemia, Tangier disease, broad beta disease, lipoprotein lipase deficiency, and lipoprotein X in patients with cholestasis.

2. Evaluate the test results.

RECOMMENDATIONS FOR CLASSIFICATION OF ADULTS' SERUM TOTAL CHOLESTEROL

<200 mg/dL (<5.17 mmol/L): desirable blood cholesterol
200–239 mg/dL (5.17–6.18 mmol/L): borderline-high blood cholesterol
≥240 mg/dL (≥6.21 mmol/L): high blood cholesterol

To use these reference ranges properly, your laboratory's results must be accurate, that is, appropriately standardized with the reference method of the CDC or the National Institute for Standards and Technology (NIST).

3.   If the serum total cholesterol concentration is below 200 mg/dL (5.17 mmol/L), remeasure within 5 years or with subsequent physical examination. In individuals with a cholesterol concentration of 200 to 239 mg/ dL (5.17 to 6.18 mmol/L), no CHD (history of myocardial infarction or angina pectoris), and not more than one additional risk factor, remeasure annually and prescribe a step-1 diet (essentially the same as the American Heart Association diet for the public). Provide dietary and risk-factor education. Consider measuring HDL cholesterol in individuals who are likely to have a low concentration.

The serum cholesterol concentration can vary with age, diet, weight, physical activity, and medications, and it is prudent to remeasure the level periodically.

Additional risk factors include the following:

- Male sex
- Family history of premature CHD (definite myocardial infarction or sudden death before 55 years of age in a parent or sibling)
- Cigarette smoking (currently smokes more than 10 cigarettes per day)
- Hypertension
- Low HDL cholesterol concentration (<35 mg/dL [<0.91 mmol/L])
- Diabetes mellitus
- History of definite cerebrovascular or occlusive peripheral vascular disease
- Severe obesity (≥30% overweight)

There are a number of causes for a low HDL cholesterol concentration, some of which are reversible: heavy cigarette smoking, obesity, lack of exercise, hypertriglyceridemia, anabolic steroids, progestational agents, antihypertensive agents, and genetic factors (e.g., primary hypoalphalipoproteinemia). If HDL cholesterol is low, try to increase it by managing the above variables. A favorable total cholesterol:HDL cholesterol ratio is 4.5:1 or lower.

Moderate drinking of alcohol appears to reduce the risk of CHD by increasing the concentrations of two types of HDL cholesterol and possibly by decreasing the concentration of low-density lipoprotein (LDL) cholesterol. A reduction in the risk of CHD occurred in those who drank more than 5 g but less than 30 g of pure alcohol daily (one drink equals approximately 10 to 15 g of alcohol). All benefits vanish and alcohol can seriously injure the heart when the daily intake exceeds 50 g.

In public screening programs all individuals with a serum cholesterol concentration of 200 mg/dL (5.17 mmol/L) or greater should be referred to their physician for remeasurement and evaluation. Remember that all serum cholesterol values should be confirmed by repeat measurements, with the average used to guide clinical decisions. Baseline lipid values are best determined by averaging two to three measurements, 1 to 8 weeks apart. If the initial serum cholesterol concentration is 200 mg/dL (5.17 mmol/L) or greater, the individual should return in 1 to 8 weeks for confirmation. If the confirmation value is within 30 mg/dL (0.78 mmol/L) of the first test result, use the average of the two results to guide subsequent decisions. If the second value differs from the first by more than 30 mg/dL (0.78 mmol/L), obtain a third test within 1 to 8 weeks and average the three values.

Lipoprotein(a), a genetic variant of LDL, is gaining acceptance as an independent risk factor for atherothrombotic cardiovascular disease. High plasma concentrations are a risk factor for premature CHD. Lipoprotein(a) should be measured in patients with premature CHD and normolipidemia.

In patients with hyperlipidemia the following abnormal blood test results may occur:

↑ **Calcium** due to an increase in the calcium bound to lipoproteins.

↓ **(Artifactual) sodium.** Pseudohyponatremia caused by lipemia (when sodium is measured with flame photometer but not with ion-specific electrode). The serum osmotic pressure is normal.

4. If serum total cholesterol is 240 mg/dL (6.21 mmol/L) or above or if it is 200 to 239 mg/dL (5.17 to 6.18 mmol/L) and the patient has CHD or two or more additional risk factors, remeasure and order a serum lipid analysis, including total cholesterol, LDL cholesterol, HDL cholesterol, and triglyceride values. The patient must fast 12 to 14 hours before blood is drawn for the repeat studies.

RECOMMENDATION FOR CLASSIFICATION OF ADULTS

Serum LDL cholesterol*

<130 mg/dL (<3.36 mmol/L): desirable LDL cholesterol
130–159 mg/dL (3.36–4.11 mmol/L): borderline-high LDL cholesterol
>160 mg/dL (>4.14 mmol/L): high LDL cholesterol

HDL cholesterol

≥35 mg/dL (≥0.91 mmol/L): desirable HDL cholesterol
≤4.5:1 desirable total cholesterol: HDL cholesterol ratio

Triglycerides

<250 mg/dL (<2.86 mmol/L): desirable triglycerides
250–500 mg/dL (2.86–5.72 mmol/L): borderline hypertriglyceridemia
≥500 mg/dL (≥5.72 mmol/L): hypertriglyceridemia

*Two measurements of LDL cholesterol after a 12- to 14-hour fast are made 1 to 8 weeks apart, and the average is used for clinical decisions unless the two values differ by more than 30 mg/dL (0.78 mmol/L), in which case a third test is carried out, and the average of all three is used. If the triglycerides are <400 mg/dL (<4.57 mmol/L), calculate LDL cholesterol as follows (all quantities are in milligrams per deciliter):

LDL cholesterol = Total cholesterol − HDL cholesterol − 0.2 × Triglycerides.

The usual serum cholesterol measurement estimates total cholesterol, which is mainly composed of LDL cholesterol and HDL cholesterol. Decreasing LDL cholesterol and increasing HDL cholesterol potentially can prevent and reverse plaque formation. Serum triglyceride values are an important part of the total lipid profile. Individuals with relatively normal serum total cholesterol concentrations but with a low HDL cholesterol value and a high triglyceride value are at significantly increased risk for CHD. Hypertriglyceridemia frequently is associated with obesity, uncontrolled diabetes mellitus, liver disease, alcohol ingestion, uremia, and the use of estrogen-containing contraceptives, steroids, isoretinoin, and some antihypertensive agents. Very high triglyceride values (>1000 mg/dL [>11.43 mmol/L]) are associated with pancreatitis. A common problem with obtaining valid serum lipid studies is failure of the patient to observe the 12- to 14-hour fast.

5.   If the serum LDL cholesterol concentration is <130 mg/dL (3.36 mmol/L), remeasure within 5 years. If it is 130 to 159 mg/dL (3.36 to 4.11 mmol/L) and there are less than two additional risk factors and no CHD, remeasure annually and prescribe a step-1 diet. Provide dietary and risk factor education.

A low serum cholesterol concentration may be a sign of good health, proper diet, and appropriate exercise. On the other hand, it may signal disease since the following disorders can be associated with low cholesterol values: acquired immunodeficiency syndrome (AIDS), severe liver damage, hyperthyroidism, malnutrition, chronic anemia, cerebral hemorrhage, and malignancy. Drugs are an additional cause of hypocholesterolemia. Nursing home residents and patients in acute care hospitals who have serum cholesterol concentrations <120 mg/dL (3.10 mmol/L) are at increased risk of premature death. Moreover, the development of hypocholesterolemia after admission to the hospital may be a unique marker for poor prognosis in older hospitalized patients. Thus reduction of total cholesterol to <150 to 160 mg/dL (3.88 to 4.14 mmol/L) may be contraindicated.

6.   If serum LDL cholesterol is 160 mg/dL (4.14 mmol/L) or above or if it is 130 to 159 mg/dL (3.36 to 4.11 mmol/L) and the patient has CHD or two or more additional risk factors, evaluate the patient for secondary hypercholesterolemia caused by diabetes mellitus, hypothyroidism, cholestasis, the nephrotic syndrome, dysproteinemia, and drugs. If a disease or drug is the cause, treat the disease or remove the drug.

The effects of selected drugs on lipid values follow:

DRUG	TOTAL CHOLESTEROL	LDL CHOLESTEROL	HDL CHOLESTEROL	TRIGLYCERIDES
Androgens	—	↑	↓	—
Antiepileptics	—	↑	↑	↑
Antihypertensives				
Thiazide diuretics	↑/—	↑	—	↑

Drug	Total Cholesterol	LDL Cholesterol	HDL Cholesterol	Triglycerides
Beta blockers	—	—	↓	↑
Alpha blockers	↓/—	↓/—	↑	↓
Corticosteroids	↑	↑	↑	↑
Cyclosporin A	↑	↑	—	—
Cyproterone acetate	↓	↓	—	—
C-19 Progestin	—	↑	↓	—
C-21 Progestin	—	—	↓	—
Oral estrogens	↓	↓	↑	↑
Phenothiazines	↑	—	↓	↑
Retinoids	↑	↑	↓	↑

Source: Adapted from Henkin Y, Como JA, Oberman A: Secondary dyslipidemia: Inadvertent effects of drugs in clinical practice. JAMA 267:961-968, 1992. Copyright 1992, American Medical Association.

7.   If a cause for secondary hypercholesterolemia is not present, consider familial dyslipidemia, including familial hypercholesterolemia (FH).

The triad of hypercholesterolemia, xanthomas, and a familial incidence is typical of FH. Other familial dyslipidemias should be considered. Because an accurate diagnosis is important for proper therapy, you may wish to refer patients suspected of having familial dyslipidemia to a lipid specialist.

8.   After considering secondary hypercholesterolemia and familial dyslipidemia, if the LDL cholesterol concentration is 160 mg/dL (4.14 mmol/L) or higher (total cholesterol of 240 mg/dL [6.21 mmol/L]) or if LDL cholesterol is 130 to 159 mg/dL (3.36 to 4.11 mmol/L) (total cholesterol of 200 to 239 mg/dL [5.17 to 6.18 mmol/L]) and the patient has CHD or two or more additional risk factors, prescribe a step-1 diet. Remeasure cholesterol in 4 to 6 weeks and at 3 months.

For individuals with less than two additional risk factors and no CHD, the goal is to reduce the serum cholesterol concentration to <240 mg/dL (6.21 mmol/L) and LDL cholesterol to <160 mg/dL (4.14 mmol/L). For individuals with CHD or two or more additional risk factors the target for serum cholesterol is <200 mg/dL (5.17 mmol/L) and for LDL cholesterol <130 mg/dL (3.36 mmol/L). Individuals with additional risk factors need to achieve lower values since, for example, the risk of a concentration of 200 mg/dL (5.17 mmol/L) in a smoker is roughly equivalent to the risk of 275 mg/dL (7.11 mmol/L) in a nonsmoker.

If goals are not achieved by 3 months, refer the individual to a registered dietitian and remeasure cholesterol in 4 to 6 weeks and at 3 months after retrial on a step-1 diet and then after trial on a step-2 diet. Continue dietary therapy under a registered dietitian for at least 6 months before considering drug treatment. Shorter periods of dietary therapy may be considered for patients with severely increased LDL cholesterol (>225 mg/dL [5.82 mmol/L]) or those with established CHD.

9.   If the serum total cholesterol goal is achieved, confirm that the LDL cholesterol goal is achieved, and monitor serum cholesterol four times in the first year and two times per year thereafter. Reinforce dietary and behavior modification.

Reducing the patient's total cholesterol concentration toward 200 mg/dL (5.17 mmol/L) helps prevent premature CHD, and reducing it toward lower values reduces the risk even further. Appropriate goals are the reduction of the serum cholesterol concentration to <180 mg/dL (4.66 mmol/L) for patients less than 30 years of age and to <200 mg/dL (5.17 mmol/L) for patients more than 30 years of age.

10.   If the serum total cholesterol and LDL cholesterol goals are not achieved after a minimum of 6 months of dietary therapy under a registered dietitian, review the medical history, continue dietary therapy, and commence drug treatment for patients with LDL cholesterol levels of 190 mg/dL (4.91 mmol/L) or higher and for patients with LDL cholesterol levels from 160 to 189 mg/dL (4.14 to 4.89 mmol/L) and CHD or two or more additional risk factors.

Remeasure LDL cholesterol in 4 to 6 weeks and at 3 months. If the LDL cholesterol goal is achieved, monitor total cholesterol every 4 months and remeasure LDL cholesterol annually. If the LDL cholesterol goal is not achieved, use another drug or combination treatment or consult with or refer the patient to a lipid specialist if drug treatment is not successful. In women a more conservative approach to drug therapy is appropriate because the absolute risk of CHD is lower in women than in men.

11.   After prescribing drug therapy, monitor the patient for possible adverse effects of cholesterol-lowering drugs.

For example, for patients taking lovastatin (Mevacor), monitor liver function tests before treatment begins and every 4 to 6 weeks during the first 15 months of therapy with lovastatin and periodically thereafter.

BIBLIOGRAPHY

Bush TL, Riedel D: Screening for total cholesterol: Do the National Cholesterol Education Program's recommendations detect individuals at high risk of coronary heart disease? Circulation 83:1287, 1991.
   Screening for low HDL cholesterol and high LDL cholesterol, not just total cholesterol, may be appropriate.
Cooper GR, Myer GL, Smith SJ, et al: Blood lipid measurements: Variations and practical utility. JAMA 267:1652, 1992.
   Highlights the problem of estimating the true cholesterol level due to biological and technical variability of cholesterol measurements and makes recommendations for physicians.
Expert Panel: Report of the National Cholesterol Education Program Expert Panel on detection, evaluation, and treatment of high blood cholesterol in adults. Arch Intern Med 148:36, 1988.

Recommendations for a national program to reduce risk of CHD by lowering serum cholesterol levels. This report constitutes the basis for most of the guidelines in treating this problem.

Gambino R, Rosen M: NIH Consensus Development Conference on triglycerides, high density lipoprotein, and coronary heart disease. Lab Report for Physicians 14:17, 1992.
Panel recommended always measuring HDL cholesterol and total cholesterol together. Triglyceride measurement is recommended in patients with diabetes, obesity, peripheral vascular disease, high blood pressure, and kidney disease.

Hancock EW: Coronary artery disease: Epidemiology and prevention. In Rubenstein E, Federman DD (eds): Scientific American. New York, Scientific American, June 1991, p 1.VIII.
Favorable serum total cholesterol/HDL cholesterol ratio is 4.5 : 1 or lower.

Hayward RSA, Steinberg EP, Ford DE, et al: Preventive care guidelines: 1991. Ann Intern Med 114:758, 1991.
Authoritative recommendations for wellness screening for hypercholesterolemia.

Kane JP, Malloy MJ, Ports TA, et al: Regression of coronary atherosclerosis during treatment of familial hypercholesterolemia with combined drug regimens. JAMA 264:3007, 1990.
Cashin-Hemphill L, Mack WJ, Pogoda JM, et al: Beneficial effects of colestipol-niacin on coronary atherosclerosis: A 4-year follow-up. JAMA 264:3013, 1990.
Aggressive therapy for lowering LDL cholesterol can cause regression of CHD.

Manninen V, Tenkanen L, Koskinen P, et al: Joint effects of serum triglyceride and LDL cholesterol and HDL cholesterol concentrations on coronary heart disease risk in the Helsinki Heart Study: Implications for treatment. Circulation 85:37, 1992.
Points out that increased triglycerides can be a risk factor for CHD.

Newman TB, Browner WS, Hulley SB: The case against childhood cholesterol screening. JAMA 264:3039, 1990.
Starc TJ, Belamarich PF, Shea S, et al: Family history fails to identify many children with severe hypercholesterolemia. Am J Dis Child 145:61, 1991.
Review the controversy about routine childhood cholesterol screening.

Noel MA, Smith TK, Ettinger WH: Characteristics and outcomes of hospitalized older patients who develop hypercholesterolemia. J Am Geriatr Soc 39:455, 1991.
Documents the poor prognosis in patients with hypocholesterolemia, especially in older patients recently admitted to the hospital.

Rimm EB, Giovannucci EL, Willett WC, et al: Prospective study of alcohol consumption and risk of coronary disease in men. Lancet 338:464, 1991.
Suh IL, Shaten J, Cutler JA, et al: Alcohol use and mortality from coronary heart disease: The role of high-density lipoprotein cholesterol. Ann Intern Med 116:881, 1992.
There is an inverse relationship between alcohol consumption and risk of CHD.

Scanu AM: Lipoprotein(a): A genetic risk factor for premature coronary heart disease. JAMA 267:3326, 1992.
Look for high lipoprotein(a) values in patients with premature CHD and normolipidemia.

Wong ND, Wilson PWF, Kannel WB: Serum cholesterol as a prognostic factor after myocardial infarction: The Framingham Study. Ann Intern Med 115:687, 1991.
After myocardial infarction, patients with increased cholesterol values should be effectively managed.

Occult Fecal Blood Testing and Colorectal Cancer

1.   To screen for colorectal cancer in average-risk men and women, perform the following studies:

- Annual digital rectal examination yearly beginning at age 40.
- Annual fecal occult blood tests beginning at age 50.
- Flexible sigmoidoscopy to 65 cm every 3 to 5 years beginning at age 50.

In addition to having annual fecal occult blood tests, persons with first-degree relatives with colorectal cancer can be offered barium enemas or colonoscopy instead of sigmoidoscopies every 3 to 5 years. Persons with inflammatory bowel disease, hereditary polyp syndromes, or a personal history of colorectal cancer or clinical findings of colorectal cancer require more aggressive diagnostic studies.

Most authorities recommend wellness screening for colorectal cancer. Approximately 150,000 new cases of and 60,900 deaths from colorectal cancer occur annually in the United States. Digital rectal examination, fecal occult blood testing, and sigmoidoscopy represent ways to detect this common cancer. A number of genes are involved in triggering the development of colorectal polyps and cancer. In the future, by testing for these genes in the stool, it may be possible to predict more accurately which patients are at increased risk for colorectal cancer.

A recent study revealed that people who regularly take aspirin cut nearly in half their risk of dying from colorectal cancer. Although more research is needed, one theory is that aspirin enhances bleeding from colorectal cancer and facilitates earlier detection of the tumor.

2. To perform fecal occult blood testing, place the individual to be tested on a diet (see below) 2 days before the first stool collection and continue this diet throughout the collection period. Instruct the individual about specimen collections. A positive test result on stool obtained via digital rectal examination should be regarded as a true positive.

For fecal occult blood testing, the individual should be instructed as follows:

- The diet should eliminate certain drugs (aspirin, nonsteroidal anti-inflammatory agents, vitamin C, iron, laxatives), rare red meat, raw fruits and vegetables high in peroxidases (broccoli, cantaloupe, cauliflower, horseradish, radish, turnips), and excessive amounts of foods moderately high in peroxidase (artichokes, cabbage, carrots, cucumbers, grapefruit, mushrooms, potatoes). Consumption of ethanol (up to three bottles of beer per day or the equivalent) should not invalidate the test. Therapeutic doses of aspirin should be withheld at least 4 days before the collection of specimens, but one aspirin or less a day should not affect the results, provided that ethanol is excluded.
- Beginning on the third day of the diet, using specimen cards, take two specimens from each of three consecutive stools. Because specimen collection is unpleasant and may adversely affect compliance, a suggested solution is to dab a small amount of stool from the toilet paper directly onto the card.
- Promptly return these three completed cards (six samples) to the laboratory.

Test samples promptly. Although most laboratories use a qualitative test such as Hemoccult II® (SmithKline Diagnostics, Inc., Philadelphia), consider using a quantitative test such as HemoQuant® (SmithKline Diagnostics, Inc., Philadelphia), which is sensitive and specific and may offer advantages over qualitative guaiac tests.

Fecal contamination by menstrual or urinary blood may cause false-positive test results.

3. Evaluate the fecal occult blood test results.

One or more positive results in any of these six samples is considered a positive test for occult blood that cannot be ignored. After a race marathon runners may have a positive fecal occult blood test. If a retrospective history of use of therapeutic nonsteroidal anti-inflammatory agents during the collection period is elicited, discontinue the agents, and perform another set of fecal occult blood tests after 3 weeks.

4. Evaluate every asymptomatic individual with a positive fecal occult blood test by flexible sigmoidoscopy and air-contrast barium enema or full colonoscopy. Full colonoscopy is preferable.

In the past sigmoidoscopy with air-contrast barium enema was often used; however, full colonoscopy is the current procedure of choice because it is more effective and less costly.

Approximately 1% to 5% of unselected persons tested with fecal occult blood tests have positive test results. Of those with positive test results, approximately 10% have cancer, and 20% to 30% have adenomas. The remainder has either a benign source of bleeding (e.g., proctitis, anal fissure, hemorrhoid) or no detectable lesion. Some individuals with a positive fecal occult blood test result and normal gastrointestinal studies may have a lesion that was not detected. These individuals should be reevaluated in the near future, perhaps in 1 or 2 months.

5. In patients with colorectal cancer the following abnormal blood test results may occur:

↓ **Hemoglobin and hematocrit** caused by iron deficiency anemia due to blood loss.

↑ **Erythrocyte sedimentation rate** caused by inflammatory complications of the tumor.

↑ **Lactate dehydrogenase** coming from the cancer.

↑ **Carcinoembryonic antigen** coming from the cancer.

↑ **Leukocytes** caused by inflammatory complications of the tumor.

↓ **Potassium** when the cancer is associated with a villous adenoma.

↑ **Creatine kinase** originating in the cancer.

↑ **Alkaline phosphatase** that may be due to the Regan isoenzyme.

BIBLIOGRAPHY

Eddy DM: Screening for colorectal cancer. Ann Intern Med 113:373, 1990.
   Guidelines for detecting early colorectal cancer based on available data and a mathematical model.
Eisner MS, Lewis JH: Diagnostic yield of a positive fecal occult blood test found on digital

rectal examination: Does the finger count? Arch Intern Med 151:2180, 1991.
Positive test result should be followed up, even if the sample was obtained by digital rectal examination.

Fleming JL, Ahlquist DA, McGill DB, et al: Influence of aspirin and ethanol on fecal blood levels as determined by using the HemoQuant assay. Mayo Clin Proc 62:159, 1987.
Discussion of the effects of two heavily used drugs, aspirin and ethanol, on tests for fecal occult blood.

Hayward RSA, Steinberg EP, Ford DE, et al: Preventive care guidelines: 1991. Ann Intern Med 114:758, 1991.
Authoritative recommendations for wellness screening for colorectal cancer.

Levine R, Tenner S, Fromm H: Prevention and early detection of colorectal cancer. Am Fam Physician 45:663, 1992.
Reviews principles of an effective program.

Mandel JS, Bond JH, Bradley M, et al: Sensitivity, specificity, and positive predictivity of the Hemoccult test in screening for colorectal cancers: The University of Minnesota's Colon Cancer Control Study. Gastroenterology 97:597, 1989.
No data are presently available on whether fecal occult blood testing reduces colorectal cancer mortality.

Matzen RN: Fecal occult blood testing: Guidelines for follow-up after positive findings. Postgrad Med 90:181, 1991.
Cleveland Clinic Foundation physician explains why full colonoscopy is today's diagnostic follow-up procedure of choice.

Nattinger AB: Colon cancer screening and detection. In Panzer RJ, Black ER, Griner PF (eds): Diagnostic Strategies for Common Medical Problems. Philadelphia, American College of Physicians, 1991, p 104.
Recommends strategies for detecting colorectal cancer with discussion of fecal occult blood testing.

Rozen P, Ron E, Fireman Z, et al: The relative value of fecal occult blood tests and flexible sigmoidoscopy in screening for large bowel neoplasia. Cancer 60:2553, 1987.
Discusses the yield in patients with positive fecal occult blood tests in terms of benign and malignant lesions.

Selby JV, Friedman GD, Quesenberry CP Jr: A case-control study of screening sigmoidoscopy and mortality from colorectal cancer. N Engl J Med 326:653, 1992.
Levin B: Screening sigmoidoscopy for colorectal cancer. N Engl J Med 326:700, 1992.
Screening sigmoidoscopy is effective in reducing colorectal cancer deaths—once every 10 years may be enough.

Thun MJ, Namboodiri MM, Heath CW Jr: Aspirin use and reduced risk of fatal colon cancer. N Engl J Med 325:1593, 1991.
Findings of a 10-year American Cancer Society study on 662,424 people that showed a lower risk of dying from colorectal cancer in people who regularly took aspirin.

Wagner JL, Herdman RC, Wadhwa S: Cost effectiveness of colorectal cancer screening in the elderly. Ann Intern Med 115:807, 1991.
Concludes that screening for colorectal cancer in persons 65 to 85 years of age is cost-effective.

Digital Rectal Examination, Prostate-Specific Antigen, and Prostate Cancer

1.   Perform an annual digital rectal examination of the prostate in men after age 40 to discover nodularity or induration that may be due to prostate

cancer. Recently, the American Cancer Society recommended annual serum prostate-specific antigen (PSA) measurements on men 50 years and older.

Most authorities recommend wellness screening for prostate cancer, using digital rectal examination; however, the American Urological Association believes that both serum PSA and digital rectal examination should be used. Approximately 120,000 new cases of and 32,000 deaths from prostate cancer occur annually in the United States. Digital rectal examination is both accurate and cost-effective for detecting prostate cancer. The role of screening with PSA and/or transrectal ultrasonography to detect prostate cancer is controversial. A recent study suggests that rectal examination plus serum PSA measurement will detect significantly more prostate cancers than rectal examination alone; but others argue that many prostate cancers never cause clinical problems and detecting these clinically silent cancers may expose patients to the risks of treatment without the potential for benefit. Moreover, approximately 30% of patients with benign prostatic hypertrophy have a high PSA concentration. Measuring the rate of change in serum PSA and correlating the PSA concentration with prostatic volume (PSA density) may improve the diagnostic sensitivity and specificity of this tumor marker. Finasteride (Proscar), a new drug for benign prostatic hypertrophy, can decrease PSA—men taking this drug should be followed with digital rectal examination as well as baseline and periodic PSA measurements.

2.   If digital rectal examination of the prostate reveals an area of nodularity or induration, establish the diagnosis using PSA and a transrectal ultrasound (TRUS)-guided biopsy. Draw a blood specimen for determining PSA (by immunoassay) and prostate acid phosphatase (PAP) (by chemical method or immunoassay) before performing the biopsy.

Measurement of both PSA and PAP is useful for three reasons: (1) some patients with prostate cancer have a high PAP but a normal PSA measurement (most of these patients were on hormone therapy); (2) the two assays should confirm one another; and (3) the two assays differ in sensitivity and specificity (e.g., PSA is more sensitive for the detection of prostate cancer, but PAP is more specific).

Assuming normal prevalence, the positive predictive value of PSA in conjunction with digital rectal examination is as follows:

	PSA RANGES ng/mL (μg/L)*		
DIGITAL RECTAL EXAMINATION	**0.0–4.0**	**4.1–10**	**>10**
Negative	9%	20%	31%
Positive	17%	45%	77%

$$\text{Positive predictive value} = \frac{\text{True positives}}{\text{True positives} + \text{False positives}}$$

Source: Oesterling JE: Prostate-specific antigen: A valuable clinical tool. Oncology 5:112, 1991.
*Tandem®—R PSA Assay

Definitive diagnosis is established by TRUS-guided biopsy and examination of prostate tissue under the microscope. Prostate biopsy but not digital rectal examination may significantly increase PSA and PAP. TRUS alone does not increase the PSA in patients with prostate cancer or benign prostatic hypertrophy. It may, however, slightly increase PSA in patients with prostatitis.

The best chemical methods for measuring serum PAP are the tartrate-inhibited fraction using p-nitrophenylphosphate or, more recently, thymolphthalein monophosphate. Ideally, immunoassays should be used for measuring both PSA and PAP. When measured chemically, PAP is very labile at room temperature; the specimen should be analyzed quickly or acid-treated and stored at 4° C until analysis.

3. Evaluate the test results and obtain other appropriate studies: CBC, lactate dehydrogenase (LD), alkaline phosphatase (ALP), and hepatic and renal function studies.

REFERENCE RANGES

TEST	SPECIMEN	CONVENTIONAL UNITS	INTERNATIONAL UNITS
Acid phosphatase: thymolphthalein monophosphate	Serum*	<0.8 U/L	<0.8 U/L
Prostate-specific antigen	Serum†	0–4 ng/ml	0–4 µg/L

*Automatic Clinical Analyzer (EI du Pont de Nemours & Co., Inc., Wilmington, Del).
†Tandem®—R PSA (Hybritech, Inc., San Diego, Calif).

Although not affected by digital rectal examination, the serum PSA level may increase twofold with prostate massage, fourfold with cystoscopy, and more than fiftyfold with needle biopsy or transurethral resection of the prostate. Since the effective half-life of PSA is 2.2 to 3.2 days, a needle biopsy requires a delay of approximately 2 to 3 weeks before measurement of PSA would be valid. Serum PSA is increased in patients with prostate cancer, benign prostate hypertrophy, and prostatitis. A PSA concentration >10 ng/mL (10 µg/L) is highly suspicious for cancer, and the higher the PSA, the greater is the likelihood of advanced disease (e.g., lymph node metastases are present in two thirds of patients with a PSA concentration >25 ng/mL [25 µg/L]). PSA values may be unreliable in patients on antiandrogen therapy. It is wise to measure baseline PSA since this measurement will be useful for comparing with future measurements of PSA to determine adequacy of surgical removal of the cancer or recurrence.

Although serum PAP is rarely increased when the cancer is confined to the gland, approximately 80% of patients with locally invasive or metastatic cancer will have sustained high values. In addition to prostate cancer, serum

PAP may be increased secondary to prostatitis, prostate infarct, prostate surgery or biopsy, Gaucher's disease, Niemann-Pick disease, some benign and malignant hematologic disorders, and other miscellaneous conditions. Prostate massage may increase serum PAP for 72 hours, but routine digital examination appears to have no effect. Values are increased in some patients with benign hypertrophy, prostatitis, or retention of urine. It is not possible to determine whether such patients also have subclinical cancer of the prostate.

Serum ALP may be high because of osteoblastic bone metastases or cholestatic liver metastases. These high ALP values may occur in individuals who have an increased or normal PAP level. In patients with metastatic cancer who have a normal PAP level, a high ALP level can suggest the presence of metastatic disease, and a CBC can detect secondary anemia. A high serum urea nitrogen and creatinine concentration and an abnormal urinalysis can detect renal dysfunction such as obstructive uropathy. Serum LD, specifically LD-5, may increase secondary to the tumor mass.

A recent study indicated that normal serum acid and alkaline phosphatase levels and absence of bone pain in patients with newly diagnosed prostate cancer have a negative predictive value for bone metastases of 99% (i.e., bone scan may be omitted in such patients).

4.   If the prostate biopsy is negative for cancer, the patient is probably free of disease, but remember that false-negative biopsy and test results can occur.

Approximately 50% of prostate nodules felt on rectal examination will be confirmed as cancer. The sensitivity of a single biopsy to detect existing prostate cancer is approximately 80%. With repeated attempts, the sensitivity increases to 90%.

Up to 90% of patients with prostate cancer metastatic to bone will have an increased serum ALP level because of osteoblastic activity. Liver metastases can also cause an increased ALP level that is secondary to cholestasis.

A negative chemistry and hematology screen—including normal serum PSA and PAP test results—does not completely exclude prostate cancer.

5.   Grade and stage the tumor using test results in the context of clinical findings and radiographic data.

Prostate cancer should be histologically graded and clinically staged so that appropriate therapy can be chosen.

6.   In addition to standard clinical procedures, use PSA to monitor the response of prostate cancer to treatment.

Measure PSA 3 weeks after treatment, then every 3 months for the first year, every 4 months for the second year, and then every 6 months.

After curative radical prostatectomy, serum PSA becomes undetectable 3 weeks after surgery. Those patients who do not achieve an undetectable PSA level by 3 months after radical prostatectomy usually never do and probably have residual disease.

During the first 12 months after radiation therapy, the PSA level decreased in 82% of patients in one study, but only 8% continued to decline beyond 1 year. Only 11% had an undetectable PSA level at a mean follow-up of 5 years. After 1 year a rising PSA level correlated with a positive prostate biopsy and metastatic disease.

After endocrine therapy PSA concentration increased as the cancer progressed, decreased during periods of remission, and fluctuated erratically when the patient was clinically stable.

7.   In men with prostate cancer the following additional abnormal blood test results may occur.

Anemia.

↑ **Carcinoembryonic antigen** originating in the tumor.

↑ **Creatine kinase** coming from the tumor.

BIBLIOGRAPHY

Barry MJ: Nonpalpable prostate cancer screening. In Panzer RJ, Black ER, Griner PF (eds): Diagnostic Strategies for Common Medical Problems. Philadelphia, American College of Physicians, 1991, p 430.
  Makes a good argument for not screening for prostate cancer with PSA.
Catalona WJ, Smith DS, Ratliff TL, et al: Measurement of prostate-specific antigen in serum as a screening test for prostate cancer. N Engl J Med 324:1156, 1991.
  Proposes PSA plus rectal examination to screen for prostate cancer.
Finasteride for benign prostatic hypertrophy. The Medical Letter 34:83, 1992.
  Suggests baseline and periodic rectal examination and PSA measurements for patients on finasteride (Proscar).
Gambino R: Prostate-specific antigen or prostatic acid phosphatase, or both? Lab Report for Physicians 12:73, 1990.
  Recommends simultaneous immunological measurements of PSA and PAP.
Gerber G, Chodak GW: Assessment of value of routine bone scans in patients with newly diagnosed prostate cancer. Urology 37:418, 1991.
  Establishes that bone scans are unnecessary in newly diagnosed patients with normal chemistry test results and absence of bone pain.
Gittes RF: Carcinoma of the prostate. N Engl J Med 324:236, 1991.
  Excellent review of pathogenesis, diagnosis, and management of prostate cancer.
Hayward RSA, Steinberg EP, Ford DE, et al: Preventive care guidelines: 1991. Ann Intern Med 114:758, 1991.
  Authoritative recommendations for wellness screening for prostate cancer.
Hughes HR, Penney MD, Gryan P, et al: Serum prostatic specific antigen: *in vitro* stability and the effect of ultrasound rectal examination *in vivo.* Ann Clin Biochem 24 (suppl): S1206, 1987.
  Reports the effects of transrectal ultrasound on serum PSA.
Littrup PJ, Lee F, Mettlin C: Prostate cancer screening: Current trends and future implications. CA Cancer J Clin 42:198, 1992.
  Screening for prostate cancer remains a clinical dilemma.
Oesterling JE: Prostate-specific antigen: A valuable clinical tool. Oncology 5:107, 1991.
  Discussion from the Mayo Clinic on the role of PSA for screening, diagnosis, and management.
Oesterling JE: Prostate-specific antigen: Improving its ability to diagnose early prostate cancer. JAMA 267:2236, 1992.

Discusses the "rate of change of PSA" and "PSA density" as promising ways to improve the value of this tumor marker.

Thomson RD, Clejan S: Digital rectal examination–associated alterations in serum prostate-specific antigen. Am J Clin Pathol 97:528, 1992.

Gillenwater JY: Digital rectal examination–associated alterations in serum prostate-specific antigen. Am J Clin Pathol 97:466, 1992.

Establishes that digital rectal examination does not significantly increase serum PSA and mentions that the American Urological Association endorses screening using digital rectal examination and PSA.

Detection of Alcohol Abuse

1.   To detect individuals with alcohol abuse, ask the CAGE questions and the Brief Michigan Alcoholism Screening Test questions, and request appropriate laboratory tests.

Some authorities have recommended case finding, education, and counseling about the appropriate use of alcohol. In the United States the combined lifetime prevalence of alcohol abuse and dependence is estimated at 11% to 16%. In hospitalized medical patients estimates range from 15% to 60%, depending on the population studied. More than 65,000 Americans lost their lives in 1990 because of alcohol abuse— 22,000 of them on the highways. The National Center for Health Statistics estimates that the financial burden of alcohol abuse will reach $150 billion by 1995 (up from $128 billion in 1986)—more than the cost of cardiovascular disease.

Helpful tests to detect alcohol abuse include a blood alcohol measurement; a CBC; red blood cell indices and examination of a Wright-stained blood smear for macrocytic red cells; and liver function tests, including serum GGT. It may be worthwhile to obtain a biochemical profile and a urinalysis since alcohol abuse affects so many analytes. Urinary alcohol determinations on daily samples collected for at least 1 week have also been recommended as an effective screening test for occult alcohol abuse. Serum carbohydrate-deficient transferrin determination is a promising new test to detect alcohol abuse. High concentrations occur in individuals drinking more than 50 to 80 g of alcohol per day for at least 1 week (one drink equals approximately 10 to 15 g of alcohol). The high values normalize slowly during abstinence, with a half-life of approximately 15 days. Other new tests that may be useful to detect alcohol abuse include evaluation of platelet monoamine oxidase inhibition by alcohol and adenylate cyclase activity in platelets and lymphocytes.

When directly questioned about their drinking habits, individuals who abuse alcohol frequently underreport the quantity of alcohol they consume. The CAGE questions are designed to detect alcohol abuse in a less confrontational way. Sometimes individuals will deny drinking altogether. In this circumstance laboratory test results and other clues such as unexplained bruises and frequent ingestion of antacids for gastritis become more important. A history of trauma can signal the presence of alcohol abuse. Also alcoholics often smoke and abuse other drugs. Exercise and physical fitness are frequently neglected. Hypertension, cardiomyopathy, and cardiac arrhythmias are additional clues. Any patient with an odor of alcohol probably has a problem with alcohol. According to the National Institute of Drug Abuse, consuming five or more drinks at one sitting constitutes abusive drinking.

The CAGE acronym focuses on *C*utting down, *A*nnoyance by criticism, *G*uilt feelings, and *E*ye-openers. The questions are as follows:

1. Have you ever felt you ought to cut down on your drinking?
2. Have people annoyed you by critizing your drinking?
3. Have you ever felt bad or guilty about your drinking?
4. Have you ever had a drink first thing in the morning to steady your nerves or get rid of a hangover (eye-opener)?

The Brief Michigan Alcoholism Test has the following questions (*Y* is a yes answer, and *N* is a no answer; the number after *Y* or *N* is the number of points for that yes or no answer).

1. Do you feel you are a normal drinker?	YES	NO	N2
2. Do friends or relatives think you are a normal drinker?	YES	NO	N2
3. Have you ever attended a meeting of Alcoholics Anonymous?	YES	NO	Y5
4. Have you ever lost friends, girlfriends, or boyfriends because of drinking?	YES	NO	Y2
5. Have you ever gotten into trouble at work because of drinking?	YES	NO	Y2
6. Have you ever neglected your obligations, your family, or your work for 2 or more days in a row because you were drinking?	YES	NO	Y2
7. Have you ever had delirium tremens (DTs), had severe shaking, heard voices, or seen things that weren't there after heavy drinking?	YES	NO	Y2
8. Have you ever gone to anyone for help about your drinking?	YES	NO	Y5
9. Have you ever been in a hospital because of drinking?	YES	NO	Y5
10. Have you ever been arrested for drunk driving or driving after drinking?	YES	NO	Y2

2.   Evaluate the questionnaires and laboratory test results.

Once ingested, ethanol is rapidly cleared from the blood, and after 24 hours it is completely gone. Changes in hematologic values, liver enzymes, and serum lipid concentrations persist for longer periods of time. Interestingly, individuals taking H_2-receptor antagonists (rantidine and cimetidine) achieve significantly higher blood alcohol concentrations for a given number of alcoholic drinks consumed—probably because these drugs interfere with the metabolism of alcohol by alcohol dehydrogenase in the gastric mucosa.

CAGE QUESTIONNAIRE

In a recent study on alcohol abuse, likelihood ratios were developed for alcoholism for the CAGE questionnaire. The gold standard was the revised criteria of the *Diagnostic and Statistical Manual of Mental Disorders—III*. The likelihood ratios were 0.14 for no positive answers, 1.5 for one positive answer, 4.5 for two positive answers, 13 for three positive answers, and 100 for four positive answers. These likelihood ratios were used to construct a table of pretest (prior) probabilities and posttest (posterior) probabilities as follows:

CAGE SCORES, PRIOR PROBABILITIES, AND ASSOCIATED POSTERIOR PROBABILITIES FOR ALCOHOLISM IN A GENERAL MEDICINE POPULATION

CAGE SCORE	POSTERIOR PROBABILITIES ACCORDING TO PRIOR PROBABILITIES					
	10%	15%	20%	24%	36%	63%
0	2%	2%	3%	4%	7%	19%
1	14%	21%	27%	32%	46%	72%
2	33%	44%	53%	59%	72%	88%
3	59%	70%	76%	81%	88%	96%
4	92%	95%	96%	97%	98%	99%

Source: Reproduced with permission Buchsbaum DG, Buchanan RG, Centor RM, et al: Screening for alcohol abuse using CAGE scores and likelihood ratios. Ann Intern Med 115:776, 1991.

Using likelihood ratios to interpret CAGE scores enables the clinician to stratify patients along a continuum of risk for alcohol abuse. This is better than simply regarding two or more positive CAGE responses as positive and no or one positive CAGE responses as negative for alcoholism. The problem with this approach is the difficulty in assigning prior probabilities in actual patient care situations.

BRIEF MICHIGAN ALCOHOLISM SCREENING QUESTIONNAIRE

A score of six or more points indicates a probable diagnosis of alcohol abuse.

U.S. NATIONAL COUNCIL ON ALCOHOLISM CRITERIA FOR ALCOHOL ABUSE

BLOOD ALCOHOL CONCENTRATION	FINDINGS
>100 mg/dL (>22 mmol/L)	At the time of routine examination by a physician
>150 mg/dL (>33 mmol/L)	Without gross evidence of intoxication
>300 mg/dL (>66 mmol/L)	At any time

3.   If the answers to the CAGE questions, the Brief Michigan Alcoholism questions, and laboratory test results are consistent with alcohol abuse, the diagnosis is supported with a level of confidence that depends on the number of consistent answers and positive test results. The CAGE questions are probably better than laboratory tests for detecting alcohol abuse.

Even without laboratory tests, a history of heavy drinking, appropriate clinical findings, and consistent answers to the CAGE questions and Brief Michigan Alcoholism Screening questions may allow you to make the diagnosis. If laboratory test results are positive, they lend support to the diagnosis. An increased red cell mean corpuscular volume, increased GGT, and increased liver enzymes are consistent with alcohol abuse. Although the CAGE questions and laboratory tests are sensitive for alcohol abuse, they are not completely specific. Occasionally positive answers and test results occur in patients who are not alcoholics. With the CAGE questions, two positive answers are usually recommended for identifying alcohol abuse; three positive answers are highly predictive for the diagnosis. Also, there are other causes for an increased GGT value such as therapy with phenytoin sodium (Dilantin) or phenobarbital and other causes for increased transaminase and ALP values such as drug-related or viral hepatitis.

4.   If the answers to the CAGE questions and the Brief Michigan Alcoholism Screening questions are negative and the laboratory test results are normal, the diagnosis of alcohol abuse is not supported by objective data.

Since the sensitivity of the CAGE questions and laboratory tests for alcohol abuse is <100%, negative answers and normal test results do not exclude the disorder with complete confidence. If clinical suspicion of alcohol abuse continues to exist, the CAGE questions, the Brief Michigan Alcoholism Screening questions, and laboratory tests should be repeated in the future.

5.   If you wish to monitor an alcoholic who is in a treatment program, measure GGT, aspartate aminotransferase (AST/SGOT), and alanine aminotransferase (ALT/SGPT). If there is an odor of alcohol, measure blood alcohol.

When a patient is in a treatment program, a measurable level of blood or urinary alcohol provides evidence of failure to abstain from drinking. Indeed, regular determination of urinary alcohol is a convenient way to follow these patients—the only potential false positives are diabetics with a urinary tract infection by a fermentor such as *Candida albicans*. Another way to detect a drinking relapse is to measure GGT, AST (SGOT), and ALT (SGPT). An increase in the serum activity of any of these enzymes—GGT of 20% or more, AST of 40% or more, and ALT of 20% or more—above an individual's baseline values after 4 weeks of abstinence indicates a return to drinking.

6.   In the alcoholic patient the following additional abnormal blood test results may occur:

Anemia from a variety of causes (e.g., iron or folate deficiency).
↓ **Leukocytes** from bone marrow suppression.
↓ **Platelets** from bone marrow suppression.
↑ **Prothrombin time (PT)** due to decreased hepatic synthesis of coagulation factors.
↑ **Activated partial thromboplastin time,** less frequent than increased PT.
Alcoholic pH changes; acidosis or alkalosis, which may be respiratory or metabolic.
↓ **Glucose** in fasting patients because of suppression of gluconeogenesis by alcohol (as little as one or two drinks can cause this effect in any person).
↓ **Glucose tolerance.**
↓ **Urea nitrogen** in severe liver diseases.
↑ **Uric acid** (often >7 mg/dL [>416 μmol/L]).
↓ **Sodium.**
↓ **Potassium.**
↓ **Calcium.**
↓ **Magnesium.**
↑ **Creatine kinase** caused by myopathy, rarely myoglobinemia, and myoglobinuria.
↑ **Lactate dehydrogenase.**
↓ **Phosphorus.**
↑ **Amylase** in patients with acute pancreatitis.

Abnormal liver function tests caused by fatty liver, alcoholic hepatitis, and/or cirrhosis.
↑ **HDL cholesterol,** which returns to baseline after 1 or 2 weeks of abstinence.
↓ **Thyroxine (T_4)** (modestly) and a marked decrease in serum triiodothyronine (T_3); return to normal after several weeks of abstinence.
↑ **Triglycerides** caused by increased hepatic production, often >180 mg/dl (>2.06 mmol/L).
↑ **Cortisol** after an alcoholic binge.
↓ **Testosterone.**
Inhibition of vasopressin at rising alcohol concentrations and the opposite at falling concentrations so that most alcoholics are often slightly overhydrated.
↑ **Carcinoembryonic antigen** in patients with alcoholic liver disease.
↑ **Serum osmotic pressure** when measured by a freezing point osmometer but not a vapor pressure osmometer; provided other osmotically active substances such as methanol or mannitol are not present in the serum, the serum ethanol concentration can be calculated, based on the osmotic gap, as follows:

Estimated blood alcohol (mg/dL)

$$= \text{Osmotic gap} \times \frac{100}{22}$$

or

Estimated blood alcohol (mmol/L) = Osmotic gap

Where osmotic gap equals measured osmolality minus calculated osmolality (all units in mOsm/kg) (see section in Chapter 10, "Classifying Fluid

Volume, Acid-Base, Electrolyte, and Osmolality Disorders by Laboratory Tests").

BIBLIOGRAPHY

Beresford TP, Blow FC, Hill E, et al: Comparison of CAGE questionnaire and computer-assisted laboratory profiles in screening for covert alcoholism. Lancet 336:482, 1990.
CAGE questions are probably better than laboratory tests for detecting alcohol abuse.
Buchsbaum DG, Buchanan RG, Centor RM, et al: Screening for alcohol abuse using CAGE scores and likelihood ratios. Ann Intern Med 115:774, 1991.
Developed likelihood ratios for stratifying the posttest probability of alcohol abuse based on how many CAGE questions are answered affirmatively.
Crowley TJ: Alcoholism: Identification, evaluation, and early treatment. West J Med 140:461, 1984.
Discusses the use of CAGE questions and the Brief Michigan Alcoholism Test to detect alcohol abuse.
DiPadova C, Roine R, Frezza M, et al: Effects of ranitidine on blood alcohol levels after ethanol ingestion: Comparison with other H_2-receptor antagonists. JAMA 267:83, 1992.
Describes the increased blood alcohol values that occur in individuals taking H_2-receptor antagonists.
Gambino R: Screening for occult alcoholism. Lab Report for Physicians 2:42, 1980.
Urinary alcohol measurements are effective for detecting alcoholism.
Gibbons B, Steinmetz G: Alcohol: The legal drug. National Geographic 181:3, 1992.
Excellent photo essay on the role of alcohol in society from biblical times to the present.
Hayward RSA, Steinberg EP, Ford DE, et al: Preventive care guidelines: 1991. Ann Intern Med 114:758, 1991.
Authoritative recommendations about programs to encourage the appropriate use of alcohol.
Irwin M, Baird S, Smith TL, et al: Use of laboratory tests to monitor heavy drinking by alcoholic men discharged from a treatment program. Am J Psychiatry 145:595, 1988.
Describes a way to use GGT, AST, and ALT tests to monitor abstinence.
Magarian GJ, Lucas LM, Kumar KL: Clinical significance in alcoholic patients of commonly encountered laboratory test results. West J Med 156:287, 1992.
Discusses abnormal test results that can occur in the alcoholic patient.
Spivak JL: Medical complications of alcoholism. In Spivak JL, Barnes HV (eds): Manual of Clinical Problems in Internal Medicine, 4th ed. Boston, Little, Brown & Co, 1990, p 533.
Summarizes alcohol's effects on many laboratory tests and includes annotated key references.
Stibler H: Carbohydrate-deficient transferrin in serum: A new marker of potentially harmful alcohol consumption reviewed. Clin Chem 37:2029, 1991.
Describes a promising new test for alcohol abuse.
Wrenn KD, Slovis CM, Minion GE, et al: The syndrome of alcoholic ketoacidosis. Am J Med 91:119, 1991.
Describes acid-base disturbances and other abnormal laboratory test results after an alcoholic binge.

Urine Screening for Drug Abuse

1.   If an individual shows clinical findings of drug abuse, if you wish to screen for drug abuse, or if you wish to monitor a known drug abuser,

obtain a urine specimen collected by a reliable observer, request appropriate tests, and maintain a chain of custody. Consult the laboratory director or supervisor for information on anabolic steroid testing.

Screening for drug abuse is controversial. It is practiced by the federal government and many private industries. The value of workplace screening has not been determined. Although some authorities have recommended education and counseling about the hazards of drug abuse, none has recommended screening for drug abuse in the context of a routine checkup.

Blood is not a good specimen for drug abuse screening. The sensitivities of laboratory methods for detecting drugs in blood are not as good as in urine. Usually the drugs that can be detected in blood are limited to aspirin, acetaminophen, anticonvulsants, barbiturates, diazepam, and volatiles such as alcohol.

For tests to have legal validity, a chain of custody is required. It involves documentation of every person who had custody of the specimen from the time it was collected to the time it was tested. Moreover, every person who had custody must have kept the specimen in a secure manner so that no one could have tampered with it.

Clinical findings of drug abuse include mental changes (delirium, dementia, depression); school difficulties, behavior problems, or unexplained medical problems in adolescents or young adults; and a newly developing psychosis or unexpected deterioration in occupational or social functioning. Known drug abusers should be tested to determine the specific drug or drugs of abuse.

A critical issue in forensic drug abuse testing is observation of collection of the urine specimen by a reliable observer to ensure that the specimen truly belongs to the subject being tested. Collection personnel can inspect the urine color and measure its temperature, pH, and specific gravity to verify specimen validity. The specimen should be accurately labeled and refrigerated and a chain of custody maintained.

Appropriate tests for drug abuse should include those for agents most prevalent in the group or class to which the individual belongs. Screening by thin-layer chromatography (TLC) is capable of detecting a wide spectrum of drugs. In contrast, screening by immunoassay detects only the individual agents included in the screening profile.

Because different drugs of abuse have different half-lives (e.g., cocaine, 40 to 80 minutes; amphetamines, 6 to 12 hours; marijuana or tetrahydrocannabinol [THC], 4 to 6 weeks), different screening schedules are necessary to detect different drugs as follows:

DETECTION LIMITS FOR URINE TESTING*

DRUG	DOSE (MG)	DETECTION TIME	SCREENING FREQUENCY
Amphetamines	30	1–120 hr	1–2/wk
Barbiturates			
Short acting	100	6–24 hr	1–2/wk
Phenobarbital	30	At least 4½ days	1–2/wk

Table continued on following page.

DETECTION LIMITS FOR URINE TESTING* Continued

DRUG	DOSE (MG)	DETECTION TIME	SCREENING FREQUENCY
Benzodiazepines			
Long acting (diazepam)	10	7 days	1/wk
Short acting (triazolam)	0.5	24 hr	2–3/wk
Cocaine	250	8–48 hr	2–3/wk
Methadone	40	7.5–56 hr	2–3/wk
Methaqualone	150	60 hr	1–2/wk
Morphine opiates (IV)	10	84 hr	1/wk
THC metabolites	†	7–34 days	1/mo
	‡	6–81 days	1/mo

Source: Saxon AJ, Calsyn DA, Haver VM, et al: Clinical evaluation and use of urine screening for drug abuse. West J Med 149:297, 1988.
*Detection time is the length of time the drug can be detected in the urine after a given dose. Screening frequency is the suggested number of times per week or per month that urine testing would be required to detect repeated use of a given drug.
†Weekly marijuana use.
‡Daily marijuana use.

2. Evaluate the test results.

Choose the most reputable laboratory available. You may wish to inquire about the laboratory's performance on outside proficiency surveys.

Laboratories use two types of tests, screening and confirmatory, for detecting and confirming drugs in urine. Initially a screening test is performed. A confirmatory test—using a more specific method—should be done to verify a positive screening test. The confirmatory test should be based on a different principle of analysis and be at least as sensitive as the screening test. Enzyme immunoassay (EIA), fluorescence polarization immunoassay (FPIA), and radioimmunoassay (RIA) are generally preferred for screening. TLC may also be used for screening. Gas chromatography (GC) and high-performance liquid chromatography (HPLC) are currently used for confirmatory analysis; however, gas chromatography–mass spectrometry (GC-MS) is the best confirmatory test.

3. Interpret test results in the context of clinical findings.

As with all clinical laboratory tests, decisions must be made about what constitutes a positive test result. In marijuana screening, for example, establishing a threshold value of 0.1 μg/mL (0.1 mg/L) of urine will minimize the possibility of a positive result for persons with only a passive exposure to cannabis. Much lower concentrations actually can be detected. Using a threshold value of 0.1 μg/mL (0.1 mg/L) reduces the incidence of false-positive results but increases the incidence of false-negative results. A combination of EIA screening and GC-MS confirmation yields virtually 100% accuracy in detection of marijuana abuse. The choice of a threshold value may be influenced by the clinical purpose of the test.

Remember that, in contrast to ethanol, there is no established correlation between concentrations of drugs of abuse in body fluids and clinical impairment.

BIBLIOGRAPHY

Davis KH, Hawks RL, Blanke RV: Assessment of laboratory quality in urine drug testing: A proficiency testing pilot study. JAMA 260:1749, 1988.
Survey of the quality of laboratory testing for drugs.
Everett WD, Linder M: Drug testing in the workplace: What primary care physicians need to know. Postgrad Med 91:287, 1992.
Guidelines for testing procedures and interpretation of results in the workplace.
Farrar HC, Kearns GL: Cocaine: Clinical pharmacology and toxicology. J Pediatr 115:665, 1989.
Reviews the pharmacology, detection, and management of cocaine intoxication.
Gerson B (ed): Clinical Toxicology I and II. Clin Lab Med 10:June and September 1990.
Two volumes, totaling 647 pages, extensively covering the field.
Giannini AJ, Miller NS: Drug abuse: A biopsychiatric model. Am Fam Physician 40:173, 1989.
Explains how different drugs exert their effects and provides a rationale for intervention.
McNagny SE, Parker RM: High prevalence of recent cocaine use and the unreliability of patient self-report in an inner-city walk-in clinic. JAMA 267:1106, 1992.
Cocaine abuse continues in epidemic proportions throughout the United States.
Moyer TP, Palmen MA, Johnson P, et al: Marijuana testing: How good is it? Mayo Clin Proc 62:413, 1987.
Demonstrates the accuracy of properly performed drug tests for marijuana.
Saxon AJ, Calsyn DA, Haver VM, et al: Clinical evaluation and use of urine screening for drug abuse. West J Med 149:296, 1988.
Good overview of detecting drug abuse.
Spivak JL: Medical complications of opiate and cocaine use. In Spivak JL, Barnes HV (eds): Manual of Clinical Problems in Internal Medicine, 4th ed. Boston, Little, Brown & Co, 1990, p 537.
Focuses on effects of opiates and cocaine and includes annotated key references.
Zwerling C, Ryan J, Orav EJ: Costs and benefits of preemployment drug screening. JAMA 267:91, 1992.
Presents a method for analyzing the costs and benefits of a preemployment drug screening program.

Hemochromatosis

1.   Consider screening individuals for hemochromatosis using fasting serum transferrin saturation—measure serum iron, transferrin, and percent transferrin saturation. If the percent of transferrin saturation is greater than 60%, measure serum ferritin, and if the ferritin concentration is high, perform a liver biopsy.

Most authorities have not made any recommendations about wellness screening for hemochromatosis. Increasingly individuals are being discovered with few or no clinical findings. Iron overload may be due to hereditary hemochromatosis or secondary to other causes such as ineffective erythropoiesis (e.g., β-thalassemia, sideroblastic anemia, aplastic anemia) in which iron absorption is increased and transfusions are frequent; chronic liver disease (e.g., alcoholic cirrhosis, conditions secondary to portacaval anastomosis, porphyria cutanea tarda); or ingestion of excessive iron. Hereditary hemochromatosis is caused by an abnormal gene on the short arm of chromosome 6, closely linked to the HLA-A locus. It affects approximately 5% of the population of the United States, Australia, and Europe, with 0.2% to 0.7% of the population homozygous and 8% to 14% heterozygous. Recently, increased iron (ferritin over 200 ng/mL [200 μg/L]) has been implicated as a risk factor for coronary heart disease.

Excessive iron deposits in the heart, liver, pancreas, adrenal glands, pituitary, hypothalamus, and joints result in congestive heart failure, arrhythmias, cirrhosis, hepatocellular carcinoma, insulin-dependent diabetes, hypogonadism, hypoaldosteronism, arthralgia, and arthritis. The disease is underdiagnosed because of lack of recognition, confusion with other diseases, minimal clinical findings, and incomplete phenotypic expression of the hereditary variety in some persons. Although expert clinicians skilled in the clinical findings of hemochromatosis may identify these patients, many patients risk not being diagnosed except by laboratory tests. The tragedy of missed diagnosis is that these patients are treatable by therapeutic phlebotomy. Individuals with hemochromatosis are at risk for infections with iron-using bacteria such as *Yersinia enterocolitica, Pasteurella pseudotuberculosis,* and *Vibrio vulnificus* (from eating raw oysters).

2. Interpret test results in the context of clinical findings.

The serum iron level is high in patients with hemochromatosis, the percent saturation of transferrin is greater than 60%, and the serum ferritin level is greater than 300 ng/ml (300 μg/L) in males and greater than 200 ng/ml (200 μg/L) in females, with levels ranging from 700 ng/ml (700 μg/L) to several thousand ng/ml (μg/L). The gold standard for diagnosis is demonstration of excessive iron deposits in liver tissue obtained by biopsy. Hepatic concentration of iron is greater than 22,000 μg/g (dry weight), with histologic evidence of severe iron deposition.

3. Monitor therapeutic phlebotomy for hemochromatosis using serial determinations of blood hemoglobin and serum iron and ferritin.

Therapeutic phlebotomy—at least weekly—should be continued until the hemoglobin level decreases and the serum iron and the serum ferritin levels fall to normal.

4. In individuals with hemochromatosis the following additional abnormal blood test results may occur:

↑ Glucose   **Abnormal liver function tests**

BIBLIOGRAPHY

Adams PC, Kertsez AE, Valberg LS: Clinical presentation of hemochromatosis: A changing scene. Am J Med 90:445, 1991.
Clinical findings of hemochromatosis are very subtle. A high index of suspicion is necessary.
Bacon BR: Causes of iron overload. N Engl J Med 326:126, 1992.
Discusses the spectrum of iron overload diseases.
Bullen JJ, Spalding PB, Ward CG, et al: Hemochromatosis, iron, and septicemia caused by *Vibrio vulnificus*. Arch Intern Med 151:1606, 1991.
The organism thrives in a high iron environment.
Edwards CQ, Kushner JP: Iron storage disorders. In Conn RB (ed): Current Diagnosis, 8th ed. Philadelphia, WB Saunders Co, 1991, p 807.
Good discussion of the clinical findings of hemochromatosis.
Salonen JT, Nyyssönen K, Korpela H, et al: High stored iron levels are associated with excess risk of myocardial infarction in Eastern Finnish men. Circulation 86:803, 1992.
Reports a correlation between high iron levels and increased risk of acute myocardial infarction.
Sheehy TW: Hemochromatosis: Early recognition of the hallmark features. Modern Medicine 60:61, 1992.
Suspicion is the key to early diagnosis of the disease.
Spivak JL: Iron overload. In Spivak JL, Barnes HV (eds): Manual of Clinical Problems in Internal Medicine, 4th ed. Boston, Little, Brown & Co, 1990, p 334.
Discusses diagnosis and management with annotated key references.
Stipp D: Is Popeye doomed? Some experts sound warnings about ingesting too much iron. *Wall Street Journal,* January 17, 1992, p B1.
Warns that increasing iron supplementation of food is potentially dangerous for patients at risk for hemochromatosis.
Weintraub LR: The many faces of hemochromatosis. Hosp Pract 26:49, 1991.
Discusses the diagnosis and management of hemochromatosis.

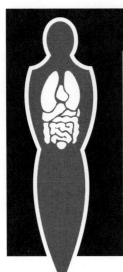

CHAPTER 2

GENERAL AND MISCELLANEOUS PROBLEMS

Human Immunodeficiency Virus Infection and
 AIDS
Lyme Disease
Sexually Transmitted Disease
Food Poisoning and the Restaurant Syndromes
Cerebrospinal Fluid Analysis
Synovial Fluid Analysis

Human Immunodeficiency Virus Infection and AIDS

1.   For patients with clinical findings of acquired immunodeficiency syndrome (AIDS) or the AIDS-related complex (ARC) or to screen for infection with the human immunodeficiency virus (HIV), request an enzyme-linked immunoabsorbent assay (ELISA) for HIV antibodies and confirm positive test results with a Western blot analysis, which identifies antibodies to specific viral proteins. Remember that ARC and AIDS are primarily clinical diagnoses and that HIV testing has significant legal, ethical, sociological, and emotional implications. In 1992 the Centers for Disease Control (CDC) proposed broadening the definition of AIDS to include any person infected with HIV with fewer than 200 CD4 lymphocytes/μL (200 $\times$ 10^6 cells/L).

Several authorities recommend against general wellness screening for HIV infection but endorse selective wellness screening for individuals at increased risk. A recent study supports the use of universal precautions but not routine determination of HIV status before elective surgery. AIDS is caused by HIV, of which there are two known types. The prototype virus, HIV-1, is responsible for most cases; however, a second virus, HIV-2, is increasingly being reported from Africa and has also been found in the United States. Although HIV-1 is present in a variety of body fluids, it has not been found in sweat.

In broadening the definition of AIDS to HIV-infected individuals with

56

fewer than 200 CD4 lymphocytes, the CDC will add approximately 173,000 people to the current caseload of more than 200,000 classified as having AIDS. The previous classification required HIV infection plus an opportunistic infection (e.g., *Pneumocystis carinii* pneumonia) and/or a neoplasm (e.g., Kaposi's sarcoma) to diagnose AIDS. ARC was diagnosed when an HIV-infected individual had clinical findings that fell short of AIDS (e.g., fever, weight loss, generalized lymphadenopathy, diarrhea, fatigue, and night sweats). The cumulative number of adult AIDS cases in the United States by transmission category through September 30, 1991, follows:

INDIVIDUALS	NO. CASES
Homosexual or bisexual males	112,812
Intravenous (IV) drug users	43,028
Homosexual males who are IV drug users	12,580
Hemophiliacs	1,622
Transfusion	4,205
Heterosexuals	10,989
Undetermined	7,170
TOTAL ADULT CASES	192,406

As of December 31, 1991, the total rose to 206,392—of those cases, 133,232 have died. Of the above categories, the fastest rising category of new cases in the United States is heterosexuals. Although women accounted for only 9% of the first 100,000 cases, they accounted for 12% of the second 100,000. Approximately 1 million Americans are currently believed HIV-infected, and 20% of them have developed AIDS. Worldwide, the World Health Organization (WHO) estimates that 10 to 12 million adults are infected with HIV: 1 million children have been infected. Approximately 90% of new adult infections result from heterosexual intercourse.

Although therapy with zidovudine (AZT) and dideoxyinosine (ddI) can prolong the lives of some patients with HIV infection, in the absence of treatment AIDS occurs approximately 10 years after the initial infection, and death usually ensues approximately 2 years after the development of AIDS.

FIRST 5 YEARS (CD4 LYMPHOCYTE CELL COUNT AROUND 1000 CELLS/μL [1000 $\times$ 10^6 CELLS/L])

- Takes approximately 6 to 8 weeks but can take up to 1 year after HIV infection for ELISA to turn positive.
- Some individuals develop an acute febrile illness resembling influenza or infectious mononucleosis, whereas other individuals have no symptoms. There follows a period when most people feel fine except perhaps for generalized lymphadenopathy.

SECOND 5 YEARS (CD4 LYMPHOCYTE CELL COUNT AROUND 500 CELLS/μL [500 × 10⁶ CELLS/L])

- In spite of decreasing CD4 lymphocyte cell counts, many people continue to feel fine.
- AZT, ddI, and other antiviral drug therapies are recommended.
- Simultaneously, cell-mediated immunity, as demonstrated by skin tests, is disintegrating.

FINAL 2 YEARS (CD4 LYMPHOCYTE CELL COUNT AROUND 200 CELLS/μL [200 × 10⁶ CELLS/L])

- Although initially asymptomatic, individuals with CD4 lymphocyte cell counts in this range are increasingly affected with infections and neoplasms. In a recent study nearly all deaths occurred in patients with CD4 counts <50 cells/μL (50 × 10⁶ cells/L).

P. carinii pneumonia is the most common life-threatening infection in AIDS patients and eventually develops in 80% or more of those not receiving primary prophylaxis. Other infections include *Toxoplasma gondii* infection of the central nervous system; diarrhea caused by *Cryptosporidium* infection; strongyloidiasis; oral candidiasis; cryptococcal meningitis; other fungal infections (histoplasmosis, coccidioidomycosis, aspergillosis); mycobacterial infections; bacterial infections such as *Nocardia, Legionella, Salmonella, Shigella, Helicobacter jejuni,* and syphilis; viral infections such as herpes simplex virus, cytomegalovirus, viral hepatitis, Epstein-Barr virus, and progressive multifocal leukoencephalopathy (papovavirus). Tuberculosis (TB) is particularly troublesome in prisons, shelters, drug treatment programs, and inner-city hospitals where HIV prevalence is high and standard TB tests (skin tests and x-ray examinations) fail to detect the disease. In HIV-positive persons with TB, 25% to 50% have negative skin tests, rising to 50% to 75% in individuals with AIDS (only 5 mm of induration is recommended for a positive purified protein derivative [PPD] skin test). Because patients with AIDS seldom have clear chest x-ray films, pulmonary TB is difficult to detect. Neoplasms include Kaposi's sarcoma, nonHodgkin's lymphoma, Hodgkin's disease, and certain carcinomas. For patients with neuropsychiatric findings, consider obtaining cerebrospinal fluid (CSF) for routine studies and viral culture. The CDC recently added tuberculosis, invasive cervical cancer, and recurrent bacterial pneumonia to the list of conditions used to classify someone as having AIDS.

2. Evaluate the tests.

Currently HIV infection is detected by a positive ELISA test and is confirmed by a positive Western blot analysis. A person is classified and notified as being HIV-1 seropositive only after blood sample test results are positive in three tests—two successive ELISAs and one confirmatory Western blot (or an equally sensitive and specific confirmatory test).

3. If the ELISA test and Western blot analysis are positive, consider the

patient as infected with HIV. Do not diagnose HIV infection solely on the basis of a positive ELISA test.

The specificity of the ELISA test may vary, and when persons come from a clinical class with a low prevalence of HIV infection, false-positive results are more likely to occur. Recently false-positive results occurred in individuals who received immunization for influenza. To exclude false-positive results, every positive ELISA test should be confirmed by a second ELISA test and a Western blot analysis. Indeterminant Western blot tests should be repeated monthly. Indeterminant patterns fall into three categories: (1) those in the early stages of HIV-1 infection; (2) those infected with a closely related retrovirus, HIV-2; and (3) truly false-positive results, that is, healthy people who are not infected with HIV-1 or with any closely related retroviruses such as HIV-2. If the diagnosis is in doubt, other tests are available: polymerase chain reaction (PCR) for HIV-1, HIV-1 antigen tests, and HIV-1 culture.

4.   If the ELISA test is negative, conclude that the patient is probably, but not necessarily, free of HIV infection.

With the ELISA test, occasional persons infected with HIV are negative for the antibody. There is a period of 6 to 8 weeks (sometimes up to 1 year or more) during a primary HIV infection when an HIV-infected person is seronegative. Interestingly, some of these patients may have an acute febrile illness resembling influenza or infectious mononucleosis. When the suspicion for infection is high, the ELISA test should be repeated periodically for at least 1 year.

Patients with a variety of other diseases may have "AIDS-like" clinical findings, including abnormal laboratory test results such as depressed helper/suppressor T-cell ratios and polyclonal gammopathy. Do not automatically conclude that these patients are infected with HIV. If they are seronegative, they probably are not infected.

5.   In patients with HIV infection periodically measure CD4 lymphocytes to monitor the course of the disease. When the CD4 lymphocyte cell count is less than 500 cells/μL (500 $\times$ 10^6 cells/L), monitor for complications of the disease.

There is a high correlation between the level of CD4 lymphocytes and the progress of the disease—the lower the count, the worse is the prognosis.

6.   In patients with HIV infection the following abnormal blood test results may occur:

↓ **Hemoglobin and hematocrit** due to normochromic, normocytic anemia.

↓ **Leukocytes** and decreased lymphocytes with decreased CD4 lymphocytes.

Abnormal liver function tests.
↑ **Lactate dehydrogenase.**
↓ **Cholesterol.**
↑ **Triglycerides.**
↓ **Cortisol and aldosterone** due to primary adrenocortical insufficiency.

↓ **Platelets,** either immune thrombocytopenic purpura or thrombotic thrombocytopenic purpura.

↑ **Erythrocyte sedimentation rate.**

↓ **Glucose.**

↑ **Glucose.**

↓ **Sodium** in up to 50% of hospitalized patients and 20% of ambulatory patients.

↑ **Cortisol.**

↑ **Gamma globulins** (IgG, IgA, IgM, IgD) and circulating immune complexes.

Lupus anticoagulant.

Positive VDRL—some may be false positive.

↓ **Blastogenesis** (phytohemagglutinin [PHA] or con A).

7. In patients with HIV infection with neurologic disorders the following CSF results may occur:

↑ **Lymphocytes,** mild.
Normal glucose.

↑ **Protein.**

HIV infection often involves the CNS, causing dementia in 40% to 60% of patients—usually those in advanced stages. There may be an associated encephalitis. CNS mass lesions may also occur in decreasing order of frequency as follows: toxoplasmosis, primary lymphoma, progressive multifocal leukoencephalopathy, other opportunistic infections, and cerebral infarctions. HIV-positive patients should be evaluated for neurosyphilis.

BIBLIOGRAPHY

Barry MJ: Human immunodeficiency virus infection. In Panzer RJ, Black ER, Griner PF (eds): Diagnostic Strategies for Common Medical Problems. Philadelphia, American College of Physicians, 1991, p 217.
Recommends strategies for detecting HIV infection.

Bylund DJ, Ziegner UHM, Hooper DG: Review of testing for human immunodeficiency virus. Clin Lab Med 12:305, 1992.
Review article about the different kinds of HIV tests, including their strengths and weaknesses.

Chalmers AC, Aprill BS, Shephard H: Cerebrospinal fluid and human immunodeficiency virus: Findings in healthy, asymptomatic, seropositive men. Arch Intern Med 150:1538, 1990.
Even asymptomatic HIV-positive persons may show CSF pleocytosis, high protein, oligoclonal bands, and positive HIV culture.

Charache P, Cameron JL, Maters AW, et al: Prevalence of infection with human immunodeficiency virus in elective surgery patients. Ann Surg 214:562, 1991.
Does not support screening before elective surgery.

Diagnostic and Therapeutic Technology Assessment (DATTA): Surrogate markers of progressive HIV disease. JAMA 267:2948, 1992. Questions and Answers.
CD4 cell count is an effective marker of progression to disease in HIV-infected individuals.

Eckholm E: Facts of life: More than inspiration is needed to fight AIDS. *New York Times,* November 17, 1991, section 4, p 1.
Current overview of the HIV problem described in straightforward terminology.

Grinspoon SK, Bilezikian JP: HIV disease and the endocrine system. N Engl J Med 327:1360, 1992.

Adrenal insufficiency is the most important abnormality, but a number of other abnormalities may occur.

Holland SM, Quinn TC: Acquired immunodeficiency syndrome. In Spivak JL, Barnes HV (eds): Manual of Clinical Problems in Internal Medicine, 4th ed. Boston, Little, Brown & Co, 1990, p 395.
Good discussion of diagnosis and management with annotated key references.

Jacobson K, Jordan GW: Primary human immunodeficiency virus infection: Will you miss the diagnosis? West J Med 156:68, 1992.
Suggests an approach to diagnosing acute HIV infection.

Kassirer JP, Kopelman RL: Case 21—Interpreting negative test results and Case 61—Learning clinical reasoning from examples. In Learning Clinical Reasoning. Baltimore, Williams & Wilkins, 1991, pp 130, 303.
Describes the clinical reasoning in two cases of patients with HIV infection.

O'Brien TR, George JR, Holmberg SD: Human immunodeficiency virus type 2 infection in the United States. JAMA 267:2775, 1992.
Summarizes current information about the epidemiology and diagnosis of HIV-2.

Rodnick JE: New guidelines for tuberculin skin test interpretation. West J Med 154:322, 1991.
CDC recommends making 5-mm induration a positive tuberculin test in groups at high risk and 15-mm induration a positive test in groups at low risk.

Rosenthal E: HIV infection thwarting efforts to detect TB and curb its spread. New York Times, December 10, 1991, p 1.
Highlights the problem of diagnosing tuberculosis in HIV-positive persons.

The second 100,000 cases of acquired immunodeficiency syndrome: United States, June, 1981—December, 1991. MMWR 41:28, 1992.
Interesting statistics on the second 100,000 cases of AIDS.

Wormser GP, Bittker S, Forseter G, et al: Absence of infectious human immunodeficiency virus type 1 in "natural" eccrine sweat. J Infect Dis 165:155, 1992.
Interesting observation about individuals infected with the HIV-1 virus.

Lyme Disease

1. In patients with clinical findings of Lyme disease, request serum tests for IgM and IgG antibodies. Do not request serologic tests in the absence of clinical findings of Lyme disease.

Lyme disease is a multisystem disorder caused by the spirochete, *Borrelia burgdorferi*, which is transmitted by tiny ixodid ticks. The size of the nymph tick form is 1-2 mm, and the adult tick is a little larger. Nearly 8000 cases were reported in 1990 alone, a sixteenfold increase since 1982, making Lyme disease the leading vector-borne disease in the United States. In 1991 reported cases jumped to 9344. The disease typically occurs from May to August, and cases are concentrated in well-established areas in northeastern, north-central, and Pacific-coast states. Exposure exists when the patient was in an incidence area less than 30 days before the onset of erythema chronicum migrans (ECM); a history of tick bite is not essential. ECM is an enlarging annular rash with a red border and a clear center. Lyme disease has three stages: stage 1, lasting approximately 4 weeks (flu-like illness or meningitis-like illness); stage 2, lasting days to months (cardiac conduction disturbances and neurological abnormalities); and stage 3, lasting months to years (chronic arthritis and chronic neurological and skin abnormalities).

The diagnosis of Lyme disease can be made either in the presence of ECM or with involvement of other organ systems and a history of exposure. Laboratory tests are useful to confirm the diagnosis.

Currently a number of tests can be used to diagnose *B. burgdorferi* infection: measurement of serum IgM and IgG antibodies, using either indirect immunofluorescence (IFA) or ELISA; Western Blot assay; the lymphocyte blast transformation test; and culture. Only the IFA and ELISA are widely used.

2. Evaluate the tests.

There is poor agreement among different laboratories about Lyme disease tests. These tests need standardization. Assays of the ELISA type are preferred because their sensitivity and reproducibility are better than those of IFA. Western blotting may aid in distinguishing true-positive from false-positive ELISA results. A highly sensitive assay for *B. burgdorferi* based on the polymerase chain reaction (PCR) is being developed. Another new test, an antigen capture–detection assay for bacterial proteins, apparently is quite sensitive and specific for the organism.

3. If the serologic titer for Lyme disease antibodies is 1:128, consider the diagnosis; if it is 1:256, make the diagnosis. The Venereal Disease Research Laboratory (VDRL) test and tests for rheumatoid factor and antinuclear antibodies are usually negative.

The CDC laboratory criteria for the diagnosis of Lyme disease are as follows: isolation of *B. burgdorferi* from a clinical specimen; demonstration of diagnostic levels of IgM and IgG antibodies to the spirochete in serum or CSF; or significant changes in IgM or IgG antibody response to *B. burgdorferi* in paired acute and convalescent serum samples.

The IgM antibody response generally first develops within 2 to 4 weeks after the onset of ECM, peaks after 6 to 8 weeks of illness, and declines to the normal range after 4 to 6 months of illness in most patients. The IgM response only occurs in 40% to 60% of patients. The IgG response quickly follows within 6 to 8 weeks after the onset of the disease and peaks after 4 to 6 months of illness. Most authorities believe that by the time of well-established stage 2 signs and symptoms, a prominent IgG response is present in all patients. This apparently is maintained, unless therapy is initiated, indefinitely. Sera from patients with other spirochetal diseases such as syphilis, yaws, pinta, leptospirosis, relapsing fever, periodontal disease, and some cases of HIV infection, infectious mononucleosis, rheumatoid arthritis, and systemic lupus erythematosus may give false-positive results. As stated previously, the minimal titer at which Lyme disease should be considered is 1:128, and 1:256 is confirmatory. These titers are much higher than those used to diagnose other infectious diseases, and although specificity is increased, sensitivity is decreased. At this time, however, this is the only way to avoid cross-reacting antibodies and false-positive test results.

4.   If the serologic titer for Lyme disease is negative, rely on clinical findings to make the diagnosis.

Since a positive antibody response may not occur for weeks to several months after infection, some patients in the early stage of the disease may test negative. Patients with a negative test result and presumptive or clinical findings of Lyme disease should receive prompt antibiotic treatment without waiting for laboratory confirmation or convalescent specimens. Patients who have a compatible systemic illness without ECM or a known tick bite should have paired acute and convalescent serum samples tested.

5.   In patients with Lyme disease the following additional abnormal blood test results may occur (especially in stage 1):

↓ **Hemoglobin and hematocrit,** mild.

↑ **Erythrocyte sedimentation rate,** moderate.

↑ **Total IgM.** Persistent increase is a predictor of later disease manifestations.

↑ **Leukocyte count** with left shift in differential.

↑ **Aspartate aminotransferase (SGOT)** in patients with prominent systemic symptoms, generally returning to normal several weeks after disease onset.

6.   In patients with Lyme disease the following abnormal urine test results may occur:

Transient microscopic hematuria and mild proteinuria in a few patients. Renal function usually is normal.

7.   In patients with Lyme disease with meningitis the following abnormal CSF test results may occur:

IgM and IgG antibodies to *B. burgdorferi* in the CSF.
Normal to low glucose.

↑ **Cells,** 25 to 450/μL (25 to 450 cells × 10^6/L), mostly lymphocytes.
Normal to high protein.

8.   In patients with Lyme disease with arthritis the following synovial fluid test results may occur:

↑ **Cells,** 500 to 110,000/μL (500 to 110,000 × 10^6/L), of which most are polymorphonuclear leukocytes.

Biopsy findings of fibrin deposits, synovial hypertrophy, vascular proliferation, and marked infiltration by lymphocytes and plasma cells.

Protein, 3 to 6 g/dL (30 to 60 g/L).

BIBLIOGRAPHY

Case definitions for public health surveillance. MMWR 39:19, 1990.
  Reviews the CDC case definition for Lyme disease.
Corpuz M, Hilton E, Lardis P, et al: Problems in the use of serologic tests for the diagnosis
  of Lyme disease. Arch Intern Med 151:1837, 1991.
  Suggests caution in the interpretation of serologic tests for Lyme disease.
Dennis DT: Lyme disease: Tracking an epidemic. JAMA 266:1269, 1991.
  Editorial that highlights the growing importance of Lyme disease.
Kaslow RA: Current perspective on Lyme borreliosis. JAMA 267:1381, 1992.
  Good case discussion from grand rounds at the Clinical Center of the National Institutes of Health.
Luft BJ, Steinman CR, Neimark HC, et al: Invasion of the central nervous system by
  Borrelia burgdorferi in acute disseminated infection. JAMA 267:1364, 1992.
  Eight of 12 patients had evidence of CNS involvement.
Neff JC: Lyme borreliosis: Notes on laboratory diagnosis. Ohio State University Reference
  Laboratory Update, Columbus, Ohio, August-September 1989.
  Practical suggestions for the laboratory diagnosis of Lyme disease.
Rahn DW, Malawista SE: Lyme disease: Recommendations for diagnosis and treatment.
  Ann Intern Med 114:472, 1991.
  Recent article discussing the fine points of diagnosis and treatment of Lyme disease.
Rahn DW, Malawista SE: Lyme disease. West J Med 154:706, 1991.
  Excellent general review of Lyme disease.
Rosa PA, Schwan TG: A specific and sensitive assay for the Lyme disease spirochete *Borrelia
  burgdorferi* using the polymerase chain reactions. J Infect Dis 160:1018, 1989.
  Promising new test using the PCR.
Sigal LH: Summary of the first 100 patients seen at a Lyme Disease Referral Center. Am
  J Med 88:577, 1990.
  *Reports that of the first 100 patients referred to the Lyme Disease Center, only 37 had Lyme
  disease. Approximately half of the 91 courses of antibiotic therapy were probably unwarranted.*
Steere AC: Lyme disease. N Engl J Med 321:586, 1989.
  Thorough review of Lyme disease by the investigator who first described it.
Zoschke DC: Is it Lyme disease? How to interpret results of laboratory testing. Postgrad
  Med 91:46, 1992.
  Guidelines for resolving problems with currently available tests.

Sexually Transmitted Disease

1.   For patients with clinical findings of sexually transmitted disease (STD), perform appropriate tests, depending on the type of lesion. Regardless of the specific STD, consider screening for HIV with an ELISA and for syphilis with either a VDRL test or a rapid plasma reagin (RPR) test.

Several authorities recommend against general wellness screening for STDs but endorse selective wellness screening for individuals at increased risk. HIV and syphilis counseling and testing for persons with STD are important parts of an HIV prevention program because patients who have acquired an STD have demonstrated the potential risk for acquiring HIV and syphilis. A positive HIV ELISA test should be repeated and confirmed with a Western blot test. A positive VDRL or RPR (nontreponemal) test should be confirmed with a treponemal test—either the microhemoagglutination *Treponema pallidum* (MHA-TP) assay or the fluorescent treponemal-antibody absorption (FTA-ABS) test. Although the VDRL and RPR are equally valid tests, RPR titers are not equivalent to VDRL titers and are often slightly higher than VDRL titers. Both the VDRL and RPR tests can be carried out as qualitative and quantitative procedures; however, the titers are not interchangeable. Although there are many infectious and noninfectious causes for false-positive VDRL and RPR tests, there are only a small number of causes for false-positive treponemal tests (i.e., Lyme disease, leprosy, malaria, infectious mononucleosis, relapsing fever, leptospirosis, systemic lupus erythematosus). Both nontreponemal and treponemal tests may become negative after treatment; thus negative test results do not necessarily exclude past syphilis infection.

2. In patients with genital ulcers or regional lymphadenopathy consider the following:

DISEASES/AGENTS	CLINICAL FINDINGS	TESTS
Herpes simplex virus infection	Painful, multiple, superficial ulcers; early lesions are vesicular	Tzanck smear and culture for herpes simplex virus
Syphilis	Painless, clean-based, indurated ulcer with painless regional lymphadenopathy	Darkfield examination, serology
Chancroid	Painful, often multiple, genital ulcers with painful inguinal lymphadenopathy	Culture
Granuloma inguinale	Mildly painful ulcer that follows a painless papule	Smear, biopsy
Lymphogranuloma venereum (LGV)	Small papular lesion	Serology, biopsy

3. In patients with lesions affecting epithelial surfaces consider the following:

DISEASES/AGENTS	CLINICAL FINDINGS	TESTS
Gonococcal infections	Urethritis and/or pelvic inflammatory disease	Culture or nucleic acid probe

Table continued on following page.

Diseases/ Agents	Clinical Findings	Tests
Chlamydial infections	Urethritis and/or pelvic inflammatory disease	Culture or nucleic acid probe
Genital warts	Exophytic genital and anal warts	Human papillomavirus (HPV) tests and biopsy of atypical, pigmented, or persistent lesions

4.   In patients with findings suggestive of bacterial STD syndromes consider the following:

Agents	Clinical Findings	Tests
C. trachomatis, Ureaplasma urealyticum, Trichomonas vaginalis, and herpes simplex virus	Nongonococcal urethritis	Culture or nucleic acid probes for *N. gonorrhoeae* and *C. trachomatis*
N. gonorrhoeae, C. trachomatis, T. vaginalis, herpes simplex, and HPV	Mucopurulent cervicitis	
N. gonorrhoeae and *C. trachomatis*	Epididymitis	Tzanck smear and culture for herpes simplex virus
N. gonorrhoeae, C. trachomatis, anaerobes, gramnegative rods, streptococci, *Mycoplasma,* and *Ureaplasma*	Pelvic inflammatory disease	Wet preparation on culture for *T. vaginalis*
N. gonorrhoeae, C. trachomatis, Campylobacter jejuni, Shigella, T. pallidum, and cytomegalovirus	Sexually transmitted enteric disease	

5.   In women with vaginal findings consider the following:

Diseases/Agents	Clinical Findings	Tests
Bacterial vaginosis (*Gardnerella*)	Homogeneous vaginal discharge and itching	Three of four criteria: discharge, pH >4.5, abnormal odor, clue cells
Trichomoniasis	Vaginal discharge and itching	Wet preparation or culture
Vulvovaginal candidiasis	Vaginal discharge and itching	Wet preparation or culture

6.   In patients with miscellaneous findings consider the following:

Diseases/Agents	Clinical Findings	Tests
Viral hepatitis (hepatitis B, delta hepatitis, and probably hepatitis C)	Constitutional and gastrointestinal symptoms, with enlarged tender liver	Liver function tests; viral serologic tests
Cytomegalovirus	Heterophile-negative mononucleosis	Culture virus in throat, blood buffy coat, or urine; serologic tests
Pediculosis pubis	Intense itching	Lice or eggs on pubic hair
Scabies	Severe itching; worse at night	Scrapings, skin biopsy

7.   Remember that syphilis has a variety of clinical presentations and test result patterns.

Syphilis has a variety of presentations that can be divided into five stages: primary stage (chancre); secondary stage (rash appearing in 1 to 4 months); latent stage (clearing of rash lasting 1 to many years); tertiary stage (gummas, neurosyphilis, cardiovascular syphilis); and congenital stage. Consult the references for additional information on diagnosing syphilis in these various stages.

BIBLIOGRAPHY

Cates W Jr, Hinman AR: Sexually transmitted diseases in the 1990's. N Engl J Med 325:1368, 1991.
   CDC experts emphasize the increased risk of HIV infection in individuals with other STDs, the rising incidence of syphilis, and the high prevalence of genital herpes simplex infections (one in six Americans) and human papillomavirus infections (one in three Americans).
Dallabetta GA, Quinn TC: Sexually transmitted disease. In Spivak JL, Barnes HV (eds):

Manual of Clinical Problems in Internal Medicine, 4th ed. Boston, Little, Brown & Co, 1990, p 453.

Good discussion of diagnosis and management, with annotated key references.

Hart G, Rothenberg RB: Syphilis tests in diagnostic and therapeutic decision making. In Sox HC Jr (ed): Common Diagnostic Tests: Use and Interpretation, 2nd ed. Philadelphia, American College of Physicians, 1990, p 302.

Reviews the use of syphilis testing in the diagnosis and management of the disease.

Hayward RSA, Steinberg EP, Ford DE, et al: Preventive care guidelines: 1991. Ann Intern Med 114:758, 1991.

Authoritative recommendations for wellness screening for HIV, syphilis, gonorrhea, and chlamydial infection.

Judson FN (ed): Sexually transmitted diseases. Clin Lab Med 9:1, 1989.

Extensive discussion of STDs with emphasis on laboratory diagnosis.

Martin DH (ed): Sexually transmitted diseases. Med Clin North Am 74:1, 1990.

Good review of sexually transmitted diseases.

Nixon SA (ed): Sexually transmitted diseases. Prim Care 17:1, 1990.

Review of most STDs.

Primary and secondary syphilis: United States, 1981-1990. MMWR 40:314, 1991.

Epidemic of primary and secondary syphilis that began in the United States in 1985 shows no signs of abating.

Romanowski B, Sutherland R, Fick GH, et al: Serologic response to treatment of infectious syphilis. Ann Intern Med 114:1005, 1991.

After treatment, nontreponemal and treponemal tests may become negative.

1989 Sexually transmitted diseases treatment guidelines. MMWR 38:1, 1989.

Authoritative summary of guidelines for the management of sexually transmitted diseases.

Shelly MA, Mushlin AI: Syphilis. In Panzer RJ, Black ER, Griner PF (eds): Diagnostic Strategies for Common Medical Problems. Philadelphia, American College of Physicians, 1991, p 227.

Recommends strategies for diagnosing syphilis.

Wooldridge WE: Syphilis: A new visit from an old enemy. Postgrad Med 89:193, 1991.

Discusses the upswing in syphilis rates with guidelines for diagnosis and management.

Food Poisoning and the Restaurant Syndromes

1.   If an illness appears related to dining (i.e., occurring during or shortly after dining), look for characteristic clinical findings and, when appropriate, obtain laboratory tests.

Illness related to dining is common. Usually recognition of the characteristic findings, symptomatic therapy, and future avoidance of the offending agent are all that is required. Occasionally laboratory tests are useful. The causes are classified as follows: bacterial food poisoning, chemical food poisoning, food poisoning caused by toxins in seafood and mushrooms, and food hypersensitivity. Certainly delayed diseases can occur from ingesting contaminated food (hepatitis A, *Salmonella, Shigella, Helicobacter, Yersinia,* and *Escherichia,* neurologic syndromes such as toxic-oil syndrome, eosinophilia-myalgia syndrome, triorthocresyl phosphate poisoning, polychlorinated biphenyls [PCBs] poisoning, pesticide poisoning, and trace mercury poisoning), but these delayed diseases are not discussed here. Mercury accumulates in large fish that live a long time (tuna, shark, swordfish). These fish should be avoided by pregnant women and young children and eaten no more than once a week by others.

2. To detect bacterial food poisoning, consider the following:

DISEASES/AGENTS	CLINICAL FINDINGS	TESTS
Staphylococcal food poisoning (toxin)	Nausea, vomiting, cramps, diarrhea 2-7 hr after a meal	Send food samples to state health laboratory if appropriate.
Bacillus cereus food poisoning (toxin)	Nausea, vomiting, cramps, diarrhea 1-16 hr after a meal	Send food samples to state health laboratory if appropriate.
Clostridium perfringens food poisoning (toxin)	Cramps, diarrhea 8-24 hrs after a meal; nausea and vomiting much less common	Send food samples to state health laboratory if appropriate.
Clostridum botulinum food poisoning (toxin)	Afebrile, neurological findings (visual problems, dysphagia, dysarthria, weakness, paralysis) and gastrointestinal findings (nausea, vomiting, cramps, diarrhea) 6 hr-8 days after a meal—especially of home-processed fruits, vegetables, meats, and seafood	Routine tests are not helpful; CSF protein level may be 50-60 mg/dl (0.5-0.6 g/L); obtain serum, which is toxic to mice; obtain food samples for testing at state health laboratory.
Traveler's diarrhea: usually enterotoxigenic *(Escherichia coli)*	Cramps and diarrhea 24-72 hr after a meal; nausea and vomiting less common; contaminated seafood recently incriminated	Send food samples to state health laboratory if appropriate.
Vibrio cholerae water or food poisoning (toxin)	Vomiting and mild-to-severe diarrhea 12-48 hr after ingestion; no cramps or fever	Culture stool.
Vibrio parahaemolyticus food poisoning (bacteria)	Nausea, vomiting, cramps, and explosive watery diarrhea 12-96 hr after eating seafood	Culture stool.
Vibrio vulnificus (bacteria)	Septicemia or gastroenteritis 24-48 hr after ingestion of raw oysters; high	Culture blood, stool, and skin lesions.

Table continued on following page.

DISEASES/AGENTS	CLINICAL FINDINGS	TESTS
Vibrio vulnificus (bacteria) cont'd	mortality rate; patients with liver disease, low gastric acid, hemochromatosis, or immunodeficiency at risk	

3.   To detect chemical food poisoning, consider the following:

DISEASES/AGENTS	CLINICAL FINDINGS	TESTS
Heavy metals: cadmium, copper, tin, zinc, mercury	Vomiting, cramps, and diarrhea less than 2 hr after ingestion	Blood and urine for heavy metals
Monosodium glutamate (MSG)—the Chinese restaurant syndrome	Flushing, paresthesias, chest pain, facial pressure and burning, dizziness, sweating, headaches, palpitation, weakness, nausea, and vomiting 10-20 min after MSG ingestion	None
Sodium nitrite—hot dog headache	Headache after ingesting smoked meats	None
Sulfites	Flushing, bronchospasm, hypotension within minutes of ingesting sulfites (e.g., salads, shrimp, dried fruit, gelatin, pickles, sausages, cheese, wine, fruit juice)	None
Wasabi (horseradish used with sushi)—the Japanese restaurant syndrome	Fainting, pallor, sweating, staggering, and confusion immediately after ingestion of wasabi	None

4.   To detect food poisoning caused by toxins in seafood or mushrooms, consider the following:

DISEASES/AGENTS	CLINICAL FINDINGS	TESTS
Ciguatera fish poisoning (ciguatoxin) resulting from contamination by the dinoflagellates	Nausea, vomiting, cramps, and diarrhea, with numbness, pruritus, paresthesias of lips few minutes-30 hr after ingesting toxic fish (e.g., barracuda, red snapper, amberjack, grouper, mullet)	Send food samples to state health laboratory; immunoassays exist but are not widely available.

DISEASES/AGENTS	CLINICAL FINDINGS	TESTS
Dungeness crab (from eating internal organs) and mussel poisoning resulting from contamination by domoic acid, a toxin produced by marine plankton	Nausea, cramps, and diarrhea; in severe cases headache, dizziness, facial grimace, disorientation, memory loss, excessive bronchial secretions, breathing problems, and even death within 48 hr	Send food samples to state health laboratory.
Paralytic shellfish poisoning (PSP); saxitoxin resulting from contamination by toxic red tides of algae of the North Atlantic and Pacific coasts and brevetoxin in the Gulf of Mexico	Paresthesias and numbness with nausea, vomiting, diarrhea, and even death 30 min after eating shellfish; PSP most common between April and October	Send food samples to state health laboratory.
Scombroid fish poisoning (histamine); most common cause of fish poisoning. Toxins formed by bacteria	Flushing, headache, dizziness, nausea, vomiting, cramps, and diarrhea (histamine-like reaction) beginning 10-30 min after ingesting fish (e.g., scombroid fish [tuna, mackerel, skipjack, bonito] and nonscombroid fish [mahi mahi, bluefish, amberjack, herring, sardines, anchovies]) or cheese; persons receiving isoniazid at risk	Send food samples to state health laboratory.
Mushroom poisoning (amatoxin and phalloidin)	Fever, abdominal pain, nausea, vomiting, and diarrhea in 6-24 hr; then hepatic and renal dysfunction in 24-48 hr; then cardiomyopathy, coagulopathy, coma, and possibly death after ingestion of *Amanita* mushrooms	Obtain CBC, coagulation tests, biochemical profile, including hepatic and renal function tests, and urinalysis; gastric aspirate, vomitus, or stool can be analyzed for toxins by thin-layer chromatography.

5. To detect food hypersensitivity, consider the following:

DISEASES/AGENTS	CLINICAL FINDINGS	TESTS
Food allergy (IgE mediated)	Anaphylactic reaction minutes-2 hr after ingesting food allergin (e.g., peanuts, walnuts, eggs, fish, crustaceans, and milk)	Positive skin test or radioallergosorbent test to offending food
Tartrazine (yellow dye)	Urticaria or angioedema and/or acute bronchospasm 1-several hr after ingesting tartrazine; sometimes a history of urticarial or bronchospastic aspirin intolerance	None

6. Interpret any test result in the context of clinical findings and treat the patient symptomatically unless specific therapy is available.

Of the above agents that cause food poisoning and the restaurant syndromes, only botulism (antitoxin available from the CDC), *V. parahaemolyticus* (tetracycline or ampicillin in protracted cases), *V. vulnificus* (tetracycline with or without gentamicin or chloramphenicol), and scombroid fish poisoning (antihistamine) have specific therapies. The other causes require symptomatic therapy and emptying the gastrointestinal tract of the offending agent. In patients with mushroom poisoning renal failure and hepatic failure can be treated by hemodialysis and liver transplantation, respectively.

BIBLIOGRAPHY

FDA says eating type of crab poses danger. *New York Times*, December 29, 1991, p Y11.
  Describes hazards of eating viscera of Dungeness crab contaminated by the toxin, domoic acid.
Foodborne illness. Lancet 336:September 22-December 29, 1990.
  Series of articles in 14 consecutive issues that review the issue of foodborne illness.
Geller RJ, Olson KR, Senécal PE: Ciguatera fish poisoning in San Francisco, California caused by imported barracuda. West J Med 155:639, 1991.
  Describes 12 cases of ciguatera fish poisoning.
Hughes JM, Potter ME: Scombroid fish poisoning: From pathogenesis to prevention. N Engl J Med 324:766, 1991.
  Good discussion of scombroid fish poisoning and other causes of food poisoning. Millions of cases of food poisoning are estimated to occur in the United States annually.
Is our fish fit to eat? Consumer Reports, February 1992, p 103.
  Survey of supermarkets and fish stores found significant contamination.
Koenig KL, Mueller J, Rose T: *Vibrio vulnificus:* Hazard on the half shell. West J Med 155:400, 1991.
  Highlights the serious risk of eating raw oysters. The infection can also be secondary to contamination of a wound in brackish waters.

Paralytic shellfish poisoning: Massachusetts and Alaska, 1990. MMWR 40:157, 1991.
  Points out a hazard of eating shellfish.
Perl TM, Bédard L, Kosatsky T, et al: An outbreak of toxic encephalopathy caused by
  eating mussels contaminated with domoic acid. N Engl J Med 322:1775, 1990.
    Teitelbaum JS, Zatorre RJ, Carpenter S, et al: Neurologic sequelae of domoic acid
      intoxication due to the ingestion of contaminated mussels. N Engl J Med 322:1781,
      1990.
    Documents domoic acid intoxication from eating mussels.
Sampson HA, Metcalfe DD: Food allergies. JAMA 268: 2840, 1992.
  Discusses the pathophysiology, diagnosis, and therapy of food allergies.
Stipp D: Toxic red tides seem to be on the rise, increasing the risks of eating shellfish.
  Wall Street Journal, November 22, 1991, p B1.
    *Describes a worldwide "epidemic" of harmful algae blooms over the past few years that includes
    recent outbreaks on both the east and west coasts of the United States.*
Swerdlow DL, Ries AA: Cholera in the Americas: Guidelines for the clinician. JAMA
  267:1495, 1992.
  Important cause of severe diarrhea.

Cerebrospinal Fluid Analysis

1.   In patients with appropriate clinical indications perform lumbar puncture and analyze the CSF.

Appropriate indications and contraindications for performing lumbar puncture follow.* A guideline used by some experienced clinicians is that if you think of a lumbar puncture during a workup, you should do it!

DIAGNOSTIC INDICATIONS

- Known or suspected meningitis and encephalitis
  - Acute: bacterial, viral
  - Subacute: tuberculous, syphilitic, fungal, neoplastic
  - Chronic: syphilitic, granulomatous, neoplastic
- Intracranial or intraspinal hemorrhage if computed tomography (CT) or magnetic resonance imaging (MRI) is not available
- Multiple sclerosis
- Acute polyneuropathy
- Suspected benign intracranial hypertension (pseudotumor) only if CT or MRI is negative

THERAPEUTIC INDICATIONS

- Intrathecal administration of antimicrobial or chemotherapeutic agents

---

*Source: Victor JD: Neurologic diagnostic procedures. In Wyngaarden JB, Smith LH, Bennett JC (eds): Cecil Textbook of Medicine, 19th ed. Philadelphia, WB Saunders, 1992, p 2035.

- CSF drainage in patient with benign intracranial hypertension or communicating hydrocephalus

CONTRAINDICATIONS

- Intracranial hypertension due to mass lesion or obstructive hydrocephalus (suggest funduscopic examination before lumbar puncture)
- Bleeding diathesis
- Local skin or epidural infections

With the patient in the lateral recumbent position and before CSF is withdrawn, measure CSF pressure (normal, 90 to 180 mm). If CSF pressure is high (>180 mm) or low (<90 mm), remove only 1 mL of fluid and carefully exclude increased intracranial pressure—a marked fall in pressure should cause concern. If CSF pressure is normal with no marked fall in pressure with removal of 1 to 2 mL, 10 to 20 mL of CSF may slowly be removed. Divide the CSF sample into three sterile tubes: (1) for chemistry and immunology (protein, glucose, lactate dehydrogenase [LD], serology), (2) for microbiology (Gram stain; bacterial, fungal, and viral cultures; india ink preparation, antigen tests), and (3) for cell count and differential. Before the needle is removed, record opening pressure, closing pressure, and the amount of fluid removed.

2. Interpret test results in the context of clinical findings.

TYPICAL CSF FINDINGS IN VARIOUS CONDITIONS

CONDITION	PRESSURE (MM CSF)	GROSS APPEARANCE	WBC/μL (WBC × 10⁶/L)	PROTEIN (MG/DL) (G/L)	GLUCOSE (MG/DL) (MMOL/L)
Normal	90-180	Clear, colorless	0-10 (0-10) lymphocytes and monocytes	<45 (<0.45)	50-80 (2.78-4.44) or ⅔ blood glucose
Acute bacterial meningitis	Increased to 200-500	Turbid, may clot	100-10,000 (100-10,000) polymorphonuclear leukocytes	50-500 (0.50-5.00)	Absent or very low
Tuberculous meningitis	Increased to 200-500	Turbid, pellicle common	10-500 (10-500) chiefly lymphocytes	50-500 (0.50-5.00)	Often under 40 (2.22)
Aseptic or viral meningitis	Increased to 200-500	Clear or slightly turbid	10-500 (10-500) chiefly lymphocytes	45-200 (0.45-2.00)	Normal
Multiple sclerosis	Normal	Clear, colorless	Normal or 10-50 (10-50) lymphocytes	Normal or 45-100 (0.45-1.00)	Normal

TYPICAL CSF FINDINGS IN VARIOUS CONDITIONS Continued

Condition	Pressure (mm CSF)	Gross Appearance	WBC/μL (WBC × 10⁶/L)	Protein (mg/dL) (g/L)	Glucose (mg/dL) (mmol/L)
Cerebral thrombosis	Usually normal to slightly increased	Clear	Usually normal	Normal or 45-100 (0.45-1.00)	Normal
Cerebral hemorrhage	Usually normal	Bloody or xanthochromic	Increased red blood count (RBC)	Increased 45-100 (0.45-1.00)	Normal
Subarachnoid hemorrhage	Increased to 200-500	Bloody or xanthochromic	Increased RBC	Increased 50-1000 (0.50-10.00)	Normal
Brain tumor	Usually increased to 200-500	Clear or xanthochromic	Normal to 50 (50) lymphocytes	Normal or slightly increased	Normal or slightly decreased

Source: Bakerman S: ABC's of Interpretive Laboratory Data, 2nd ed. Greenville, NC, Interpretive Laboratory Data, Inc., 1984, p 113.

MENINGITIS

A Gram stain (sensitivity, approximately 60% to 90%), acid-fast stain (sensitivity, approximately 40%), and india ink preparation (sensitivity, approximately 25% to 50%) are invaluable for determining the cause of an infectious process. C-reactive protein may be useful to distinguish bacterial infection (increased values) from other causes of meningitis. Antigen tests may be useful. They are usually not as sensitive as cultures but are fairly specific, if positive.

For syphilis the CSF VDRL and CSF fluorescent treponemal antibody with absorption (CSF FTA-ABS) tests are appropriate. Cultures are the gold standard for diagnosing infections.

Rarely, aseptic meningitis is drug induced (e.g., trimethoprim, sulfadiazine, ibuprofen, immune globulins, azathioprine). Results of lumbar puncture usually show an increased opening pressure and CSF pleocytosis. The condition rapidly resolves (24 to 48 hours) after cessation of the offending medication.

NEUROLOGIC DISORDERS

Besides its use for determining the white blood cell (WBC) differential count, a Wright-stained preparation of CSF is useful to determine the presence of leukemia, tumor cells, and other elements.

The CSF IgG index and IgG synthesis rate help diagnose multiple sclerosis (MS) (approximately 90% of patients have an IgG index >0.77 or a synthesis rate >3 mg/day or both; specificity, 80% to 90%). Increased values may also occur with many other CNS inflammatory conditions. CSF immunoelectrophoresis detects oligoclonal bands of IgG, which are found in patients with MS (sensitivity, 70% to 90%; specificity, 70% to 90%); however, they may also be present in other inflammatory and neoplastic conditions. Myelin basic protein is another protein that is elevated in patients with MS (sensitivity, 90%), but it too is not specific and is high in a number of other conditions.

CSF lactate may be high with any condition associated with CNS anoxia. It is also increased in patients with bacterial, tuberculous, and fungal meningitis—more so than in viral meningitis.

Recently determination of CSF LD and LD isoenzymes has been advocated during the first hours after a stroke: significantly higher values occur in patients with stroke (40.9 ± 14.5 U/L) than in patients with transient ischemic attacks (11.8 ± 2.9 U/L). Also, the CSF LD-1:LD-2 ratio may provide an early sensitive test for the differential diagnosis of brain tumors: a ratio <1 indicates carcinomatous meningitis or cerebral metastases; whereas a ratio >1 indicates a primary benign or malignant CNS tumor.

BIBLIOGRAPHY

Aseptic meningitis: New York State and United States, weeks 1-36, 1991. MMWR 40:773, 1991.
   Aseptic meningitis is on the rise.
Barnes HV: Aseptic meningitis and bacterial meningitis, and Spivak JL: Tuberculous meningitis. In Spivak JL, Barnes HV (eds): Manual of Clinical Problems in Internal Medicine, 4th ed. Boston, Little, Brown & Co, 1990, pp 402, 404, 463.
   Good discussion of differential diagnosis with annotated references.
Chaudhry HJ, Cunha BA: Drug-induced aseptic meningitis. Postgrad Med 90:65, 1991.
   Highlights a rare cause of aseptic meningitis.
Hall CD, Snyder CR, Robertson KR, et al: Cerebrospinal fluid analysis in human immunodeficiency virus infection. Ann Clin Lab Sci 22:139, 1992.
   Reviews the cerebrospinal fluid changes in 59 HIV-infected patients.
Kleine TO, Hackler R, Meyer-Rienecker H: Classical and modern methods of cerebrospinal fluid analysis. Eur J Clin Chem Clin Biochem 29:705, 1991.
   Reviews new developments in the analysis of cerebrospinal fluid.
Kjeldsberg CR, Knight JA: Body Fluids, 2nd ed. Chicago, American Society of Clinical Pathologists, 1986.
   Contains excellent colored photographs of various kinds of Wright-stained cells in the CSF fluid.
Lampl Y, Paniri Y, Eshel Y, et al: Cerebrospinal fluid lactate dehydrogenase levels in early stroke and transient ischemic attacks. Stroke 21:854, 1990.
   Suggests CSF lactate dehydrogenase to distinguish a stroke from a transient ischemic attack.
Lampl Y, Paniri Y, Eshel Y, et al: LDH isoenzymes in cerebrospinal fluid in various brain tumors. J Neurol Neurosurg Psychiatry 53:697, 1990.
   Suggests CSF LD-1 : LD-2 ratio to distinguish primary brain tumors from metastatic brain tumors.
Whiting AS, Johnson LN: Papilledema: Clinical clues and differential diagnosis. Am Fam Physician 45:1125, 1992.
   Papilledema is a sign of increased intracranial pressure.

Synovial Fluid Analysis

1.   In patients with synovial effusion obtain radiographic studies and consider an arthrocentesis. Request synovial fluid (SF) analysis, including Gram stain, cultures, crystal analysis, cell count, and differential.

The cause of acute monoarticular arthritis with synovial effusion can often be diagnosed by synovial fluid analysis, particularly when the arthritis is due to gout, pseudogout, or septic arthritis.

Record the total volume and appearance of the removed SF and estimate viscosity by allowing the SF to form a string when dripping from a syringe with the needle removed (normal SF forms a 4- to 6-cm string). Strings <3 cm indicate low viscosity because of depolymerization of hyaluronate, which is compatible with inflammatory conditions such as septic arthritis, gouty arthritis, and rheumatoid arthritis. A false-positive string test can occur with a rapid effusion after trauma. Alternatively, a poor mucin clot within 1 minute of adding a few drops of synovial fluid to 20 ml of 5% acetic acid indicates depolymerization of hyaluronate (Ropes test). Hemorrhagic effusions occur with trauma, fracture, neurotropic arthropathy, tumor, pigmented villonodular synovitis, hemorrhagic diathesis, and septic arthritis. Remember that more than one disease can occur simultaneously in the same joint (e.g., septic arthritis and lupus erythematosus; septic arthritis and gout; gout and rheumatoid arthritis; and septic arthritis and rheumatoid arthritis). Likewise several different crystals can occur together (e.g., urate and pyrophosphate crystals; apatite and pyrophosphate crystals; and urate and apatite crystals). In patients with monoarticular effusions consider bacterial infection (e.g., tuberculous or gonococcal arthritis).

In 100 consecutive patients undergoing joint aspiration the diagnoses were as follows:

DIAGNOSIS	NO. OF PATIENTS
Noninflammatory disease	
• Osteoarthritis	14
• Trauma	11
Inflammatory disease	
• Rheumatoid arthritis	11
• Crystal-induced arthritis	25
• Septic arthritis*	8
Miscellaneous diagnoses†	5
No diagnosis	26

Source: Shmerling RH, Delbanco TL, Tosteson ANA, et al: Synovial fluid tests: What should be ordered? JAMA 264:1009-1014, 1990. Copyright 1990, American Medical Association.

*Includes five patients with probable septic arthritis.

†Includes two patients with sickle cell anemia and one patient each with systemic lupus erythematosus, mixed connective tissue disease, and hepatitis B.

2.   Interpret test results in the context of clinical findings.

With the exception of tests for crystals and infectious agents, most other studies are relatively nonspecific. Therefore it is particularly important that tests for crystals and infectious agents are done well.

Normal synovial fluid is clear and pale yellow in appearance, has a WBC count of 0 to 200 μ/L (0 to 200 × 10⁶/L), of which less than 10% are neutrophils, and contains no abnormal elements.

CATEGORIES OF SYNOVIAL FLUID FINDINGS

	GROUP I (NONINFLAMMATORY)	GROUP II (MILDLY INFLAMMATORY)
Diagnosis	Osteoarthritis	Systemic lupus erythematosus Scleroderma
Appearance	Clear to slightly turbid	Clear to slightly turbid
WBC/μL (WBC × 10⁶/L)	50-2000 (50-2000)	0-9000 (0-9000)
Neutrophils	<30%	<20%
Other	Cartilage fragments	—

	GROUP III (SEVERELY INFLAMMATORY)			GROUP IV (INFECTIOUS)	
Diagnosis	Gout	Pseudo-gout	Rheumatoid arthritis	Acute bacterial arthritis	Tuberculous arthritis
Appearance	Turbid	Turbid	Turbid	Very turbid	Turbid
WBC/μL (WBC × 10⁶/L)	100-160,000 (100-160,000)	50-75,000 (50-75,000)	250-80,000 (250-80,000)	150-250,000 (150-250,000)	2500-100,000 (2500-100,000)
Neutrophils	Approximately 70%	Approximately 70%	Approximately 70%	Approximately 90%	Approximately 60%
Other	Monosodium urate crystals	Calcium pyrophosphate dihydrate crystals	—	Culture positive	Culture often negative

Source: Arnold WJ, Ike RW: Specialized procedures in the management of patients with rheumatic diseases. In Wyngaarden JB, Smith LH, Bennett JC (eds): Cecil Textbook of Medicine, 19th ed. Philadelphia, WB Saunders, 1992, p 1504.

SYNOVIAL FLUID CRYSTALS

CRYSTAL	POLARIZATION MICROSCOPY	OTHER IDENTIFICATION
Monosodium urate	Strong negative birefringence,* needle shaped, long	Uricase digestion X-ray diffraction
Calcium pyrophosphate dihydrate (CPPD)	Weak positive birefringence, rhomboid or small rods, pleomorphic	X-ray diffraction
Calcium phosphate (hydroxyapatite)	Not easily visualized	Electron microscopy X-ray diffraction
Cholesterol	Rhombic or platelike, notched corners, multicolored, occasionally small and needlelike	Chemical determination
Corticosteroids	Pleomorphic, variable birefringence	Follows intra-articular steroid treatment

Source: Cohen AS: Specialized diagnostic procedures in the rheumatic diseases. In Wyngaarden JB, Smith LH (eds): Cecil Textbook of Medicine, 18th ed. Philadelphia, WB Saunders, 1988, p 1994.
*Birefringence refers to crystals that are doubly refractive in plane-polarized light.

SEPTIC ARTHRITIS

The most important diagnosis to distinguish from other causes of arthritis is septic arthritis. Synovial fluid leukocyte count (WBC) and % neutrophils are the most accurate and useful tests for diagnosing the cause of joint effusions, and glucose and protein measurements are less useful. In more than 80% of cases the SF WBC and SF % neutrophils values are increased in inflammatory disease and are normal in noninflammatory disease.

A Gram stain is positive in approximately 75% of patients with staphylococcal infections, in 50% of patients with gram-negative septic arthritis, and in less than 25% of patients with gonococcal arthritis. If tuberculosis is suspected, perform an acid-fast stain (sensitivity, approximately 20%). Synovial biopsy is recommended for the rapid diagnosis of tuberculosis. Cultures are usually positive in most cases of septic arthritis; however, the yield may be less than 50% in purulent joints of patients with disseminated gonococcal infection and approximately 80% in patients with tuberculosis arthritis.

BIBLIOGRAPHY

Gatter RA, Schumacher HR: A Practical Handbook of Joint Fluid Analysis, 2nd ed. Philadelphia, Lea & Febiger, 1991.
Excellent monograph on the subject.

Kjeldsberg CR, Knight JA: Body Fluids, 2nd ed. Chicago, American Society of Clinical Pathologists, 1986.

Contains excellent colored photographs of various kinds of Wright-stained cells in synovial fluid.

Marino C, McDonald E: Diagnostic joint aspiration: When is it necessary? Emergency Medicine 24:67, 1992.

Acute monoarticular arthritis often needs aspiration—particularly to diagnose gout, pseudogout, and septic arthritis.

Rosenthal J: Acute monarticular arthritis: Sleuthing out the cause. Postgrad Med 89:79, 1991.

Provides a strategy for diagnosing the cause of monoarticular arthritis.

Shmerling RH, Delbanco TL, Tosteson ANA, et al: Synovial fluid tests: What should be ordered? JAMA 264:1009, 1990.

Critical review of the diagnostic yield of synovial fluid laboratory tests.

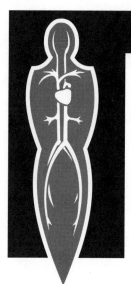

CHAPTER 3

CARDIOVASCULAR DISEASES

Acute Myocardial Infarction
Congestive Heart Failure
Hypertension
Digoxin Monitoring

Acute Myocardial Infarction

1.   For ambulatory patients who are seen in the emergency department with clinical findings of acute myocardial infarction (AMI), decide on hospital admission by using the history, physical examination, and electrocardiogram (ECG). Although a single serum creatine kinase (CK) and CK-MB test has limited use, serial measurements performed in an observation unit can be very helpful.

In the United States AMI affects approximately 1.5 million Americans every year, and 500,000 patients with AMI die annually. Up to 7 million Americans have chronic coronary artery disease. Moreover, up to 25% of AMIs are silent—these silent or painless infarcts are more common in diabetics and after cardiac transplantation.

Hospital coronary care units represent the standard level of care in the United States for patients who are thought to have an AMI because the mortality rate during the 72 hours after infarction is only 6% in these units versus 25% at home. These coronary care units are expensive; since only approximately 30% of patients admitted to these units have an AMI, being able to decide whether a patient with clinical findings suggestive of an AMI actually has an AMI before admitting the patient to such a unit would be useful. Because blood specimens are often drawn too early to detect the rise in enzymes, single measurements of CK and CK-MB isoenzymes in the emergency department are not sufficiently sensitive to exclude a diagnosis of AMI, and the decision to hospitalize the patient must be made on clinical and ECG findings. An additional complicating factor is the long turnaround times for conventional CK-MB tests. Using single test results in patients with chest pain in the emergency department, the CK was elevated in only 38% and the CK-MB in only 34%. On the other hand, if the clinical findings do not suggest an AMI, a single serum CK and CK-MB test can sometimes detect an AMI; however, false-positive results may be high. Because a single CK and CK-MB test has low sensitivity and specificity for AMI compared with serial samples, an observation period with a second set of measurements may be useful in deciding whether to admit the patient. The recent development of rapid turnaround time CK-MB tests has already proved useful in identifying patients with AMI who had negative initial ECGs and who would have otherwise been discharged. See the Introduction of this book for a discussion of different laboratory test-related clinical decisions for AMI.

Specimen collection and handling are important. An intramuscular injection can increase total CK (not CK-MB) two to three times. Once the specimen is drawn, CK-MB starts to deteriorate within hours but with refrigeration is stable up to 24 hours. If more than 2 hours may pass before CK isoenzymes will be assayed, the serum sample should be preserved on ice. Lactate dehydrogenase (LD) will last for days at room temperature. Hemolysis interferes with LD measurements because red blood cells contain 150 times more LD than serum, mainly LD_1.

2. For patients admitted to the hospital with clinical findings of AMI, request serial measurements of CK and CK isoenzymes. Serial measurements of LD and LD isoenzymes may be helpful. Serum transaminase measurements are unnecessary. When CK measurements are delayed more than 2 hours, the specimen should be refrigerated or placed on ice.

Although many clinicians measure serum CK and CK-MB more frequently, sampling at 0, 12, and 24 hours is adequate for diagnosis. Because some patients with AMI can show a rise in CK-MB, even though the total CK remains within the normal range, CK-MB should be measured; however, some experts still recommend routinely measuring CK-MB only if the total CK level is above 150 U/L. Failure to detect an increased total CK level may be caused by inappropriate sampling times. The rise and subsequent fall of CK and CK-MB levels in a patient with AMI are characteristic. Commonly LD and LD isoenzymes have been measured at 0 hours and every 24 hours for 2 to 3 days. Recent studies suggest that LD studies are confirmatory, are not always necessary, and may be required only if the patient's admission has been delayed more than 24 hours or if the CK studies fail to show an abnormality. If the serum total LD level is normal, LD isoenzyme measurements may not be needed. If chest pain recurs after admission, a new set of CK and CK-MB measurements are indicated at 0, 12, and 24 hours.

Serum CK rises within 3 hours of the onset of pain in a typical case of AMI. The peak value is reached approximately 24 hours later, followed by a decline to normal after another 48 to 72 hours. The duration of the rise and fall of the CK-MB fraction is similar to that of the total CK level. Serum LD rises in 8 to 12 hours, peaks in 48 to 72 hours, and becomes normal after 8 to 14 days. An increased $LD_1:LD_2$ ratio (>1) usually appears in 12 to 24 hours, peaks in 48 hours, and is present in less than 50% of patients after 1 week.

3.   Evaluate the tests and the results.

Some serum CK-MB assays are qualitative and measure only the presence or absence of CK-MB, whereas others are quantitative and express the CK-MB level in terms of its percentage of total CK, with upper reference limits for CK-MB ranging from 3% to 6%. Electrophoretic methods for measuring CK-MB have been particularly satisfactory, giving good separation of isoenzymes and clinically reliable results. When compared with determination of CK-MB by electrophoresis, chemical methods for measuring CK-MB may give values that are more sensitive but less specific.

In the future analysis of CK isoforms, myosin light chains, or troponin T may enable us to detect AMI within 1 hour after onset. Earlier diagnosis of AMI will be helpful, especially for patients with equivocal clinical and ECG findings in the emergency department or for whom thrombolytic therapy is being considered. At present, these newer tests are not generally available.

A CK value >1800 U/L is most often seen in pathological entities other than AMI such as rhabdomyolysis, delirium tremens, and status epilepticus, and an LD value >500 U/L is most often seen in patients with megaloblastic anemia, acute leukemia, metastatic carcinoma, trauma, and shock liver.

4.   If the test results show a characteristic rise and subsequent fall of CK and CK-MB in the context of appropriate clinical findings, conclude that the diagnosis is AMI. An increased $LD_1:LD_2$ ratio is confirmatory and, by itself, can occur in other disorders.

An increased serum CK-MB level is the best method for diagnosing AMI; and in patients whose CK-MB levels are increased within 24 hours of the onset of chest pain, the sensitivity approaches 100%, and the specificity is very high. The rise and fall of CK-MB are characteristic. The sequence of an increased serum CK-MB level followed in time by an increased serum LD level with an increased $LD_1:LD_2$ ratio is unique for AMI. An increased $LD_1:LD_2$ ratio above 1 is 81% sensitive for AMI and above 0.76 is 92% sensitive. The $LD_1:LD_2$ ratio may flip back and forth around 1 several times. Failure to detect an increased $LD_1:LD_2$ ratio in a patient with AMI may be a result of inappropriate sampling times. An isomorphic LD isoenzyme pattern (all isoenzyme values increased) may indicate shock, an increased LD_3 level may indicate pulmonary edema, and an increased LD_5 level may indicate congestive heart failure (CHF).

The guidelines for interpreting serum CK and CK-MB test results for the diagnosis of AMI after noncardiac surgery are essentially the same as for the medical patient; however, after cardiac surgery the guidelines are different. Surgical manipulation of the heart during cardiac surgery causes an increase of CK and CK-MB at the time of surgery, which falls to normal over the next 12 to 18 hours. Persistently increased values after cardiac surgery suggest AMI.

Numerous diseases other than AMI can cause increased CK and CK-MB. Cardiovascular causes include myocarditis, pericarditis, myocardial puncture or trauma, and acute dissection of the aorta. Systemic diseases (e.g., muscular dystrophy, hypothermia, hyperthermia, and Reye's syndrome) with cardiac involvement can also cause increased values. Peripheral sources of high values include myositis, rhabdomyolysis, athletic activity, prostate surgery, cesarean delivery, gastrointestinal surgery, and tumors. Miscellaneous causes include renal failure, subarachnoid hemorrhage, and hypothyroidism. An increased $LD_1 : LD_2$ ratio without increased CK-MB can occur with hemolysis and renal infarction.

Consider macro creatine kinase (macro CK) when the increased CK iso-enzyme values do not fit the clinical picture. An autoantibody to CK-BB (macro CK, type 1) is a possible cause of macro CK, but macro CK also is caused by release of mitochondrial CK into the serum (macro CK, type 2). Macro CK, type 1, is found in the sera of healthy persons and hos-pitalized persons, but macro CK, type 2, is found in severely ill persons of all ages, mainly those with various malignant tumors, including small cell carcinoma of the lung, cirrhosis of the liver, myocardial damage, and shock. In addition to macro CK, increased CK-MB, and especially CK-BB have been described in patients with certain malignant tumors: lung, pros-tate, bladder, colorectal, gastric, hepatoma, breast, ovarian, sarcoma, and lymphoma.

5.   If serial measurements for serum CK, CK-MB, and LD are normal in a patient seen early after the onset of clinical findings of AMI, exclude AMI.

Serial measurements of CK, CK-MB, LD, and LD isoenzymes are im-portant for excluding AMI. If the values are normal and no other significant disease is present, the patient may be discharged.

6.   In patients with AMI estimate the infarct size by the magnitude of increase of serum enzymes, but remember that the prognostic information may not be very good.

There is a relationship between the peak serum concentrations of CK, CK-MB, and LD and the size of an AMI, with larger infarcts producing higher values. This relationship is stronger with CK and CK-MB than with LD. Infarct size can also be estimated from the time interval to peak CK, with longer times indicating larger infarcts. Frequent sampling (e.g., every 4 hours) is necessary to detect true enzyme peaks. Since there are a number of other variables, prognostic information is not very good. Routine mea-surements taken more often than 0, 12, and 24 hours are not indicated.

7.   In patients with clinical findings of AMI begin thrombolytic therapy as early as possible without waiting for enzyme and isoenzyme results. Measure serial levels of serum CK and CK-MB to monitor therapy.

Because the goal of thrombolytic therapy is to reopen an occluded artery as soon as possible, the decision to attempt thrombolysis should be based on the clinical history and ECG rather than waiting for increased enzyme values.

Ideally, in individuals without contraindications thrombolytic agents should be used within 2 to 3 hours of the onset of findings. Waiting more than 4 to 6 hours is too long. Earlier and higher peak CK values have been observed in both spontaneous and therapeutic reperfusion of an infarct.

8.   In patients with AMI the following additional abnormal blood test results may occur:

↑ **Hematocrit.** May show a small early increase related to decreased blood volume, followed by a small decrease later.

↑ **Leukocytes, increased erythrocyte sedimentation rate, and C-reactive protein** caused by the inflammatory response associated with the infarct. Leukocytosis appears within hours of onset of pain, persists for 1 to 2 weeks, and often reaches 12 to 15 × 10^3 cells/μL (12 to 15 × 10^9 cells/L). Erythrocyte sedimentation rate rises more slowly than leukocyte levels, peaks during the first week, and sometimes remains increased for 1 to 2 weeks.

↓ **pH** with metabolic acidosis caused by tissue hypoxia.

↓ **Partial pressure of oxygen (PO₂)** from cardiopulmonary dysfunction. Mild hypoxemia can occur even without complications.

↑ **Glucose** related to diabetes mellitus as a predisposing risk factor or simply secondary to the stress of the infarct. In stress hyperglycemia, hemoglobin A1C is normal. In nondiabetics mortality rate of 3.4% at admission glucose levels <120 mg/dL (<6.7 mmol/L) rises to 42.9% at levels >180 mg/dL (>10.0 mmol/L).

↑ **Urea nitrogen and creatinine** related to decreased renal perfusion.

↓ **Sodium.**

↓ **Potassium** caused by either a high level of circulating catecholamines or previous diuretic therapy. Potassium value <3.6 mEq/L (<3.6 mmol/L) during admission is a risk factor for ventricular arrhythmia within 6 hours after admission.

↑ **Aspartate aminotransferase (SGOT)** from infarct and possibly from hepatic congestion.

↑ **Alanine aminotransferase (SGPT) and LD₅** may occur from congestion and poor perfusion of the liver secondary to heart failure.

↓ **Albumin** caused by hepatic congestion.

↑ **Bilirubin** with severe heart failure from hepatic failure.

↑ **Lactate** (>32 mg/dL [>3.6 mmol/L]) occurs in 60% of patients the day before the development of shock.

↑ **Triglycerides:** peak in 3 weeks; increase may persist for 1 year.

↑ **Cholesterol,** which may constitute a predisposing risk factor for coronary heart disease. If cholesterol level can be measured within the first 24 hours of infarction, it is statistically the same as the preinfarction level.

BIBLIOGRAPHY

Bellodi G, Manicardi V, Malavasi V, et al: Hyperglycemia and prognosis of acute myocardial infarction in patients without diabetes mellitus. Am J Cardiol 64:885, 1989.
Correlates increasing admission glucose values in nondiabetics with increasing mortality.

Clausen TG, Brocks K, Ibsen H: Hypokalemia and ventricular arrhythmias in acute myocardial infarction. Acta Med Scand 224:531, 1988.
Hypokalemia during admission, whether spontaneous or diuretic induced, correlates with an increased incidence of ventricular arrhythmia.

Eng C, Skolnick AE, Come SE: Elevated creatine kinase and malignancy. Hosp Pract 25:123, 1990.
Reviews various malignancies that are associated with increased creatine kinase.

Hohnloser SH, Zabel M, Kasper W, et al: Assessment of coronary artery patency after thrombolytic therapy: Accurate prediction utilizing the combined analysis of three noninvasive markers. J Am Coll Cardiol 18:44, 1991.
Early peak CK predicts successful thrombolysis.

Kassirer JP, Kopelman RI: Case 54—Memory: How we overcome its limitations. In Learning Clinical Reasoning. Baltimore, Williams & Wilkins, 1991, p 271.
Discusses the clinical reasoning in a patient with AMI and methemoglobinemia caused by too much nitroglycerin.

Knudsen J, Steenstrup B, Bryjalsen I, et al: At what level of serum total creatine kinase activity can measurement of serum creatine kinase MB isoenzyme activity be omitted in suspected myocardial infarction? Scand J Clin Lab Invest 49:661, 1989.
Suggests measuring CK-MB only if the total CK is greater than 150 U/L.

Lee TH: Chest pain in the emergency department: Uncertainty and the test of time. Mayo Clin Proc 66:963, 1991.
Concludes that current tests in the emergency department (CK-MB and lipid studies) are not very useful to identify patients with AMI and that the use of short-term observation units may be the best alternative.

Lee TH, Goldman L: Serum enzyme assays in the diagnosis of acute myocardial infarction: Recommendations based on a quantitative analysis. In Sox HC Jr (ed): Common Diagnostic Tests: Use and Interpretation, 2nd ed. Philadelphia, American College of Physicians, 1990, p 35.
Reviews the use of serum enzymes for the diagnosis of AMI.

Litin SC, O'Brien JF, Pruett S, et al: Macroenzyme as a cause of unexplained elevation of aspartate aminotransferase. Mayo Clin Proc 62:681, 1987.
Discusses macroenzyme formation as a cause for unexplained high enzyme values.

Marin MM, Teichman SL: Use of rapid serial sampling of creatine kinase MB for very early detection of myocardial infarction in patients with acute chest pain. Am Heart J 123:354, 1992.
Serial hourly measurements of serum CK-MB can be used to diagnose AMI within 2 to 4 hours of arrival at a hospital.

Martin LJ, Knight JA: Mitochondrial creatine kinase. American Society of Clinical Pathologists, Chicago, Clinical Chemistry No. CC 88-10 (CC-198), 1988.
Discusses various forms of macro creatine kinase and their clinical significance.

Mavrić Z, Zaputović L, Zager D, et al: Usefulness of blood lactate as a predictor of shock development in acute myocardial infarction. Am J Cardiol 67:565, 1991.
In patients who were not in shock during admission, high blood lactate correlates with risk of shock in the next 24 hours.

Sullebarger JT, Greenland P: Myocardial infarction. In Panzer RJ, Black ER, Griner PF (eds): Diagnostic Strategies for Common Medical Problems. Philadelphia, American College of Physicians, 1991, p 55.
Recommends strategies for the diagnosis of myocardial infarction.

Congestive Heart Failure

1. In patients with clinical findings of congestive heart failure assess organ dysfunction by requesting determinations of serum electrolytes, glucose, urea nitrogen, creatinine, and liver function, arterial blood gas analysis, and a urinalysis.

Each year congestive heart failure (CHF), a syndrome affecting approximately 3 million persons or 1% of the population, develops in approximately 400,000 Americans. The leading cause is myocardial infarction. For individuals older than age 75, the prevalence of the syndrome rises to approximately 10%.

Although serum electrolyte values are generally normal before treatment, diuretic therapy and sodium restriction can cause abnormalities. Reductions in renal blood flow can increase serum urea nitrogen and creatinine concentrations, and congestion of the liver and poor cardiac output can cause abnormal liver function test results. Congestion of the lungs can cause pulmonary edema and affect arterial blood gas values. Pleural and pericardial effusions may occur. Ascites is a late manifestation.

2. Interpret test results in the context of the clinical findings.

Hypoglycemia may occur in the presence of severe, prolonged hepatic congestion and severely compromised cardiac output. Hyperglycemia is common, probably related to stress.

The serum urea nitrogen, creatinine, and uric acid values may be increased secondary to reductions in renal blood flow and glomerular filtration rate. Urea nitrogen values may be as high as 80 to 100 mg/dL (13.3 to 16.7 mmol/L) and are disproportionately high relative to those for creatinine. This prerenal azotemia is usually characterized by a urea:creatinine ratio >15:1.

Prolonged rigid sodium restriction coupled with intensive diuretic therapy and the inability to excrete water may lead to hypervolemic hyponatremia, which occurs despite an increase in total body sodium in the context of an expanded extracellular fluid volume. Prolonged administration of kaliuretic diuretics such as the thiazides or loop diuretics may cause hypokalemia. Hypokalemia is associated with a poor prognosis as a result of ventricular arrhythmias. Triamterene is often administered with thiazides for its potassium-sparing effect. In patients with terminal heart failure hyperkalemia may occur.

In failure of the right side of the heart, acute congestive hepatomegaly can cause a significant increase of serum transaminase (AST [SGOT] and ALT [SGPT]) values to several thousand units, which may resemble the findings with acute viral hepatitis. Low cardiac output is often present. A differential clue is that, in contrast to those with viral hepatitis, the increased transaminase values of heart failure can be rapidly reversed by successful treatment. In a patient with AMI the AST (SGOT) level is increased, but in one with AMI with CHF both the AST (SGOT) and ALT (SGPT) levels are increased. Other liver function test results may be increased. They include serum alkaline phosphatase (ALP), LD (especially isoenzyme LD_5), and total and conjugated bilirubin. In fact, frank jaundice may occur. The prothrombin time may be prolonged. Rarely, acute hepatic decompensation can occur, with hepatic coma and an increased blood ammonia concentration.

A recent study categorized chronic CHF as mild, moderate, or severe. The mean values for the liver function test results in patients in the mild and moderate groups were normal or mainly normal. Patients in the severe group had significantly higher activities of AST (SGOT; 65 ± 82 U/L), ALT (SGPT; 77 ± 102 U/L), and LD (282 ± 91 U/L), and an increased total bilirubin concentration (1.7 ± 0.8 mg/dL [29 ± 14 μmol/L]). In patients with chronic congestive hepatomegaly serum albumin may be decreased not only because of liver dysfunction, but also because of protein-losing enteropathy (a rare occurrence).

In failure of the left side of the heart with acute pulmonary edema, arterial blood gas determinations can help assess decreased oxygenation (decreased Po_2 with normal to decreased partial pressure of carbon dioxide [Pco_2]). Cyanosis is seen with greater than 5 g/dL (50 g/L) of reduced hemoglobin.

Oliguria is characteristic of failure of the right side of the heart, and urinary specific gravity may increase above 1.020. During periods of diuresis the specific gravity may be low. Mild albuminuria (<1 g/day) is common, and the urinary sediment may show isolated red blood cells, white blood cells, and casts (hyaline and granular). With acute oliguria, the urinary sodium concentration in a CHF patient is generally less than 20 mEq/L (20 mmol/L), whereas in a patient with acute renal failure caused by intrinsic renal disease or postrenal obstruction, the urinary sodium concentration is typically greater than 40 mEq/L (40 mmol/L).

3.   In patients with congestive heart failure receiving drug therapy, monitor the patient for possible adverse effects of drugs.

For example, thiazides and loop diuretics can cause alkalosis, decreased serum potassium, magnesium, glomerular filtration rate, and lithium clearance (in patients receiving lithium therapy), and increased serum glucose, uric acid, calcium, total cholesterol, low-density lipoprotein (LDL) cholesterol, triglycerides, and possibly plasma renin activity. The hypercholesterolemic effect of diuretics may abate with continued administration of the drug. Uncommon effects include inappropriate antidiuretic hormone (ADH) secretion and decreased red blood cells, white blood cells, and platelets.

Potassium-sparing diuretics (e.g., triamterene) can cause megaloblastic anemia, increased potassium and plasma renin activity, and decreased glomerular filtration.

To determine which drug increases or decreases serum lipid values, wait until the patient has been taking the drug for at least 6 to 8 weeks before measuring lipids. See the discussion of serum cholesterol in Chapter 1 for a table of drug effects on serum lipids.

In a recent study serum electrolyte determinations were the most common laboratory studies performed in patients with CHF, and they were measured at median intervals of 3 to 5 months. The digoxin level was the next most common laboratory test.

4. In patients with CHF the following additional abnormal blood test results may occur:

↓ **Hematocrit,** mild, even when red blood cell mass is increased.

↓ **Erythrocyte sedimentation rate.**

↑ **Erythrocyte sedimentation rate.**

↓ **Magnesium** caused by anorexia, malabsorption, and excessive use of diuretic agents; when less than 1.6 mEq/L (0.80 mmol/L), associated with worse prognosis related to ventricular arrhythmia and sudden death.

↑ **Magnesium** associated with worse prognosis related to severity of disease and poor organ function.

↓ **Cholesterol** possible with severe congestion of the liver.

BIBLIOGRAPHY

Cohen JA, Kaplan MM: Left-sided heart failure presenting as hepatitis. Gastroenterology 74:583, 1978.
  Points out that liver enzyme values may be very high in CHF and may simulate hepatitis.
Fleg JL, Hinton PC, Lakatta EG, et al: Physician utilization of laboratory procedures to monitor outpatients with congestive heart failure. Arch Intern Med 149:393, 1989.
  Describes the most common tests that physicians use to monitor outpatients with CHF.
Gottlieb S, Baruch L, Kukin ML, et al: Prognostic importance of the serum magnesium concentration in patients with congestive heart failure. J Am Coll Cardiol 16:827, 1990.
  Correlates hypomagnesemia and hypermagnesemia with a worse prognosis.
Haber HL, Leavy JA, Kessler PD, et al: The erythrocyte sedimentation rate in congestive heart failure. N Engl J Med 324:353, 1991.
  The erythrocyte sedimentation rate in patients with CHF may be high or low and is of limited clinical value.
Kubo SH, Walter BA, John DHA, et al: Liver function abnormalities in chronic heart failure: Influence of systemic hemodynamics. Arch Intern Med 147:1227, 1987.
  Quantifies liver function test abnormalities based on the severity of liver dysfunction.
Lardinois CK, Neuman SL: The effects of antihypertensive agents on serum lipids and lipoproteins. Arch Intern Med 148:1280, 1988.
  Describes the adverse effects of diuretics in CHF.
Parmley WW, Chatterjee K, Francis GS, et al: Congestive heart failure: New frontiers. West J Med 154:427, 1991.
  Good review of CHF.
Powers ER, Bergin JD: Recent advances in evaluating and managing congestive heart failure. Modern Medicine 60:54, 1992.
  Discusses the diagnosis and management of patients with CHF.

Hypertension

1.   For patients with hypertension request a complete blood count, determinations of serum glucose (fasting), urea nitrogen, creatinine, potassium, calcium, uric acid, cholesterol, and high-density lipoprotein [HDL] cholesterol, and a urinalysis. Sometimes these tests can be ordered as part of less costly batteries or profiles.

Although certainly not the sole explanation, aggressive detection and treatment of hypertension have coincided with a decline in coronary artery disease mortality of roughly 40% and a decline in stroke of approximately 57%.

Hemoglobin and hematocrit values are useful in detecting anemia, which can further stress the heart, and a baseline white blood cell count and platelet count may assist in monitoring drug therapy. An increase in the fasting serum glucose level can detect diabetes mellitus, which may be associated with accelerated atherosclerosis, renal vascular disease, and diabetic nephropathy. Additionally, hyperglycemia can signal the presence of adrenal hyperfunction, Cushing's syndrome, and pheochromocytoma. Glucose concentrations may also be affected by therapy. Serum determinations of urea nitrogen and creatinine and a urinalysis are useful in excluding renal parenchymal disease and assessing renal function. Serum potassium measurements serve not only as a screen for mineralocorticoid-induced hypertension but also as a baseline measurement before initiating drug therapy. Serum uric acid concentration may be affected by drugs and is often increased in patients with renal and essential hypertension. Hypercholesterolemia is another important risk factor for accelerated atherosclerosis, and serum cholesterol may be increased by antihypertensive drugs such as thiazide diuretics.

2.   Interpret test results in the context of clinical findings.

For most hypertensive patients the laboratory evaluation at this point will be complete. Baseline data will be in place, and target organ damage will be assessed. Patients with a high serum total cholesterol concentration or low HDL cholesterol concentration should be studied further to determine LDL cholesterol and triglyceride concentrations and whether the hypercholesterolemia is primary or secondary. Physicians may select additional tests, based on their clinical judgment. Type and frequency of repeated laboratory tests should be based on the severity of target organ damage and the effects of the selected treatment program. If a specific form of secondary hypertension is suspected because of certain clinical and laboratory clues, commence studies for coarctation, Cushing's syndrome, pheochromocytoma, primary aldosteronism, and renovascular hypertension. Additional diagnostic testing should be reserved for cases in which potentially correctable causes of hypertension are suspected, including patients whose age at onset of hypertension is less than 30 years or more than 60 years and patients who respond poorly to aggressive medical treatment.

a.   To diagnose coarctation of the aorta, request appropriate radiographic studies in the context of consistent physical and electrocardiographic findings.

Greater systolic pressure between the right arm and the legs, decreased pulses in the legs, left ventricular hypertrophy, and left atrial enlargement can be demonstrated by physical findings and electrocardiography. The chest radiograph may show prominence of the aorta, enlarged left ventricle and left atrium, and rib notching. The diagnosis can be confirmed by aortography.

b.   To diagnose Cushing's syndrome (hypertension, central obesity, glucose intolerance, weakness [hypokalemia], depression), measure a 24-hour urine free cortisol level or perform an overnight dexamethasone suppression test.

The 24-hour urine free cortisol test is nearly 100% sensitive and specific for diagnosing Cushing's syndrome: false-negative test results are rare, and except when stress leads to an increased cortisol excretion or with chronic alcoholism, false-positive urine free cortisol values are seldom seen. Always refer to the reference range of the laboratory you use; but, in general, a 24-hour urine cortisol concentration <100 µg/24 hours (276 nmol/24 hours) excludes the diagnosis, whereas a level >150 µg/24 hours (414 nmol/24 hours) strongly suggests the diagnosis.

Perform the overnight dexamethasone suppression test by giving the patient an oral dose of 1 mg of dexamethasone at 10:00 P.M. and measuring the serum:plasma cortisol concentration at 8:00 A.M. the next morning. A level <5 µg/dL (138 nmol/L), typically 1 to 2 µg/dL (28 to 55 nmol/L), is present in most normal patients, whereas a value >10 µg/dL (280 nmol/L) is typical of Cushing's syndrome.

If the clinical findings are suggestive but the laboratory test results are normal or equivocal or if the reverse is true, Liddle's low-dose dexamethasone suppression test may be helpful. In difficult cases consult an endocrinologist.

c.   To diagnose pheochromocytoma (hypertension, weight loss, glucose intolerance, "spells" of palpitations, perspiration, pounding headache, and pallor [the "four *ps*"], tremor, and nervousness), measure 24-hour urinary metanephrine excretion or a 12-hour overnight urine collection for metanephrine and creatinine.

In unstressed patients the 24-hour metanephrine test is nearly 100% sensitive and has almost no false-negative results. Increased values occur in times of severe stress, but results are usually normal when the test is repeated. Although the 24-hour urine test is preferable, the 12-hour metanephrine test is satisfactory when combined with a test for creatinine. A normal urinary metanephrine:creatinine ratio is <1.2 µg metanephrine per milligram of creatinine (0.69 mmol/mol creatinine)—patients with the disease will have higher ratios. If spells are part of the clinical presentation, a 2-, 4-, or 6-hour urine collection for determining metanephrine and creatinine values during a spell should be done.

If the clinical findings are suggestive and the urinary metanephrine test results are normal or equivocal, consider measuring urinary vanillylmandelic acid (VMA) or catecholamines or both. These measurements are more specific (fewer false-positive results) and less sensitive (more false-negative results) but are also more subject to drug interferences than metanephrine determinations. Measurement of plasma catecholamines may be helpful. In difficult cases consult an endocrinologist.

    d. To diagnose primary hyperaldosteronism (hypertension and hypokalemia), determine whether the urinary potassium level is high when the serum potassium level is low. If this is the case, measure plasma renin activity.

It is important to begin by measuring urinary potassium levels when the serum potassium level is low because a urinary potassium level <30 mEq/L (30 mmol/L) excludes hyperaldosteronism. Plasma renin activity (PRA) is a good initial screening test for primary hyperaldosteronism. Low PRA is highly suggestive of primary hyperaldosteronism. Once low PRA has been found in a patient with hypokalemia caused by renal potassium wasting, aldosterone should be measured, which is typically high.

    e. To diagnose renovascular hypertension, measure PRA.

A high PRA level is consistent with renovascular hypertension or pheochromocytoma (secondary hyperaldosteronism). When measuring PRA to diagnose either hyperaldosteronism or renovascular hypertension, remember to exclude other factors that alter PRA such as drugs (e.g., caffeine, diuretics, and estrogens increase PRA; whereas beta-adrenergic blockers, digoxin, and testosterone decrease PRA).

3. In patients with hypertension who are on drug therapy, monitor the patients for possible adverse effects of drugs.

For example, beta blockers can cause high serum potassium and triglyceride concentrations and decreased HDL cholesterol concentration, glomerular filtration rate, and PRA. A rare effect is a positive antinuclear antibody determination. To assess the effects of a drug on serum lipid values, wait until the patient has been taking the drug for at least 6 to 8 weeks before measuring serum lipids.

BIBLIOGRAPHY

Alderman MH: Which antihypertensive drugs first—and why! JAMA 267:2786, 1992.
    Describes the impressive declines in coronary artery disease and stroke associated with aggressive detection and treatment of hypertension.
Black ER: Secondary hypertension; and Black ER, Mushlin AI: Hypercortisolism: Cushing syndrome. In Panzer RJ, Black ER, Griner PF (eds): Diagnostic Strategies for Common

Medical Problems. Philadelphia, American College of Physicians, 1991, pp 66, 364.
Recommends strategies for the differential diagnosis of the cause of secondary hypertension.
Cryer PE: Pheochromocytoma. West J Med 156:399, 1992.
Reviews the pathophysiology, diagnosis, and management of pheochromocytoma.
Gifford RW Jr, Kirkendall W, O'Connor DT: Office evaluation of hypertension: A statement for health professionals by a writing group of the Council for High Blood Pressure Research, American Heart Association. Circulation 79:721, 1989.
Useful recommendations for the office workup of hypertension.
1988 Joint National Committee: The 1988 report of the Joint National Committee on Detection, Evaluation, and Treatment of High Blood Pressure. Arch Intern Med 148:1023, 1988.
Documents the case for early diagnosis and treatment of hypertension.
Lardinois CK, Neuman SL: The effects of antihypertensive agents on serum lipids and lipoproteins. Arch Intern Med 148:1280, 1988.
Describes the effects of antihypertensive drugs on lipids.

Digoxin Monitoring

1. Monitor the serum concentration of digoxin in the following circumstances: to assess patient compliance, to tailor an optimal dosing schedule, and to confirm a clinical impression of toxicity. Routine measurement of serum digoxin concentration is inappropriate.

For monitoring digoxin, draw the sample at least 12 hours after the last dose and after four to five half-lives (6 to 7 days with normal renal function) after a dosage change. In a group of hospitalized patients receiving digoxin, the incidence of toxicity was approximately 15%, with another 3% to 5% of patients showing symptoms suggestive of toxicity.

2. Evaluate the test.

Digoxin can be measured by immunoassay or high-performance liquid chromatography. Either method is acceptable.

REFERENCE RANGE

TEST	SPECIMEN	CONVENTIONAL UNITS	INTERNATIONAL UNITS
Digoxin	Serum or plasma (heparin or ethylenedi-amine-tetraacetic acid [EDTA]); trough (>12 hr after dose)	For CHF: 0.8-1.5 ng/mL	1.0-1.9 nmol/L
		For arrhythmias: 1.5-2.0 ng/mL	1.9-2.6 nmol/L
		Toxic: >2.5 ng/mL	>3.2 nmol/L

3. Interpret test results in the context of clinical findings.

Most patients will experience the maximal increase in cardiac contractivity at a serum concentration of 1.4 ng/mL (1.8 nmol/L), with little increase at higher serum values. Toxicity typically is associated with a serum concentration of at least 1 ng/mL (1.2 nmol/L). With serum concentrations approaching or above 2 ng/mL (2.6 nmol/L), the risk of toxicity becomes unacceptably high. Thus the toxic-to-therapeutic ratio is narrow, and digoxin monitoring is quite helpful.

When serum concentrations of digitalis glycosides are excessive, consider these reasons*:

1. A dose too large for age group
2. Improved bioavailability of a new product
3. Renal insufficiency
4. Interaction with other drugs: quinidine, verapamil, amiodarone, indomethacin
5. Presence of endogenous digoxin-like factors
6. Poisoning: accidental, children, old people; suicide attempt; intentional (homicidal); or iatrogenic (medication error)
7. Inappropriate sampling time

---

*Source: Koren G, Soldin SJ: Cardiac glycosides. In Gerson B (ed): Therapeutic Drug Monitoring—II: Patient Care and Applications. Clin Lab Med 7:601, 1987.

When determining individual sensitivity to digitalis, consider these factors†:

• Type and severity of underlying cardiac disease
• Serum electrolyte derangement
  • Hypokalemia or hyperkalemia
  • Hypomagnesemia
  • Hypercalcemia
  • Hyponatremia
• Acid-base imbalance
• Concomitant drug administration
  • Anesthetics
  • Catecholamines and sympathomimetics
  • Antiarrhythmic agents
• Thyroid status
• Renal function
• Autonomic nervous system tone
• Respiratory disease

---

†Source: Smith TW: Heart failure. In Wyngaarden JB, Smith LH, Bennett JC (eds): Cecil Textbook of Medicine, 19th ed. Philadelphia, WB Saunders, 1992, p 204.

4.   In patients with life-threatening digoxin intoxication administration of digoxin-specific Fab antibody fragments is rapidly effective.

After administration of Fab fragments, total serum digoxin concentrations are no longer meaningful. Free (unbound) digoxin can be measured when monitoring of serum values is required.

BIBLIOGRAPHY

Kelly DP, Fry ETA: Heart failure. In Woodley M, Whelan A (eds): Manual of Medical Therapeutics, 27th ed. Boston, Little, Brown & Co, 1992, p 105.
  Discusses the use of digoxin-specific Fab antibody fragments for managing digoxin intoxication.
Kelly RA, Smith TW: Use and misuse of digitalis blood levels. Heart Disease and Stroke 1:117, 1992.
  Recent guidelines for digoxin monitoring.
Keys PW, Stafford RW: Digoxin: Therapeutic use and serum concentration monitoring. In Taylor WJ, Finn AL (eds): Individualizing Drug Therapy: Practical Applications of Drug Monitoring, vol. 3. New York, Gross, Townsend, Frank, Inc, 1981.
  Good discussion of practical issues.
Koren G, Soldin SJ: Cardiac glycosides. In Gerson B (ed): Therapeutic Drug Monitoring– II: Patient Care and Applications. Clin Lab Med 7:587, 1987.
  Resource for digoxin therapy in patient care.
Matzuk MM, Shlomchik M, Shaw LM: Making digoxin therapeutic drug monitoring more effective. Ther Drug Monit 13:215, 1991.
  Emphasizes sampling at least 12 hours after the last dose and four to five half-lives after a dosage change.
Mooradian AD: Digitalis: An update of clinical pharmacokinetics, therapeutic monitoring techniques, and treatment recommendations. Clin Pharmacokinet 15:165, 1988.
  Useful theoretical and practical information.

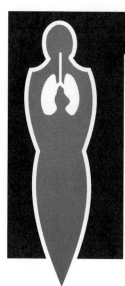

CHAPTER 4

RESPIRATORY TRACT DISEASES

Acute Pharyngitis
Allergic Rhinitis
Community-Acquired Pneumonia
Pulmonary Embolism
Chronic Obstructive Pulmonary Disease
Pleural Fluid Analysis

Acute Pharyngitis

1. In adult patients (>18 years) with a sore throat, determine their management by the presence or absence of four key clinical findings: (1) temperature >100° F (37.8° C); (2) tonsillar exudate; (3) anterior cervical lymphadenopathy; and (4) lack of cough.

- When all four findings are present, treat immediately without a rapid streptococcal antigen test or throat culture. Only three findings must be present for treatment in the emergency department.
- When all four findings are absent, a rapid test or throat culture is not required unless the patient has special risk factors.
- When some of these findings are present, obtain a rapid streptococcal antigen test or throat culture. If the rapid test is negative, obtain a throat culture.

For children always obtain a rapid streptococcal antigen test or throat culture. If the rapid test is negative, obtain a throat culture.

Leukocyte count, C-reactive protein, erythrocyte sedimentation rate, antistreptolysin O titer, and other laboratory tests are not helpful.

When the probability of group A streptococcal infection is high (>40%), it is prudent to treat adult patients immediately with antibiotics. Relying on throat culture test results in this group is inappropriate since, even in the best circumstances, the sensitivity is only approximately 90%. Rapid diagnostic tests are even less sensitive. On the other hand, in adult patients when the probability of group A streptococcal infection is low, the risks of antibiotic therapy (drug reaction and fatal anaphylaxis) approximate the risks of streptococcal pharyngitis and its complications. In this situation it is appropriate to withhold antibiotics and obtain a throat culture or rapid diagnostic test. When the probability of group A streptococcal infection is very low (<3%), a rapid test or throat culture is not required unless the patient has special risk factors.

In children the presence or absence of the organism must be documented. Early treatment with antibiotics can prevent acute rheumatic fever (ARF) and may shorten the course of the illness, reducing fever and local and systemic symptoms.

Although rapid diagnostic tests can assist in the initial decision to treat or observe, they are not as sensitive as a culture, and negative rapid diagnostic tests should be followed with a throat culture. Rapid diagnostic tests are not essential for the proper management of acute pharyngitis. If they are used, their sensitivity should be greater than 80%.

Consider the possibilities of mycoplasmal, gonococcal, or *Chlamydia trachomatis* pharyngitis in patients with persistent pharyngitis and a negative culture for group A streptococci or in patients with a positive culture who are not responding to penicillin. Consider infectious mononucleosis in patients with persistent systemic illness, lymphadenopathy, and splenomegaly. Consider diphtheria in unvaccinated populations, and look for a gray membrane that is firmly adherent to the tonsillar of pharyngeal mucosa. Specimens from both throat and nasopharynx should be submitted for culture confirmation of diphtheria. The most common and important respiratory viruses that can produce pharyngitis are rhinovirus, influenza virus, parainfluenza virus, adenovirus, the enteroviruses, cytomegalovirus, Epstein-Barr virus, and herpes simplex virus. Antibiotic therapy in patients with nonstreptococcal pharyngitis is often inappropriate.

2. Use good technique when obtaining a throat culture and performing laboratory tests.

When obtaining a throat culture, use a Dacron swab (cotton fibers may inhibit *Neisseria*) and vigorously rub the posterior pharynx, the tonsils or tonsillar pillars, and areas of purulence, exudation, or ulceration. Using a tongue blade will help prevent contamination with buccal organisms. Use of a self-contained collection or transport system such as the Culturette® (Marion Scientific, Kansas City) makes collection and transport of throat cultures relatively simple and convenient. With good specimens and high-quality laboratory tests, the sensitivity for group A streptococci nears 90%. With poor specimens and poor quality tests, the sensitivity may be as low as 30%. If you suspect gonococcal pharyngitis or the meningococcal carrier state, the swab is best inoculated onto a previously warmed JEMBEC plate (or other suitable medium) as soon as the culture is obtained. Inoculated plates should be incubated overnight at 95° F (35° C) in an atmosphere of 5% to 10% carbon dioxide before shipment to a laboratory. Immediate shipment will kill *Neisseria* if present. Another option when *Neisseria* is suspected is to place the swab in a transport medium before sending it to the laboratory. Perform a test for heterophil antibody (Monospot test) if you suspect infectious mononucleosis.

A positive rapid diagnostic test or throat culture for group A streptococci may reflect infection or an asymptomatic carrier state (false positive). In children the carrier rate can be up to 15%. At present there is no accurate way to distinguish between true streptococcal infection and the carrier state at the time of initial presentation. In infected patients the false-negative rate of a well-performed single throat culture is approximately 10%. A Gram stain of exudative material that shows gram-positive cocci in chains strongly suggests streptococcal infection.

3. Perform follow-up cultures in patients with persistent clinical findings or with unusually high risk of acute rheumatic fever.

Routine follow-up cultures are not required.

BIBLIOGRAPHY

Barnes HV: Streptococcal infections. In Spivak JL, Barnes HV (eds): Manual of Clinical Problems in Internal Medicine, 4th ed. Boston, Little, Brown & Co, 1990, p 460.
Good discussion of diagnosis and management with annotated key references.
Bisno AL: Group A streptococcal infections and acute rheumatic fever. N Engl J Med 325:783, 1991.
Even today, physicians should be alert to the possibility of acute rheumatic fever.
Centor RM, Meier FA, Dalton HP: Throat cultures and rapid tests for diagnosis of group A streptococcal pharyngitis in adults. In Sox HC Jr (ed): Common Diagnostic Tests: Use and Interpretation, 2nd ed. Philadelphia, American College of Physicians, 1990, p 245.
Good review of group A streptococcal pharyngitis with recommendations for management.
Dippel DWJ, Touw-Otten F, Habbema JDF: Management of children with acute pharyngitis: A decision analysis. J Fam Pract 34:149, 1992.
Suggests using a rapid antigen test and prompt penicillin therapy in children with a high probability of streptococcal pharyngitis.
Hedges JR, Singal BM, Estep JL: The impact of a rapid screen for streptococcal pharyngitis on clinical decision making in the emergency department. Med Decis Making 11:119, 1991.
Rapid diagnostic tests have done little to improve the overall quality of care.
Komaroff AL: Sore throat in adult patients. In Panzer RJ, Black ER, Griner PF (eds): Diagnostic Strategies for Common Medical Problems. Philadelphia, American College of Physicians, 1991, p 186.
When key clinical findings are absent, the probability of streptococcal pharyngitis is very low (<3%), and a throat culture is unnecessary unless the patient has special risk factors.
Ohio State Faculty: Acute pharyngitis. Columbus, Ohio, The Ohio State University Health Plan Clinical Notes, vol 1, no 2, Spring 1991.
Medical practice guidelines for acute pharyngitis.
Rapid diagnostic tests for group A streptococcal pharyngitis. Med Lett Drugs Ther 33:40, 1991.
Summarizes available rapid diagnostic test kits and compares their costs.
Slawson DC, Baer LJ, Richardson MD: Antibiotic use in the treatment of non-streptococcal pharyngitis. Fam Med 23:198, 1991.
Suggests that antibiotic therapy in patients with nonstreptococcal pharyngitis is often inappropriate.
Tenjarla G, Kumar A, Dyke JW: TestPack Strep A kit for the rapid detection of group A streptococci on 11,088 throat swabs in a clinical pathology laboratory. Am J Clin Pathol 96:759, 1991.
Patients with negative rapid antigen tests should be cultured.

Wegner DL, Witte DL, Schrantz RD: Insensitivity of rapid antigen detection methods and single blood agar plate culture for diagnosing streptococcal pharyngitis. JAMA 267:695, 1992.
Commercial antigen tests are less sensitive than cultures.

Allergic Rhinitis

1.   If the diagnosis of allergic rhinitis cannot be made from clinical findings, consider examining a nasal smear for eosinophils, measuring the total serum IgE level, skin testing, and performing radioallergosorbent tests (RASTs). The blood eosinophil count is not helpful.

Allergic rhinitis affects 15% to 20% of the population and accounts for 9% of outpatient visits for The Ohio State University Health Plan.

The differential diagnosis of seasonal allergic rhinitis includes viral infection; abuse of nose drops and sprays; drugs such as ovarian hormones, reserpine, hydralazine, and aspirin and other nonsteroidal anti-inflammatory agents; and premenstrual or pregnancy-related hormonal rhinitis.

The differential diagnosis of perennial allergic rhinitis includes nasal abnormalities such as deviated septum, endocrine abnormalities such as hypothyroidism, nasal mastocytosis, and idiopathic perennial nonallergic rhinitis (vasomotor rhinitis). Symptoms from nasopharyngeal masses can mimic those of allergies.

Nasal secretions should be examined for eosinophilia, even if the blood eosinophil count is normal. The specimen may be collected as follows: having the patient blow the nose onto waxed paper or cellophane, placing a swab in the nose for 2 or 3 minutes, or aspirating the specimen with a small rubber bulb syringe. The specimen is transferred to a slide, dried, and stained with Wright's stain. The blood eosinophil count is not useful since it may be normal or increased in either allergic or nonallergic rhinitis. A positive test for nasal eosinophilia provides the same support for a diagnosis of allergic rhinitis as does an increased total serum IgE level.

Skin tests are of value only in patients with clinical findings and should not be used for screening asymptomatic patients since positive reactions will occur in many individuals who have no symptoms. In practice, skin tests are used either to advise patients about avoidance therapy or to help select antigens for use in therapy. Skin tests are the quickest and least expensive way to identify specific allergens.

RAST measures allergen-specific serum IgE antibody titers, and the results correlate well with skin testing. RAST is useful in patients in whom skin testing is inappropriate because of extensive eczema, marked dermatographism, or interfering medications.

2.   Evaluate the tests.

A positive nasal smear in a patient with allergic rhinitis shows large numbers of eosinophils (usually more than 25% of all cells present).

A serum total IgE level that is normal practically rules out atopy, whereas one that is high markedly increases the likelihood of this diagnosis.

RAST is usually considered safer, more expensive, less sensitive, but perhaps more specific than skin testing; however, a recent study found the sensitivity and specificity of RAST and skin tests are almost identical. Although RAST may give false-negative results, it rarely gives false-positive results. Unlike skin tests, it is not affected when the patient is taking antihistamine or sympathomimetic drugs.

3.   If the test results are positive, they support the diagnosis, but the diagnosis must be made by considering the test results together with the clinical features.

A positive nasal smear for eosinophilia and increased serum total IgE support the diagnosis of allergic rhinitis, but they are not diagnostic. Eosinophils can also be found in the syndrome of nonallergic rhinitis with eosinophilia (NARES). Large numbers of neutrophils in the nasal smear suggest infection rather than allergic rhinitis. The manifestations of upper respiratory tract infection usually last no longer than a week and include fever, pain, and the presence of neutrophils in secretions.

4.   If the test results are negative, do not necessarily conclude that the patient does not have allergic rhinitis or that the allergen tested is not responsible.

The tests for allergic rhinitis are not 100% sensitive. For example, positive nasal smears for eosinophilia are not found in every patient with proved allergic rhinitis, and the serum total IgE level is not always increased in patients with allergic rhinitis. Achieving relief of symptoms by avoiding the suspected allergen is the best method of diagnosis.

BIBLIOGRAPHY

Kaliner M, Lemanske R: Rhinitis and asthma. JAMA 268:2807, 1992.
    Discusses the diagnosis and management of allergic rhinitis.
McGeady SJ, Mansmann HC: Rhinitis. In Conn RB (ed): Current Diagnosis, 8th ed. Philadelphia, WB Saunders Co, 1991, p 1240.
    Discusses the differential diagnosis of rhinitis.
Ohio State Faculty: Allergic rhinitis. Columbus, Ohio, The Ohio State University Health Plan Clinical Notes, vol 1, no 4, Spring 1991.
    Medical practice guidelines for allergic rhinitis.
VanArsdel PP Jr, Larson EB: Diagnostic tests for patients with suspected allergic disease: Utility and limitations. Ann Intern Med 110:304, 1989.
    Discusses strategies for the diagnosis of allergic rhinitis.

Community-Acquired Pneumonia

1.   For patients with clinical findings of pneumonia request a chest radiograph, complete blood count (CBC), and leukocyte differential count.

If sputum is available, consider obtaining a Gram stain and culture. If the clinical findings are severe enough to require hospitalization, consider obtaining two blood cultures, serology, and arterial blood gas analysis.

Some authorities recommend that for community-acquired pneumonia only severely ill patients should have routine studies (blood culture, sputum examination, acute phase serology) and one should not wait for the results before starting antibiotic treatment. For the mildly ill patient only blood cultures are recommended, with possible storage of a frozen acute serum specimen for comparison to convalescent serum in the absence of clinical improvement. In these cases posttreatment sputum cultures may also be helpful.

Findings that favor hospitalization include serious comorbid illness, preexisting lung disease, multilobar lung involvement revealed by x-ray examination, observed or likely aspiration, and symptom duration of less than 7 or more than 28 days.

Although a Gram stain and a culture of sputum are often useful, a Gram stain and a culture of saliva are always useless. The patient should thoroughly rinse his or her mouth with water several times, take some deep breaths and hold them several times, and then attempt to bring up sputum from deep in the bronchial tree. Inhalation of a warmed 3% to 10% saline solution aerosol may be helpful. Sputum can be distinguished from saliva by microscopically evaluating the specimen under low power. More than 25 neutrophils and less than 10 squamous epithelial cells per low-power field indicate an adequate sputum sample. No specimen containing more than 25 squamous epithelial cells per low-power field should be cultured because it is heavily contaminated by oropharyngeal secretions. The Gram stain can be helpful in choosing a good specimen for a culture and selecting antibiotics.

Other techniques are available to examine sputum: digestion with 10% potassium hydroxide to identify fungi; immunological techniques for respiratory syncytial virus and for *Streptococcus pneumoniae;* and direct fluorescent antibody studies to diagnose *Legionella* species, viruses, and *Pneumocystis carinii.*

Traditionally physicians have drawn simultaneous blood cultures from two different sites. Since the increased sensitivity from drawing two blood cultures appears related to the increased volume of blood rather than the two different sites, it does not matter whether the two blood cultures are drawn from the same site or different sites. Blood cultures should be inoculated with the same needle that is used for the venipuncture. An advantage of using two different sites is that chance contamination with skin flora is less likely to occur in two different sites. If a single site is contaminated, all cultures will be contaminated from that site.

2. Consider mycoplasmal pneumonia, Legionnaires' disease, influenza, primary tuberculosis, *Chlamydia pneumoniae* (strain TWAR), and other causes of atypical pneumonias in patients with the following clinical findings:

1. Occurrence in young adults
2. Onset over several days

3. Mild fever; patient not apparently severely ill
4. No or small amounts of mucopurulent sputum
5. Minimal pleurisy; small or no effusion
6. Normal to slightly increased white blood cell count
7. Patchy "pneumonitis" or nonhomogeneous segmental infiltrate on radiograph

3. Consider pneumococcal pneumonia, *Haemophilus influenzae*, staphylococcal pneumonia, gram-negative bacillary pneumonia, and suppurative pulmonary disease in patients with the following clinical findings:

1. Patient more often elderly or chronically ill
2. Abrupt onset
3. High fevers; chills; patient possibly weak, cyanotic, or confused
4. Purulent sputum
5. Pleurisy and pleural effusion common
6. Leukocytosis
7. Lobar or segmental consolidation on radiograph

4. In debilitated elderly persons and patients with predisposing conditions probable causative bacteria are as follows:

1. Chronic obstructive pulmonary disease (COPD): *S. pneumoniae* and *H. influenzae*.
2. Chronic alcoholism: *S. pneumoniae*, anaerobic bacteria (aspiration pneumonia), *H. influenzae*, *Klebsiella pneumoniae*, *Staphylococcus aureus*, and *Mycobacterium tuberculosis*.
3. Postinfluenza bacterial pneumonia: *S. pneumoniae*, *S. aureus*, and *H. influenzae*.
4. Elderly nursing home patients: *S. pneumoniae*, *S. aureus*, *K. pneumoniae*, and *H. influenzae*.
5. Patients with mental obtundation, swallowing problems, esophageal disorders, seizure disorders, and poor dental hygiene: usually mixed aerobic and anaerobic bacteria (aspiration pneumonia).
6. Cystic fibrosis: *Pseudomonas aeruginosa* and *S. aureus*.
7. Immunocompromised hosts: multiple causes, including gram-negative bacilli (e.g., *Escherichia coli*, *K. pneumoniae*, *P. aeruginosa*), *S. aureus*, and other bacteria, and viral (e.g., cytomegalovirus), fungal (e.g., *Aspergillus*), and protozoal pathogens. The likely spectrum of causative organisms will vary, depending on the cause of the immunodeficiency (e.g., *S. aureus*, aerobic gram-negative bacilli, and *Aspergillus* are likely pathogens in neutropenic patients). Mycobacterial infection is a growing problem, especially in HIV-infected patients. Although any single test must be interpreted with caution, increasing serum lactate dehydrogenase (LD) activity, particularly more than 450 U/L, is suspicious for *P. carinii* in HIV-infected patients with pulmonary disease. Also, the LD activity and Apache II severity-of-illness score are highly predictive of response to therapy and mortality.

5.   In patients with mycoplasmal pneumonia, Legionnaires' disease, influenza, primary tuberculosis, and other causes of atypical pneumonias, laboratory test results are as follows.

MYCOPLASMAL PNEUMONIA

Hemolytic anemia caused by cold agglutinins may occur with mycoplasmal pneumonia, but clinically significant hemolysis is rare. A positive direct Coombs' test result occurs in up to 83% of patients. The leukocyte count may be normal to slightly increased, with a minimal left shift and possible mild lymphopenia. The erythrocyte sedimentation rate (ESR) increases to more than 40 mm/hour in at least two thirds of cases. In the sputum mononuclear cells predominate over neutrophils in a ratio of approximately 60:40 (occasionally neutrophils predominate), and a Gram stain shows no bacteria—there may be some erythrocytes. The organism can be cultured from the sputum or posterior pharynx but takes 2 to 3 weeks to grow. A nucleic acid probe for *Mycoplasma pneumoniae* is available but is not always positive in a patient with disease. An enzyme-linked immunosorbent assay (ELISA) test for *M. pneumoniae* antibody is also available, but acute and convalescent sera are required. A diagnosis can be made by demonstrating a specific IgM titer of 1:4 or greater or by a single complement-fixing antibody titer of 1:256 or greater. Approximately 50% to 60% of patients show a fourfold or greater rise in the cold agglutinin titer for human type O erythrocytes or a single titer of 1:128 or greater. In more critically ill patients cold agglutinins are more likely. Titers of 1:32 or lower can occur in patients with infectious mononucleosis and pneumonia caused by adenovirus or influenza.

LEGIONNAIRES' DISEASE

The leukocyte count is normal to moderately increased with a left shift in patients with Legionnaires' disease. There is moderate neutrophilia in the sputum, and a Gram stain shows weakly staining gram-negative bacteria. The organism can be cultured from sputum, lung tissue, or pleural fluid and can be directly identified in secretions and tissues using an immunofluorescent technique (for sputum the sensitivity of the immunofluorescent technique varies from 30% to 70%). A nucleic acid probe detects 50% of infections. Using acute and convalescent sera, 80% of patients have a fourfold rise in titer to 1:128 in 2 to 6 weeks. A single titer of 1:256 or more is also significant. In patients with Legionnaires' disease an increased aspartate aminotransferase (AST; SGOT) level occurs in 90% of patients.

INFLUENZA

The diagnosis of influenza depends on the clinical findings. Viral culture requires 7 to 10 days. Secondary bacterial pneumonias can be caused by pneumococci, staphylococci, *H. influenzae*, and gram-negative bacteria, especially *P. aeruginosa*.

PRIMARY TUBERCULOSIS

In 1990 new cases of tuberculosis rose to 26,000 nationwide, and new strains of tuberculosis resistant to multiple drugs have emerged in at least 17 states. The diagnosis of primary tuberculosis depends on clinical findings, radiographs, and results of the tuberculin skin test. Sputum cultures fail to confirm the diagnosis in many adults with mild primary tuberculosis. The diagnosis of tuberculosis in HIV-infected patients is problematic because of undependable skin reactions and nondiagnostic chest radiographs. Watch for the availability of new diagnostic techniques such as (1) specific antigen detection by ELISA or antibody-sensitized latex particles; (2) detection of DNA sequences by probes and polymerase chain reaction; and (3) demonstration of tuberculostearic acid by chromatography and mass spectrometry.

OTHER ATYPICAL PNEUMONIAS

Many viral agents, particularly adenoviruses, can mimic mycoplasmal pneumonia. Rare causes include Q fever, psittacosis, tularemia, plague, primary histoplasmosis, and primary coccidioidomycosis. *C. pneumoniae* is a relatively common cause of atypical pneumonia. Cultures and serological tests for that organism are available only in regional laboratories at the present time.

6.   In patients with pneumococcal pneumonia, staphylococcal pneumonia, meningococcal pneumonia, pneumonia caused by *H. influenzae*, *Branhamella catarrhalis*, and gram-negative bacilli, laboratory test results are as follows.

PNEUMOCOCCAL PNEUMONIA

Pneumococcal pneumonia accounts for approximately two thirds of the cases of bacterial pneumonia. In patients with pneumococcal pneumonia the leukocyte count is usually increased to 15 to 30 × 10^3 cells/μL (15 to 30 × 10^9 cells/L), with a left shift and often toxic granulation. The white blood cell (WBC) count may also be normal or low. In the sputum neutrophils are numerous, and the predominant organisms are gram-positive, lancet-shaped diplococci, which can be cultured. The blood culture is positive in 20% to 30% of patients. If anemia is present, it probably represents a preexisting condition. Hypernatremia may occur, caused by loss of free water secondary to fever and sweating.

STAPHYLOCOCCAL PNEUMONIA

In patients with staphylococcal pneumonia the leukocyte count is increased, with a left shift, and the sputum smear shows numerous neutrophils and gram-positive cocci in clumps, which may be cultured. Blood cultures may be positive.

MENINGOCOCCAL PNEUMONIA

In patients with meningococcal pneumonia neutrophilic leukocytosis is usual. The sputum smear shows gram-negative diplococci that are often present in the cytoplasm of neutrophils. Blood cultures may be positive.

PNEUMONIA CAUSED BY *HAEMOPHILUS INFLUENZAE*

In pneumonia caused by *H. influenzae* there is a neutrophilic leukocytosis, and the sputum smear shows abundant pleomorphic gram-negative organisms, often in neutrophils. Approximately 20% of patients have positive blood cultures.

BRANHAMELLA (NEISSERIA) CATARRHALIS

Formerly regarded as a contaminant, *B. catarrhalis* has emerged as a true pathogen. Patients with COPD are susceptible. The organism can be recovered from respiratory secretions either in pure culture or occasionally in association with other potential pathogens such as *S. pneumoniae*. Many strains of *B. catarrhalis* are β-lactamase positive.

GRAM-NEGATIVE BACILLARY PNEUMONIAS

In patients with gram-negative bacillary pneumonias, neutrophilic leukocytosis is typical, but there may be neutropenia. Numerous gram-negative bacilli are present in the sputum, and they can be cultured. Approximately 20% to 30% of patients have positive blood cultures.

7.   In monitoring patients hospitalized for community-acquired pneumonia, follow the respiratory rate, diastolic blood pressure, and serum urea nitrogen level to evaluate prognosis.

A rate of 30 respirations per minute or more, a diastolic blood pressure of 60 mmHg or less, and a serum urea nitrogen level of more than 42 mg/dL (7 mmol/L) are predictive of mortality. In one study the presence of any two of these three criteria predicted death with 88% sensitivity and 79% specificity.

8.   In patients with viral, mycoplasmal, or other miscellaneous types of pneumonia, the following additional abnormal blood test results may occur:

↓ **Hemoglobin and hematocrit.**
↑ **Leukocytes.**
Although an **increased ESR** occurs in patients with mycoplasmal pneumonia, increased acute-phase reactants are more characteristic of bacterial pneumonia than viral pneumonia (e.g., an **increased C-reactive protein** level is useful to distinguish bacterial from viral pneumonia).

↓ **Partial pressure of oxygen (Po$_2$)** caused by pneumonia.
Abnormal total carbon dioxide caused by change in bicarbonate in compensation for abnormal partial pressure of carbon dioxide (Pco$_2$).
↑ **Aspartate aminotransferase (SGOT), lactate dehydrogenase,** and **alkaline phosphate.**

9.   In patients with bacterial pneumonia the following additional abnormal blood test results may occur:

↓ **Hemoglobin and hematocrit.**

↑ **Leukocytes,** characteristically neutrophilic.

↓ **Leukocytes** (e.g., in fulminating pneumococcal pneumonia in alcoholics).

↑ **ESR and C-reactive protein.**

Abnormal total carbon dioxide caused by change in bicarbonate in compensation for abnormal P_{CO_2}.

↑ **Aspartate aminotransferase** and **lactate dehydrogenase.**

↓ **Albumin.**

↑ **Bilirubin.**

BIBLIOGRAPHY

American Medical Association Department of Drugs, Division of Drugs and Technology: Drug Evaluations, 6th ed. Chicago, American Medical Association, 1986, p 1238.
Concise approach to the diagnosis of community-acquired pneumonia.

Benson CA, Spear J, Hines D, et al: Combined APACHE II score and serum lactate dehydrogenase as predictors of in-hospital mortality caused by first episode *Pneumocystis carinii* pneumonia in patients with acquired immunodeficiency syndrome. Am Rev Respir Dis 144:319, 1991.
Describes an effective way to predict response to therapy and mortality.

Black ER, Mushlin AI, Griner PF, et al: Predicting the need for hospitalization of ambulatory patients with pneumonia. J Gen Intern Med 6:394, 1991.
Identifies factors that predict the need for hospitalization.

Farr BM, Sloman AJ, Fisch MJ: Predicting death in patients hospitalized for community acquired pneumonia. Ann Intern Med 115:428, 1991.
Tachypnea, diastolic hypotension, and an increased serum urea nitrogen level were independently associated with death.

Leisure MK, Moore DM, Schwartzman JD, et al: Changing the needle when inoculating blood cultures: A no-benefit and high-risk procedure. JAMA 264:2111, 1990.
There is not much benefit and a lot of risk in changing needles before inoculating blood cultures.

National action plan to combat multidrug-resistant tuberculosis. MMWR 41:3, 1992.
Highlights the surge in new cases of tuberculosis, of which many have drug-resistant strains.

Woodhead MA, Arrowsmith J, Chamberlain-Webber R, et al: The value of routine microbial investigation in community-acquired pneumonia. Respir Med 85:313, 1991.
Mildly ill patients need only an initial blood culture.

Pulmonary Embolism

1.   In patients with clinical findings of or predisposing factors for pulmonary embolism, request a CBC, arterial blood gas analysis, an electrocardiogram (ECG), and a chest radiograph. Consider obtaining a lung scan and pulmonary angiography. Other laboratory studies such as enzymes or fibrin degradation products are not useful.

The most sensitive clinical findings are chest pain, dyspnea, and tachypnea, and the most sensitive laboratory test is the arterial P_{O_2}. In the past the triad of high serum bilirubin, high lactate dehydrogenase, and normal transaminase levels has been used, but this triad is only approximately 15% sensitive and therefore not useful. A chest radiograph and an ECG may be helpful, but a lung scan and pulmonary angiography are the definitive studies.

2.   Evaluate the tests.

A lung scan can be either a perfusion lung scan (Q lung scan) alone or a combined ventilation-perfusion lung scan (V/Q lung scan). In the Q lung scan pulmonary blood flow is assessed, using intravenous technetium-99m–labeled macroaggregated albumin. In the combined V/Q lung scan the Q lung scan is coupled with a V lung scan, using xenon 133. Although the Q lung scan alone is sensitive for pulmonary embolism, it lacks specificity. The V lung scan increases the specificity of the Q lung scan.

3.   If the results of a V/Q lung scan and/or pulmonary angiography are consistent, the diagnosis of pulmonary embolism is confirmed. Decreased arterial PO_2 and compatible Q lung scan are sensitive but not specific for pulmonary embolism.

Pulmonary angiography is the definitive test for the diagnosis of pulmonary embolism, and with some patterns of V/Q lung scans (high-probability lung scans), the diagnosis can be made with virtual certainty. Only rare patients with normal V/Q lung scans have pulmonary embolic disease. A Q lung scan is sensitive for pulmonary embolism (i.e., rarely gives false-negative results) but is not specific (i.e., false-positive results in patients with COPD, asthma, pneumonia, lung cysts, bronchiectasis, and atelectasis).

Decreased arterial PO_2 is 87% sensitive for pulmonary embolism but is not specific. The main purpose of the ECG is to exclude acute myocardial infarction. The most common finding in patients with pulmonary embolism is sinus tachycardia. A normal chest radiograph is uncommon in pulmonary embolism patients, but the changes are nonspecific. Neutral fat droplets in bronchoalveolar lavage fluid are useful for the diagnosis of fat embolism.

4.   A normal lung scan excludes pulmonary embolism, but normal arterial PO_2 does not.

Although an unequivocally normal lung scan effectively excludes pulmonary embolism, 13% of patients with proven pulmonary embolism have PO_2 >80 mmHg.

5.   In patients with pulmonary embolism the following additional abnormal blood test results may occur:

↑ **Leukocytes** with pulmonary infarction.

↓ **Platelets.**

↑ **ESR.**

↓ PCO_2, less than 35 mmHg (4.66 kPa) or decreasing PCO_2 in patients with known carbon dioxide retention.

↑ **Bilirubin.**

↑ **Lactate dehydrogenase.**

BIBLIOGRAPHY

Barnes HV: Pulmonary embolism. In Spivak JL, Barnes HV (eds): Manual of Clinical Problems in Internal Medicine, 4th ed. Boston, Little, Brown & Co, 1990, p 16.
Good discussion of diagnosis and management with annotated key references.

Bone RC, Leibovitch E: Pulmonary embolism: An algorithm for diagnosis. Modern Medicine 59:40, 1991.
Discusses the diagnosis of pulmonary embolism and points out that measurements of enzymes and fibrin degradation products are of no value.

Bounameaux H, Cirafici P, DeMoerloose P, et al: Measurement of D-dimer in plasma as diagnostic aid in suspected pulmonary embolism. Lancet 337:196, 1991.
Plasma D-dimer is suggested as a new screening test for pulmonary embolism.

Carson JL, Kelley MA, Duff A, et al: The clinical course of pulmonary embolism. N Engl J Med 326:1240, 1992.
When properly diagnosed and treated, clinically apparent pulmonary embolism was an uncommon cause of death.

Chastre J, Fagon J-Y, Soler P, et al: Bronchoalveolar lavage for rapid diagnosis of the fat embolism syndrome in trauma patients. Ann Intern Med 113:583, 1990.
Increased numbers of cells with neutral fat droplets in bronchoalveolar lavage fluid is a rapid specific test for fat embolism.

Coffman JD: Venous thrombosis and the diagnosis of pulmonary emboli. Hosp Pract 27:99, 1992.
Discusses diagnostic strategy using a case report.

Kassirer JP, Kopelman RI: Case 43—Treat: Or keep testing? In Learning Clinical Reasoning. Baltimore, Williams & Wilkins, 1991, p 217.
Discusses the clinical reasoning in a patient with pulmonary embolism.

Kerr CP, Yan L: Pulmonary embolism: Clinical decision making to increase diagnostic accuracy. Postgrad Med 91:73, 1992.
Criteria for diagnosing and treating pulmonary embolism.

Mayewski RJ: Pulmonary embolism. In Panzer RJ, Black ER, Griner PF (eds): Diagnostic Strategies for Common Medical Problems. Phildelphia, American College of Physicians, 1991, p 260.
Recommends strategies for the diagnosis of pulmonary embolism.

Monreal M, Lafoz E, Casals A, et al: Platelet count and venous thromboembolism: A useful test for suspected pulmonary embolism. Chest 100:1493, 1991.
Decreased platelet count can be a clue to pulmonary embolism.

Sherman S: Pulmonary embolism update: Lessons for the '90s. Postgrad Med 89:195, 1991.
Newer concepts in diagnosis, management, and prevention of pulmonary embolism.

Stein PD, Athanasoulis C, Alavi A, et al: Complications and validity of pulmonary angiography in acute pulmonary embolism. Circulation 85:462, 1992.
Confirms the low risk and high accuracy of angiography in most patients.

Stein PD, Gottschalk A, Saltzman HA, et al: Diagnosis of acute pulmonary embolism in the elderly. J Am Coll Cardiol 18:1452, 1991.
Clinical features of acute pulmonary embolism do not differ with age.

Chronic Obstructive Pulmonary Disease

1.   In patients with clinical findings of COPD, perform pulmonary function tests and request a chest radiograph, an ECG, and a CBC. Consider α_1-antitrypsin deficiency.

Pulmonary function tests are not recommended for the asymptomatic, cigarette-smoking patient. However, the presence of clinical findings (e.g., productive cough in a cigarette smoker, occurring at least 3 months per year for 2 consecutive years) is suggestive of COPD, and pulmonary function tests are appropriate. In individuals with a family history of COPD test for α_1-antitrypsin deficiency.

Patients with COPD are most commonly seen initially between 55 and 65 years of age. The disease is much more common in males than females (ratio, 9:1), but this may reflect only differences in smoking habits. Approximately 75,000 persons per year die of COPD in the United States, approximately one half the number of individuals dying annually of lung cancer. Young patients in their twenties and thirties rarely have accumulated enough years of smoking exposure to have COPD. If these young patients have presenting symptoms of severe dyspnea, other diagnoses such as bronchiectasis, asthma, α_1-antitrypsin deficiency, and cystic fibrosis should be considered.

In the average patient with chronic obstructive bronchitis, there is a loss of forced expiratory volume in 1 second (FEV_1), in the range of 50 to 75 mL per year, two to three times the average rate of decline for nonsmokers. Continued smoking accelerates the deterioration. The best guide to prognosis is the amount of predicted FEV_1 obtained after administration of a bronchodilator.

2.   Evaluate the tests.

The FEV_1, forced vital capacity (FVC), $FEV_1:FVC$ ratio, and midmaximal expiratory flow rate (MMEFR) are useful spirometric tests of pulmonary function.

Tests for α_1-antitrypsin deficiency include serum protein electrophoresis, α_1-antitrypsin quantitation by rate nephelometry, and isoelectric focusing for phenotyping.

3.   Interpret test results in the context of clinical findings.

In young, minimally symptomatic smokers the FEV_1, $FEV_1:FVC$ ratio, and MMEFR are not very sensitive for COPD (FEV_1, approximately 10%; MMEFR, approximately 20%); however, in older, more symptomatic patients the sensitivity increases to 30% to 40%. In both young and old groups the specificity is much higher (80% to 95%).

The chest radiograph is not very useful for diagnosing COPD. Its main value is to exclude other conditions such as infection, malignancy, or bullous disease that can mimic the findings of COPD.

Early in the disease the ECG usually is normal. Later there may be changes consistent with pulmonary artery hypertension and cor pulmonale.

The CBC is usually normal except for an increased hemoglobin and hematocrit values in some COPD patients with hypoxemia. When eosinophilia is present, consider an asthmatic-bronchitic component that may be reversible.

Laboratory confirmation of homozygous α_1-antitrypsin deficiency includes almost complete absence of α_1-globulin by serum protein electrophoresis, specifically by a pure Z phenotype. Two M genes (Pi MM phenotype) are present in normal individuals. Individuals homozygous for the disorder (approximately 1 in 4000 persons) have the Pi ZZ phenotype and severely reduced concentrations of α_1-antitrypsin (<50 mg/dL [<0.50 g/L]). Heterozygous individuals (3% to 5% of the population) have reduced antiproteolytic activity but are not at risk for COPD.

4. In patients with COPD the following additional abnormal blood test results may occur:

↓ **Hemoglobin and hematocrit** related to high incidence of bleeding peptic ulcer.

↑ **Leukocytes** due to pulmonary inflammation or infection.

↓ **pH** with respiratory acidosis.

↓ **Po₂** with pulmonary insufficiency.

↑ **Pco₂** with respiratory acidosis.

↑ **Potassium** with acidosis.

↓ **Chloride** with chronic respiratory acidosis.

↑ **Bicarbonate** with chronic respiratory acidosis.

↓ **Phosphate,** particularly those patients receiving mechanical ventilation.

5. In patients with α_1-antitrypsin deficiency the following additional abnormal blood test results may occur:

↓ **Hemoglobin and hematocrit** with hypersplenism.

↓ **Leukocytes** with hypersplenism.

↓ **Platelets** with hypersplenism.

Abnormal liver function tests.

BIBLIOGRAPHY

Mayewski RJ: Chronic obstructive lung disease. In Panzer RJ, Black ER, Griner PF (eds): Diagnostic Strategies for Common Medical Problems. Philadelphia, American College of Physicians, 1991, p 301.
Suggests strategies for the diagnosis of COPD.

Smith JG, George RB: Chronic obstructive pulmonary disease. In Conn RB (ed): Current Diagnosis, 8th ed. Philadelphia, WB Saunders Co, 1991, p 343.
Discusses the differential diagnosis of COPD.

Zaloga GP: Hypophosphatemia in COPD: How serious—And what to do? J Crit Illness 7:364, 1992.
Patients with COPD—particularly those receiving mechanical ventilation—are vulnerable to hypophosphatemia.

Pleural Fluid Analysis

1. In patients with a pleural effusion, to diagnose the cause of the effusion, perform thoracentesis and request pleural fluid total protein and lactate dehydrogenase (LD) determinations, together with serum total protein and LD determinations.

The appearance of the pleural fluid may be a clue to its cause. For example, transudates are usually clear and straw colored, whereas exudates can be turbid, purulent, or bloody. It takes approximately 10,000 red blood cells/μL to impart a pink color to the fluid. A milky appearance suggests a chylous effusion. Protein and LD measurements are useful to distinguish pleural fluid exudates from transudates.

Collect pleural fluid and venous blood as follows: (1) pleural fluid for chemistry tests—10 mL, heparinized (glucose concentration may decrease if the fluid is not frozen or preserved with fluoride); (2) venous blood for chemistry tests—one clot tube; (3) pleural fluid for cytology—25 to 50 mL, heparinized; (4) pleural fluid for bacterial cultures—10 mL, heparinized; (5) pleural fluid for acid-fast and fungal cultures—10 mL, heparinized (a larger quantity, [i.e., 50 mL] increases the sensitivity for culturing acid-fast bacilli); (6) pleural fluid for hematology tests—one ethylenediaminetetra-acetic acid (EDTA) tube; (7) pleural fluid for pH—several milliliters collected anaerobically in a syringe, iced, and quickly sent to the laboratory; and (8) pleural fluid for miscellaneous tests—10 mL, heparinized. These samples should be delivered to the laboratory immediately.

2.   Evaluate the tests.

SENSITIVITY AND SPECIFICITY OF TESTS USED FOR CLASSIFICATION OF PLEURAL EFFUSION

TEST	EXUDATE	SENSITIVITY (%)	SPECIFICITY (%)
1. Specific gravity	>1.016	78	89
2. Pleural fluid protein	>3 g/dL (30g/L)	93	85
3. Pleural fluid/serum protein	>0.5	92	93
4. Pleural fluid/LD*	>200 U/L	72	100
5. Pleural fluid/serum LD	>0.6	88	96
Test 3 or 5 positive	—	99	89
Tests 3 and 5 positive	—	81	100

Source: Skendzel LP: A practical approach to the chemical and microscopic study of pleural and peritoneal fluids. Lab Medica V (1):16, 1988.
*LD method with a reference range >300 U/L. Current LD methods may not be comparable.

Other studies have been used to distinguish transudates from exudates. The leukocyte count is usually less than 1000/μL (1000 $\times$ 10^6/L) in transudates. More than 80% of transudates but less than 20% of exudates have leukocyte counts below 1000. A pleural fluid cholesterol level >55 mg/dL (1.45 mmol/L) and a pleural fluid cholesterol:serum cholesterol ratio >0.3 correctly identifies pleural exudates. A gradient between serum albumin and pleural fluid albumin $\leq$1.2 g/dL (12 g/L) indicates an exudate. A pleural fluid to serum bilirubin ratio >0.6 indicates an exudate.

3.   If the pleural fluid:serum protein and pleural fluid:serum LD ratios indicate that the fluid is a transudate, no further testing usually is necessary.

A recent study of 533 pleural fluid specimens from 340 patients showed that an average of eight to nine tests were performed on each fluid, including WBC, WBC differential, and other specific studies. Although these tests may prove useful when the fluid is an exudate, they are of little use when the fluid is a transudate, and further testing is not required.

4.   If the pleural fluid:serum protein and/or pleural fluid:serum LD ratios indicate that the fluid is an exudate, perform cytologic studies and cultures. The following additional tests may prove useful.

USEFUL TESTS IN PLEURAL FLUID EXUDATES

TEST	DISEASES
Red blood cell count >100,000/µL (>0.1/L)	Trauma, malignancy, pulmonary embolism
WBC count >50-100 × 10^3 cells/µL (>50-100 × 10^9 cells/L)	Empyema (grossly visible pus)
>50% polymorpho-nuclear leukocytes	Inflammation
>50% lymphocytes	Neoplasm or tuberculosis
Eosinophilia	Nonspecific finding
pH <7.2	Infection, malignancy, rheu-matoid arthritis, esophageal rupture
Glucose <60 mg/dL (<3.33 mmol/L)	Infection, malignancy, rheuma-toid arthritis
Amylase increased	Pancreatitis, esophageal rupture, amylase-secreting neoplasm
Triglycerides >100 mg/dL (>1.14 mmol/L)	Chylous effusion seen in trauma, malignancy
Rheumatoid factor, antinuclear anti-bodies, lupus ery-thematosus cells, decreased comple-ment	Collagen vascular disease, lupus erythematosus, rheumatoid arthritis

Cytologic studies should include both Wright-Giemsa– and Papanico-laou-stained preparations. Pleural biopsy may be helpful. Cytologic study has a higher diagnostic yield than pleural biopsy in patients with malignant disease of the pleura but a lower yield than pleural biopsy in patients with tuberculous disease of the pleura. With tuberculous pleuritis acid-fast smears are 20% to 40% sensitive, a biopsy is 70% sensitive, and a culture is 75% sensitive; all three studies together have a combined sensitivity of 90% to 95%.

BIBLIOGRAPHY

Barnes HV: Pleural effusion. In Spivak JL, Barnes HV (eds): Manual of Clinical Problems in Internal Medicine, 4th ed. Boston, Little, Brown & Co, 1990, p 514.
  Good discussion of diagnosis and management with annotated key references.
Devuyst O, Lambert M, Scheiff JM, et al: High amylase activity in pleural fluid and primary bronchogenic adenocarcinoma. Eur Respir J 3:1217, 1990.
  In the absence of pancreatitis and esophageal perforation, high pleural fluid amylase (salivary type) values are consistent with bronchogenic adenocarcinoma.
Gottehrer A, Taryle DA, Reed CE, et al: Pleural fluid analysis in malignant mesothelioma: Prognostic implications. Chest 100:1003, 1991.
  Low pleural fluid pH and glucose indicate reduced survival time.
Iber C, Ingraham RH: Disorders of the pleura, hila, and mediastinum. In Rubenstein E, Federman DD (eds): Scientific American. New York, Scientific American, Inc, November 1991, 14.IX.
  Good discussion of laboratory tests.
Light RW: Pleural Disease. Philadelphia, Lea & Febiger, 1983.
  Excellent general reference that includes a discussion of Light's indices.
Light RW: Pleural diseases. Disease-a-Month 38(5):1, 1992.
  Reviews differential diagnosis of pleural diseases.
Meisel S, Shamiss A, Thaler M, et al: Pleural fluid to serum bilirubin concentration ratio for the separation of transudates from exudates. Chest 98:141, 1990.
  Pleural fluid to serum bilirubin ratio can be used to distinguish exudates from transudates.
Peterman TA, Speicher CE: Evaluating pleural effusions: A two-stage laboratory approach. JAMA 252:1051, 1984.
  Light's criteria effectively separate transudates from exudates, making further evaluation of transudates unnecessary.
Roth BJ, O'Meara TF, Cragun WH: The serum-effusion albumin gradient in the evaluation of pleural effusions. Chest 98:546, 1990.
  Gradient between pleural fluid albumin and serum albumin is useful to distinguish exudates from transudates.
Valdés L, Pose A, Suàrez J, et al: Cholesterol: A useful parameter for distinguishing between pleural exudates and transudates. Chest 99:1097, 1991.
  Pleural fluid cholesterol level <55 mg/dL (1.45 mmol/L) and a pleural fluid cholesterol:serum cholesterol ratio of 0.3 or less correctly identify transudates.
Wahl GW, Hall WJ: Pleural effusions. In Panzer RJ, Black ER, Griner PF (eds): Diagnostic Strategies for Common Medical Problems. Philadelphia, American College of Physicians, 1991, p 279.
  Suggests strategies for the differential diagnosis of pleural effusions.

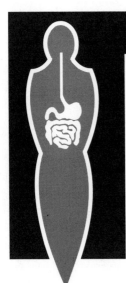

CHAPTER 5

GASTROINTESTINAL DISEASES

Acute Abdominal Pain
Acute Diarrhea
Intestinal Malabsorption
Ascites

Acute Abdominal Pain

1.   For patients with abdominal pain obtain appropriate radiographic studies and laboratory tests.

The differential diagnosis of abdominal pain is long, and the reader is referred to other texts for discussions of the various disorders. Although the correct diagnosis of these disorders is primarily a clinical exercise, radiographic studies and laboratory tests may be useful if they are carefully selected and their pitfalls and limitations are understood. Several common disorders are discussed in which laboratory tests may be useful: appendicitis, acute pancreatitis, acute cholecystitis, peptic ulcer, and acute intermittent porphyria.

Useful laboratory tests to consider include a complete blood count (CBC) with differential; determinations of serum glucose, urea nitrogen, creatinine, electrolytes, amylase, and lipase; urinalysis; porphyria tests (urine δ-aminolevulinic acid [ALA] and porphobilinogen [PBG]); and peptic ulcer tests (gastric acid secretion, *Helicobacter pylori,* serum gastrin). The use of serial serum human chorionic gonadotropin measurements to diagnose ectopic pregnancy is discussed in Chapter 1, and urinalysis for urinary tract disorders is discussed in Chapter 7.

2.   Evaluate the tests.

Recent developments in the methodology for serum lipase and tests for porphyrins and peptic ulcer require comment.

For diagnosing acute pancreatitis, the importance of improved lipase methods has been recently elucidated. These newer methods such as the Kodak Ektachem lipase method, which incorporate colipase, result in higher test results and an increased sensitivity for pancreatitis. Appropriate reference ranges should be used.

For diagnosing acute intermittent porphyria, the Watson-Schwartz test for PBG may be used, but it is subject to false-negative and false-positive results—quantitative methods for determining ALA and PBG are preferable.

For diagnosing peptic ulcer disease, determination of gastric acid secretion is usually unnecessary. *H. pylori* can be detected by biopsy of antral mucosa, bacterial culture, immunological tests, and tests based on bacterial metabolism such as the ^{13}C-urea breath test. Serum gastrin can be measured in the fasting state and after secretin or calcium stimulation.

3. Interpret test results in the context of clinical findings.

APPENDICITIS

The clinical findings of appendicitis include pain (epigastic, then right iliac); vomiting, nausea, acute loss of appetite; local tenderness; and sometimes local rigidity of muscle.

Consistent laboratory findings include polymorphonuclear leukocytosis with a "left shift." Increased hematocrit and serum urea nitrogen values may reflect dehydration, often caused by vomiting and a low fluid intake. Normal results from a urinalysis are important for excluding urinary tract disease; however, 20% of patients with acute appendicitis have a few scattered red blood cells (RBCs) and white blood cells (WBCs) in the urinary sediment. Normal WBC and neutrophil counts are the best tests for excluding appendicitis; according to a recent report, the addition of a normal C-reactive protein value can increase the negative predictive value to 100%.

ACUTE PANCREATITIS

The clinical findings of acute pancreatitis include pain, shock, vomiting, fever, tenderness, and rigidity.

Serum amylase and lipase tests should be ordered together and then performed two to three times daily during the first 48 hours. Ultrasound and computed tomography (CT) studies may be useful. Serum amylase values increase 2 to 3 hours after the onset of acute pancreatitis and return to normal in approximately 4 to 7 days. Serum lipase values increase simultaneously and take longer to return to normal. Slightly increased amylase values are present in many disorders, but values greater than two to three times the upper limit of normal most often indicate acute pancreatitis. High amylase values in the absence of acute pancreatitis occur with renal failure and macroamylasemia. A normal amylase value does not exclude acute pancreatitis. Serum lipase tests (using newer methods) are more sensitive and specific than those for amylase in determining the diagnosis. In asymptomatic alcoholics lipase values up to three times the upper limit of normal may occur; however, once the value exceeds fives times the upper limit of normal, it indicates acute pancreatitis. Serum lipase is a better test than serum amylase to diagnose acute alcoholic pancreatitis.

Other consistent test results include leukocytosis, hyperglycemia, hypocalcemia, hyperbilirubinemia, hypertriglyceridemia, and hypoxemia.

ACUTE CHOLECYSTITIS

The clinical findings of cholecystitis include pain, vomiting, nausea, loss of appetite; jaundice (sometimes); fever; palpable or visibly distended gallbladder; and tenderness and rigidity.

The diagnosis of cholecystitis is established by clinical findings and radiographic studies such as ultrasonography, oral cholecystography, and isotope scanning. Laboratory tests are ancillary and consist mainly of detecting polymorphonuclear leukocytosis with a left shift and excluding other conditions such as urinary tract disease. Liver function tests such as for serum bilirubin, alkaline phosphatase, and gamma-glutamyl transferase are helpful since they may detect cholestasis secondary to cholelithiasis.

PEPTIC ULCER

Clinical findings include gnawing epigastic pain relieved by food or antacids. Complications include perforation, bleeding, and obstruction. The symptoms and signs of perforation vary according to the time that has elapsed since the rupture occurred. Within the first 2 hours great and generalized abdominal pain occurs.

The definitive diagnosis of a peptic ulcer depends on visualizing the ulcer crater by radiographic or endoscopic studies. In the absence of hypergastrinemia, measurement of gastric acid secretion is usually unnecessary. The significance of *H. pylori* in the diagnosis and management of peptic ulcer disease is controversial. Serological tests for decreasing IgG, IgA, and IgM antibodies can be used to monitor the success of eradication of *H. pylori*. Since the prevalence of the Zollinger-Ellison syndrome is less than 1%, routine measurement of serum gastrin is unnecessary. However, do obtain serum gastrin determinations for patients at increased risk (e.g., family history of peptic ulcer, ulcer associated with hypercalcemia, manifestations of multiple endocrine neoplasia type 1, or multiple peptic ulcers).

PORPHYRIA

Clinical findings of acute intermittent porphyria include a family history of intermittent abdominal pain with episodes precipitated by certain drugs, crash dieting, and infections. In porphyric women the attacks may be menstrually related. A history of repeated attacks of pain, sometimes with surgery and normal pathological findings, may be elicited.

During an attack of acute intermittent porphyria PBG excretion is in the range of 50 to 200 mg/day (220 to 880 mmol/day [reference range, 0 to 2 mg/day]) and ALA excretion in the range of 20 to 100 mg/day (152 to 763 μmol/day [reference range, 1.5 to 7.5 mg/day]).

Porphyrias may be divided into two general categories: cutaneous photosensitivity and neurological abnormalities. Patients may have cutaneous photosensitivity (e.g., porphyria cutanea tarda), neurological abnormalities (e.g., intermittent porphyria), or both. Neurological abnormalities are associated with increased urinary excretion of the porphyria precursors PBG and ALA. Cutaneous hypersensitivity is characterized by excess uroporphyrins in a 24-hour urine collection.

BIBLIOGRAPHY

Altman LK: How tools of medicine get in the way. *New York Times*, May 12, 1992, p B6.
  Fascinating account of how medical technology interfered with the diagnosis of acute appendicitis.
Araki T, Ueda M, Taketa K, et al: Pancreatic-type hyperamylasemia in end-stage renal disease. Dig Dis Sci 34:1425, 1989.
  Serum amylase is commonly increased in patients with renal insufficiency.
Berg CL, Wolfe MM: Zollinger-Ellison syndrome. Med Clin North Am 75:903, 1991.
  Reviews the pathophysiology, diagnosis, and management of the Zollinger-Ellison syndrome.
Clearfield HR: *Helicobacter pylori:* Aggressor or innocent bystander? Med Clin North Am 75:815, 1991.
  Suggests that for most patients the organism is an innocent bystander, but for some patients it facilitates the development and relapse of peptic ulcer disease.
Cooperman AM, Fuhrman SA: Patient with abdominal pain; Shedlofsky SI: Young woman with recurrent abdominal pain; and Henderson AR, Shedlofsky SI: Severe epigastic pain. In Tietz NW, Conn RB, Pruden EL (eds): Applied Laboratory Medicine. Philadelphia, WB Saunders Co, 1992, pp 85, 89, 99.
  Discusses three causes of abdominal pain: cholelithiasis, acute intermittent porphyria, and acute pancreatitis.
Corsetti JP, Arvan DA: Acute pancreatitis; and Greene RA, Griner PF: Cholelithiasis and acute cholecystitis. In Panzer RJ, Black ER, Griner PF (eds): Diagnostic Strategies for Common Medical Tests. Philadelphia, American College of Physicians, 1991, pp 160, 121.
  Recommended strategies for diagnosing acute abdominal pain.
Dueholm S, Bagi P, Bud M: Laboratory aid in the diagnosis of acute appendicitis: A blinded, prospective trial concerning diagnostic value of leukocyte count, neutrophil differential count, and C-reactive protein. Dis Colon Rectum 32:855, 1989.
  Most efficient test combination for excluding appendicitis consists of a WBC count, a neutrophil count, and a C-reactive protein measurement—negative predictive value of 100%.
Frey CF, Gerzof SG, Vennes JA: Progress in acute pancreatitis. Patient Care 26:258, 1992.
  Alcohol-related disease or gallstones are common causes. Discusses false-positive and false-negative serum amylase results.
Frucht H, Howard JM, Slaff JI, et al: Secretin and calcium provocative tests in the Zollinger-Ellison syndrome: A prospective study. Ann Intern Med 111:713, 1989.
  Calcium provocative test is appropriate for patients with strong clinical suspicion for the Zollinger-Ellison syndrome and a negative secretin test result.
Gumaste V, Dave P, Sereny G: Serum lipase: A better test to diagnose acute alcoholic pancreatitis. Am J Med 92:239, 1992.
  Serum lipase is a better test than amylase for diagnosing acute pancreatitis.
Kosunen TU, Seppala K, Sarna S, et al: Diagnostic value of decreasing IgG, IgA, and IgM antibody titers after eradication of *Helicobacter pylori*. Lancet 339:893, 1992.
  Serological tests may be used to monitor eradication of H. pylori.
Kushner JP: Laboratory diagnosis of the porphyrias. N Engl J Med 324:1432, 1991.
  Concise discussion of the porphyrias with strategies for laboratory diagnosis.

Panteghini M, Pagani F: Clinical evaluation of an algorithm for the interpretation of hyperamylasemia. Arch Pathol Lab Med 115:355, 1991; and Lott JA: The value of clinical laboratory studies in acute pancreatitis. Arch Pathol Lab Med 115:325, 1991.
Article and editorial that discuss strategies for diagnosing acute pancreatitis.
Silen W: Cope's Early Diagnosis of the Acute Abdomen, 18th ed. New York, Oxford University Press, 1991.
Classic treatise on the differential diagnosis of acute abdominal pain.

Acute Diarrhea

1. In patients with acute diarrhea that persists for more than several days in whom toxicity and fecal blood are absent, examine a fecal smear for polymorphonuclear leukocytes to distinguish the clinical syndromes of noninflammatory diarrhea from the inflammatory types of diarrhea. Occult blood testing may be helpful.

Acute diarrhea is diarrhea of less than a week's duration that is characterized by an increase in daily stool weight of more than 250 g, liquidity, and a frequency of more than three bowel movements per day. It is usually self-limited and requires no treatment; however, it may be prolonged and reflect serious disease, that is, dysentery. Dysentery refers to severe inflammation of the intestine, usually the colon, associated with blood, pus, and mucus in the stool.

Apply a thin layer of feces or mucus to a slide, mix with one drop of Löffler's methylene blue stain, seal with a coverslip, and examine for polymorphonuclear leukocytes (Wright's stain may also be used). More than five leukocytes per high-power field in five or more fields is considered positive for inflammatory diarrhea. The presence of erythrocytes or occult blood suggests an inflammatory cause, but there are exceptions such as ischemia.

Acute diarrhea is divided into two types, noninflammatory and inflammatory, on the basis of whether or not there are polymorphonuclear leukocytes in the feces. This is a clinically relevant classification since in the United States noninflammatory disease usually is self-limited and is associated with cramping, bloating, periumbilical pain, and large-volume, watery stools. Fever, leukocytosis, and constitutional symptoms are absent. In contrast, inflammatory diarrhea or dysentery is associated with mucosal invasion and commonly is accompanied by fever, other constitutional symptoms, lower abdominal pain, and tenesmus. Stools may be small in volume and often are bloody or mucoid.

2. If the fecal smear shows five or less polymorphonuclear leukocytes per high-power field, the diarrhea is probably noninflammatory, and the illness will usually be self-limited.

In the United States Norwalk virus and other viral agents are the most common causes of noninflammatory diarrhea in adults. The diarrhea is explosive and lasts approximately 24 to 48 hours. Rotavirus infection predominates in infants and young children and produces severely watery diarrhea of 5 to 8 days' duration. Other causes of noninflammatory diarrhea include enterotoxigenic *Escherichia coli, Vibrio cholerae, Bacillus cereus, Cryptosporidium, Giardia lamblia,* and bacterial toxins associated with food poisoning (*Staphylococcus* and *Clostridium perfringens*). These organisms or toxins do not invade the mucosa but induce a secretory, watery diarrhea; thus fecal leukocytes are typically absent.

Some inflammatory diarrheas will not show more than five polymorphonuclear leukocytes per high-power field; thus they can appear to be noninflammatory diarrhea. For example, this happens with approximately 30% of *Shigella* infections, and similar results have been reported for *Campylobacter* infections. In antibiotic-associated colitis (especially with clindamycin, lincomycin, ampicillin, and cephalosporins) leukocytes are few or absent when the process is limited but are common in diffuse disease. Likewise, *Entamoeba histolytica, Salmonella, Yersinia enterocolitica,* and *Vibrio parahaemolyticus* infections produce variable findings, and the presence of leukocytes depends on the degree of colonic invasion.

There are a number of noninfectious causes of noninflammatory diarrhea. Drugs that can cause diarrhea include laxatives, warfarin, thyroid hormones, magnesium-containing antacids, quinidine, colchicine, cholestyramine, digoxin, and antimetabolites. Diarrhea can occur with toxins such as heavy metals (lead, zinc, cadmium, copper), poisonous fish (ciguatoxin, scombrotoxin, puffer fish, shellfish), monosodium glutamate, botulism, and mushroom poisoning. Fecal impaction is an additional cause. Some patients with an irritable bowel or an inflamed rectum pass several loose bowel movements each day that do not exceed a total of 250 g. Diabetic diarrhea is common in patients with diabetic peripheral and autonomic neuropathy, and bacterial overgrowth may play a role.

When the cause of diarrhea is noninflammatory and noninfectious, for diagnostic purposes it may be useful to distinguish osmotic diarrhea from secretory diarrhea. Osmotic diarrhea is caused by the accumulation in the gut lumen of nonabsorbable solutes (e.g., divalent or trivalent ions [Mg^{++}, $PO^=$, $SO^=$]) from saline solution laxatives and of lactose secondary to disaccharidase deficiency. In contrast, secretory diarrhea (usually >1000 mL/day) is caused by a net luminal gain of secretions, that is, electrolytes and water. Examples of secretory diarrhea include enterotoxin-induced diarrhea, pancreatic cholera syndrome, carcinoid syndrome, glucagonoma, Zollinger-Ellison syndrome (tumor can be demonstrated by CT scan or gastrin assay), and surreptitious ingestion of cathartic agents such as phenolphthalein (pink color of alkalinized stool). Osmotic diarrhea can be distinguished from secretory diarrhea by calculating the stool osmotic gap as follows:

$$\text{Stool osmotic gap} = \text{Measured stool osmolality} - 2[(Na^+) + (K^+)]$$

If the stool osmotic gap is high (commonly >160 mOsm/kg), it indicates osmotic diarrhea. If it is approximately zero or negative (may be negative because of multivalent anions), it indicates secretory diarrhea. The stool sample must be fresh or stored at 39.2° F (4° C). Measured osmolality of diarrheal stool is normally 285 to 330 mOsm/kg. Alternatively, in secretory diarrhea the fecal Na$^+$ and K$^+$ equal approximately one half of the stool osmolality. Osmotic diarrhea typically stops after a 24-hour fast, whereas secretory diarrhea persists.

Watery diarrhea can also occur with other chronic conditions: irritable bowel syndrome, inflammatory bowel disease, villous adenoma, ischemic colitis, and mesenteric thrombosis.

3.   If the fecal smear shows more than five polymorphonuclear leukocytes per high-power field, the diarrhea is probably inflammatory, and the cause should be determined. The presence of erythrocytes or occult blood suggests an inflammatory cause.

Polymorphonuclear leukocytes are specific for colonic inflammation and suggest infection from *Shigella, Salmonella, Yersinia, Campylobacter,* invasive *E. coli,* or *Giardia* or antibiotic-associated colitis, ulcerative colitis, or ischemic colitis. During the summer months or if seafood has been eaten, consider *V. parahaemolyticus* as a cause. Fecal occult blood testing is not as useful as examination for leukocytes, but when combined with leukocyte testing, it can increase the positive predictive value for bacterial infection. Chronic inflammatory disease of the colon (ulcerative colitis and Crohn's disease) yields low-volume diarrhea (<1000 mL/day) containing many leukocytes.

4.   Perform stool cultures and examination for ova and parasites in the following situations: fecal blood (gross or occult), fecal leukocytes, temperature above 101° F (38.3° C), admission to the hospital, food handlers, persistent diarrhea, diarrhea associated with debilitation, travelers with a history of exposure, and with epidemiological considerations. Avoid barium enema examination.

Stool cultures and examination for ova and parasites are not appropriate for inpatients who develop diarrhea more than 3 days after admission to the hospital.

If *Campylobacter jejuni* or *V. parahaemolyticus* is suspected, request selective culture techniques. Request gonorrheal identification in homosexual men, and remember that homosexual men are at increased risk for infections with *Salmonella, Shigella, Campylobacter, G. lamblia, E. histolytica, Chlamydia trachomatis,* and herpes simplex virus. Consider parasitic infection with this clinical history: undiagnosed diarrhea for longer than 1 week, history of travel exposure, and homosexual exposure to amebiasis or giardiasis. At least 90% of enteric pathogens are detected in the first stool sample; testing up to two additional samples is appropriate if the first sample is negative. Avoid barium enema examination, enemas, laxatives, and antibiotics since they can obscure the diagnosis. In patients in whom clinical suspicion of parasitism persists and all three stool examinations are negative, additional specimens should be examined. In addition to the usual infections, patients with acquired immunodeficiency syndrome (AIDS) are susceptible to infections with cytomegalovirus, adenovirus, herpes simplex virus, *Candida albicans, Histoplasma capsulatum, Cryptosporidium* species, *Isospora belli,* and *Mycobacterium avium-intracellulare.*

5.   Perform proctosigmoidoscopy in patients with toxicity, bloody diarrhea, antibiotic-associated diarrhea, or prolonged diarrhea.

Sigmoidoscopy reveals the yellow-gray plaques of antibiotic-associated colitis, and the diagnosis can be confirmed by rectal biopsy, measuring *Clostridium difficile* toxin, or anaerobic culture of *C. difficile*. In a patient with antibiotic-associated diarrhea and negative studies for *C. difficile*, consider *Candida*. In a patient with amebiasis there will be colonic ulcerations containing amebas, and serological tests using gel diffusion precipitin or indirect hemagglutination tests are positive in 85% to 95% of patients. In patients with ulcerative colitis the rectal and colonic mucosa will be diffusely red and friable, and cultures will be negative. Consider ischemic colitis in older patients with atherosclerotic vascular disease and with diarrhea. A barium enema examination may be useful to diagnose ischemic colitis, even though it is ordinarily not part of the evaluation of acute diarrhea.

6.   In patients with acute diarrhea the following additional abnormal blood test results may occur:

- ↑ **Hemoglobin and hematocrit** caused by loss of salt and water with contraction of the extracellular compartment and hemoconcentration.
- ↑ **Leukocytes** with inflammatory diarrhea.
- **Metabolic acidosis.**
- ↑ **Urea and creatinine** associated with prerenal azotemia.

- ↑ **Sodium and chloride** with dehydration related to water loss. (With diarrhea, ↓ **electrolytes** may occur if water is replaced and not electrolytes.)
- ↑ **Albumin and calcium** (bound to albumin) with dehydration.
- ↑ **Alkaline phosphatase** (intestinal type) in ulcerative lesions of the intestine such as with ulcerative colitis.

BIBLIOGRAPHY

Community outbreaks of shigellosis—United States. MMWR 39:509, 1990.
  Incidence of shigellosis is increasing. Physicians should suspect shigellosis in community outbreaks of diarrheal illness that involve young children especially.
Danna PL, Urban C, Bellin E, et al: Role of candida in pathogenesis of antibiotic-associated diarrhea in elderly inpatients. Lancet 337:511, 1991.
  In antibiotic-associated diarrhea and negative assays for C. difficile, *consider* Candida.
Guerrant RL, Bobak DA: Bacterial and protozoal gastroenteritis. N Engl J Med 325:327, 1991.
  Excellent review with an algorithm for patient management.
Lee LA, Taylor J, Carter GP, et al: *Yersinia enterocolitica* 0:3: An emerging cause of pediatric gastroenteritis in the United States. J Infect Dis 163:660, 1991.
  Y. enterocolitica *infections are increasing. Eating raw chitterlings (pork intestines) can cause the disease.*
Massey BT, Suchman AL: Acute diarrhea. In Panzer RJ, Black ER, Griner PF (eds): Diagnostic Strategies for Common Medical Problems. Philadelphia, American College of Physicians, 1991, p 113.
  Recommends strategies for the diagnosis of acute diarrhea.

Senay H, MacPherson D: Parasitology: Diagnostic yield of stool examination. Can Med Assoc J 140:1329, 1989.

At least 90% of enteric parasites are detected in the first stool sample. Obtaining up to two additional samples is appropriate if the first sample is negative.

Shiau Y-F, Feldman GM, Resnick MA, et al: Stool electrolyte and osmolality measurements in the evaluation of diarrheal disorders. Ann Intern Med 102:773, 1985.

Stool osmotic gap in patients with osmotic diarrhea is substantially higher than previously reported—commonly >160 mOsm/kg.

Siegel DL, Edelstein PH, Nachamkin I: Inappropriate testing for diarrheal diseases in the hospital. JAMA 263:979, 1990.

With rare exceptions, routine stool culture and examination for ova and parasites are not appropriate for inpatients who develop diarrhea more than 3 days after admission.

Smith PD, Quinn TC, Strober W, et al: Gastrointestinal infections in AIDS. Ann Intern Med 116:63, 1992.

National Institutes of Health conference on the gastrointestinal pathogens in HIV-infected patients.

Update: *Salmonella enteritidis* infections and Grade A shell eggs—United States, 1989. MMWR 38:877, 1990.

Salmonellosis is increasing. Consumers should be advised to avoid eating raw or undercooked eggs.

Intestinal Malabsorption

1.   In patients with clinical findings of steatorrhea obtain a 72-hour stool collection for quantitative fecal fat analysis. To perform a 72-hour fecal fat analysis, start the individual on an 80 to 100 g/day fat diet and continue this diet during the collection period. Microscopic examination of a random stool sample may be used as a qualitative screening test. Serum carotene and vitamin A concentrations may be helpful.

Intestinal malabsorption, or steatorrhea, is a type of chronic diarrhea that must be distinguished from other causes of chronic diarrhea such as irritable bowel and inflammatory bowel disease (Crohn' disease and ulcerative colitis). *Malabsorption* is a term used to indicate defective absorption of nutrients by the small intestine.

A key feature is the marked difficulty the patient describes in flushing stool down the toilet because of increased stool volume and fat content (when fecal fat is approximately 20 g/day, at least two flushings are required to clear the toilet water).

Although microscopic examination of a random stool sample may be used as a screening test, quantitative documentation of increased fecal fat over a 3-day period is the best method for diagnosing intestinal malabsorption. Serum carotene and vitamin A concentrations may be decreased, but these tests are not reliable enough to use as diagnostic tests.

For a 72-hour quantitative fecal fat study, the individual should be instructed as follows: avoid castor, mineral, or nut oils and the use of suppositories. After 3 to 5 days of the diet, begin a 72-hour stool collection for quantitative fecal fat analysis. Collect the specimens in glass or plastic containers (clean paint cans work well). Wax-coated containers should not be used. During the collection period the fecal specimens should be refrigerated, and contamination of feces with urine should be avoided. Any obvious foreign matter should be removed before proceeding with the analysis.

2. To perform a microscopic examination for increased fecal fat, obtain a random stool sample and proceed in the following manner.

When done properly, the Sudan stain has an 80% to 90% sensitivity for detecting clinically significant steatorrhea.

1. Place a small amount of stool (size of one half of a split pea) on a glass slide. If stool is not liquid, add several drops of water or saline solution and make a homogenate by using applicator stick as a pestle.
2. Add 2 or 3 drops of glacial acetic acid and 4 or 5 drops of alcoholic solution of Sudan stain, mix, and add coverslip.
3. Heat with alcohol lamp or burner to boiling to facilitate hydrolysis of soaps to free fatty acids and to facilitate staining.
4. Examine under a microscope while slide is warm, using low power to locate stained fat droplets and high power to examine droplets.
   Normal: A few small droplets should be noticeable and represent normal fat excretion; they reassure the examiner that the slide has been prepared properly.
   Abnormal: A much larger number and size of reddish-colored round droplets indicate steatorrhea.
5. Pitfalls: The skillful examiner gains experience by comparing examination of stool from patients with steatorrhea with that from healthy individuals. False-positive results can occur in patients receiving castor oil, mineral oil, and oil-based suppositories. False-negative results can result from barium's diluting the stool. Failure to examine the slide while warm can result in conversion of the stained melted fat droplets to unstained needlelike crystals. If this occurs, the slide should be reheated and reexamined.

3. Evaluate the tests.

In addition to fecal fat and serum beta carotene and vitamin A concentration, the ^{14}C-triolein breath test also screens for steatorrhea.

REFERENCE RANGES

Test	Specimen	Conventional Units	International Units
Fat, fecal	Feces (72 hr)	<6 g/day	<6 g/day
Beta carotene	Serum	60-200 μg/dL	1.12-3.72 μmol/L
Vitamin A	Serum	30-65 μg/dL	1.05-2.27 μmol/L

Test	Normal Fat Excreters (<6 g/24 hr)	Abnormal Fat Excreters (>6 g/24 hr)
Number of microscopic fat droplets per high-lower field	2.5 ± 0.8	26.6 ± 4

Compared with the quantitative fecal fat test, the ^{14}C-triolein breath test has a sensitivity of 85% to 100% and a specificity of 93% to 96%. False-positive results with the breath test can occur in patients with obesity, gastric retention, and chronic liver disease.

4. If fecal fat is increased, the patient has malabsorption. Perform a xylose absorption test to differentiate maldigestion (pancreatic disease) from malassimilation (intestinal disease). A small bowel series is appropriate.

The degree of increase of fecal fat is not useful in differentiating between pancreatic and intestinal disease. To perform the xylose absorption test, the patient ingests 25 g of xylose and collects urine for the next 5 hours. The patient must drink 500 ml of water during the first 3 hours of the collection period to ensure adequate urinary filtration of the xylose. A normal xylose absorption test shows 10 to 20 mg/dL/1.73 m^2 (0.67 to 1.33 mmol/L/1.73 m^2) of body surface area increase of the serum concentration within 60 to 75 minutes after ingestion of xylose or 5 g or more of xylose in the urine within 5 hours. False-positive xylose absorption tests occasionally occur in the following situations:

1. Decreased renal function in patients more than 60 years of age or patients of any age with renal disease (false-positive urine test, but serum test is valid).
2. Patients with increased extracellular fluid, particularly with ascites or massive edema.
3. Patients with delayed gastric emptying (can be overcome by instilling the test dose through a tube directly into the proximal intestine).

In patients with decreased renal function only serum values should be used in the interpretation of xylose absorption.

A small bowel series may be used to detect the presence of malabsorption and may help to differentiate intraluminal maldigestion from malassimilation.

5. If fecal fat is increased and the xylose absorption test result is abnormal, consider intestinal disease.

In this circumstance a small bowel biopsy may diagnose such intestinal diseases as celiac sprue, Whipple's disease, hypogammaglobulinemia (IgA), lymphangiectasia, and lymphoma. A recent study suggests that the xylose absorption test is not useful to diagnose adult celiac disease or to monitor the effect of dietary treatment. A normal biopsy result suggests bacterial overgrowth. The most common disorders of the small bowel that lead to malabsorption (other than bowel resection) are celiac disease, tropical sprue, and bacterial overgrowth.

6.   If fecal fat is increased and the xylose absorption test result is normal, consider biliary or pancreatic disease. Evaluate the patient for diabetes mellitus and perform appropriate radiographic and endoscopic studies.

Pancreatic diabetes occurs in one third of all patients with chronic pancreatitis and in approximately twice this number of patients with calcific pancreatitis. Radiographic and sometimes endoscopic studies are necessary to evaluate the patient adequately. Although the secretin, cholecystokinin stimulation, and Lundh tests are useful, they are not commonly performed because they require intubation, which is time-consuming and cumbersome. The bentiromide assay is a noninvasive test (85% to 97% sensitive) for detecting advanced chronic pancreatitis or cancer of the pancreatic head with ductal obstruction. When 500 mg of bentiromide is ingested, patients with normal amounts of trypsin excrete at least 50% of the bentiromide as *P*-aminobenzoic acid (PABA) in the urine within 6 hours. Patients with pancreatic disease excrete less. Determination of fasting serum trypsinogen levels is another test to detect chronic pancreatitis or cancer of the pancreatic head causing ductal obstruction. Serum trypsinogen is decreased in patients with these disorders. Also decreased values of other serum analytes such as pancreatic isoamylase, lipase, and pancreatic polypeptide may be used to detect chronic pancreatitis. Unfortunately, the noninvasive tests of pancreatic function usually are positive only in patients with severe pancreatic insufficiency but not with milder forms of the disease.

7.   If the fecal fat excretion is normal, intestinal malabsorption is ruled out; however, fecal fat excretion may be normal in patients with specific absorption defects such as disaccharidase deficiency.

Disaccharidase deficiency, which can be caused by giardiasis, can be diagnosed by an assay of tissue from the small intestine by peroral biopsy. Usually this is not necessary because the clinical findings can be produced by ingestion of 50 g of the sugar and because dramatic improvement results when milk products are eliminated from the diet. During the oral lactose tolerance test in a fasting patient, a healthy individual will show a 20 to 30 mg/dL (1.11 to 1.67 mmol/L) increase in serum glucose in the first 2 hours after ingesting 50 g of lactose. A lactose breath test is also available.

8.   In patients with intestinal malabsorption the following additional abnormal blood test results may occur:

↑ **Hematocrit** suggests dehydration.

↓ **Hematocrit** suggests blood loss or anemia caused by malabsorption (e.g., iron, folate, vitamin B_{12}).*

↓ **Lymphocytes** may indicate excessive leakage of lymph into the gut.

↑ **Sodium and urea nitrogen** suggest dehydration.

↓ **Potassium and sodium** may be caused by diarrhea.

↓ **Calcium** related to hypoalbuminemia and/or vitamin D deficiency with decreased calcium absorption; rare in pancreatic insufficiency.*

↑ **Eosinophils** suggests parasites or eosinophilic gastroenteritis.

↑ **Platelets** suggests ulcerative colitis, Whipple's disease, and celiac sprue.

↑ **Prothrombin time** may be caused by impaired absorption of vitamin K.*

Chronic diarrhea can cause metabolic acidosis or metabolic alkalosis with ↓ **or** ↑ **bicarbonate,** with reciprocal changes in chloride.

↑ **Glucose** from pancreatic diabetes.

↓ **Glucose and urea nitrogen** may be caused by malabsorption of glucose and protein.

↓ **Magnesium;** rare in pancreatic insufficiency.

↑ **Lactate dehydrogenase and aspartate aminotransferase (SGOT)** from ↓ **vitamin B$_{12}$** absorption with megaloblastic anemia and intramedullary death of megaloblasts.

↑ **Alkaline phosphatase** caused by vitamin D deficiency with ↓ **calcium** absorption causing osteomalacia.

↓ **albumin.**

↓ **bilirubin** related to hypoalbuminemia.

↓ **cholesterol.**

---

*Since the absorption of carotene, vitamin K, vitamin D, folate, and iron is independent of pancreatic enzyme digestion, the presence of a low serum carotene value, hypocalcemia, hypoprothrombinemia, or anemia suggests a small bowel disorder rather than a pancreatic disorder.

BIBLIOGRAPHY

Barnes HV: Malabsorption. In Spivak JL, Barnes HV (eds): Manual of Clinical Problems in Internal Medicine, 4th ed. Boston, Little, Brown & Co, 1990, p 264.
  Good discussion of diagnosis, with annotated key references.
Binder HJ: Chronic diarrhea and malabsorption in adults. In Conn RB (ed): Current Diagnosis, 8th ed. Philadelphia, WB Saunders Co, 1991, p 672.
  Discusses the diagnosis of chronic diarrhea, emphasizing clinical findings and pathophysiological principles.
Gambino R: Fecal fat. Lab Report for Physicians 3:57, 1981.
  Compares microscopic stool examination for fecal fat with quantification of fecal fat for 24 hours.
Simko V: Fecal fat microscopy: Acceptable predictive value in screening for steatorrhea. Am J Gastroenterol 75:204, 1981.
  Found microscopic stool examination for fecal fat is useful.
Trier JS: Celiac sprue. N Engl J Med 325:1709, 1991.
  Reviews pathogenesis, diagnosis, and management of the disorder.
Trier JS: Intestinal malabsorption: Differentiation of cause. Hosp Pract 23:195, 1988.
  Discusses the differential diagnosis of intestinal malabsorption.

Ascites

1.   In patients with ascites, to diagnose the cause of the ascites, perform paracentesis and measure ascitic-fluid albumin, total protein, lactate de-

hydrogenase (LD), and WBC levels together with serum albumin, total protein, and LD levels.

Clinical findings for ruling out ascites include negative histories of ankle swelling or increased abdominal girth plus lack of bulging flanks, flank dullness, or shifting dullness. The presence of a positive fluid wave, shifting dullness, or peripheral edema supports the diagnosis of ascites. The term *pseudoascites* denotes the clinical impression of ascites when, in fact, free fluid is not present within the peritoneal cavity.

The gradient (difference) between the serum albumin and ascitic-fluid albumin levels accurately reflects the oncotic pressure of ascitic fluid and has real pathophysiological significance. It provides a new way to categorize patients with ascites.

2.   Evaluate the tests.

The reference ranges and the sensitivity and specificity of the tests are important.

REFERENCE RANGES FOR GRADIENT OF SERUM ALBUMIN MINUS ASCITIC-FLUID ALBUMIN (ALBs-a)

ASCITES	CONVENTIONAL UNITS	INTERNATIONAL UNITS
With portal hypertension	≥1.1 g/dL	≥11 g/L
Without portal hypertension	<1.1 g/dL	<11 g/L

SENSITIVITY AND SPECIFICITY OF TESTS FOR DIFFERENTIATING BETWEEN TRANSUDATIVE AND EXUDATIVE ASCITIC EFFUSIONS

TEST	EXUDATE CRITERIA	SENSITIVITY (%)	SPECIFICITY (%)
1. Total protein	>3 g/dL (>30 g/L)	86	83
2. Ascitic fluid/serum protein ratio	>0.5	93	85
3. Ascitic fluid/serum LD ratio	>0.6	79	92
4. LD	>400 Sigma units (SU) (normal serum range, 200-500 SU)	57	100
5. WBC	>500/mm³	—	90
6. Serum albumin minus ascitic-fluid albumin	<1.1 g/dL (<11 g/L)	87	78
2, 3, and 4 positive		57	100

Source: Skendzel LP: A practical approach to the chemical and microscopic study of pleural and peritoneal fluids. Lab Medica V(1):19, 1988.

3.   If the Albs-a gradient is equal to or greater than 1.1 g/dL (11 g/L), conclude that portal hypertension (transudative ascites) is present, a condition consistent with the presence of cirrhosis or cardiac disease.

Occasional exceptions arise when the Albs-a gradient is 1.1 g/dL (11 g/L) or greater without portal vein hypertension—notably the presence of extensive liver metastases or portal vein thrombosis. An Albs-a gradient of 1.1 g/dL (11 g/L) or greater is maintained in patients with cirrhosis, even when a complicating process such as peritoneal tuberculosis develops. The presence of positive exudate criteria such as an increased ascitic-fluid WBC in a patient with portal hypertension and an Albs-a gradient of 1.1 g/dL (11 g/L) or greater suggests a second process such as peritoneal tuberculosis.

4.   If the Albs-a gradient is less than 1.1 g/dL (11 g/L), conclude that portal hypertension is absent (exudative ascites) and consider other causes for ascites.

Rarely low-grade portal hypertension in patients with cirrhosis produces an Albs-a gradient <1.1 g/dL (11 g/L). In most instances a low gradient suggests causes not associated with portal hypertension such as nonalcoholic liver disease, leaking ducts (thoracic, pancreatic, biliary), peritoneal disease (cancer or tuberculosis), myxedema, systemic lupus erythematous, certain benign ovarian diseases, and severe hypoalbuminemia. Positive exudate criteria are characteristic of a number of the above disorders.

Useful diagnostic studies for ascites without portal hypertension (exudative ascites) include cytology and cultures. High-protein, exudative ascites with negative cytology suggests an infection such as tuberculosis or fungal disease. In patients with tuberculous peritonitis smears are usually negative, and cultures take 4 to 6 weeks to grow the organism—biopsy can provide a rapid diagnosis.

BIBLIOGRAPHY

Albillos A, Cuervas-Mons V, Millán I, et al: Ascitic fluid polymorphonuclear cell count and serum to ascites albumin gradient in the diagnosis of bacterial peritonitis. Gastroenterology 98:134, 1990.
  Suggests a polymorphonuclear cell count >0.5 × 10³ cells/L (0.5 × 10⁹ cells/L) for diagnosing spontaneous bacterial peritonitis and a serum ascites albumin gradient <1.1 g/dL (11 g/L) for diagnosing malignancy.
Antillon MR, Runyon BA: Effect of marked peripheral leukocytosis on the leukocyte count in ascites. Arch Intern Med 151:509, 1991.
  Increased ascites fluid neutrophil count indicates a peritoneal inflammation regardless of the peripheral blood leukocyte count.
D'Amelio LF, Rhodes M: A reassessment of the peritoneal lavage leukocyte count in blunt abdominal trauma. J Trauma 30:1291, 1990.
  Grossly clear peritoneal lavage fluid after blunt abdominal trauma indicates that serious intraperitoneal injury is extremely unlikely.
Fiedorek SC, Casteel HB, Reddy G, et al: The etiology and clinical significance of pseudoascites. J Gen Intern Med 6:77, 1991.
  Discusses the differential diagnosis of pseudoascites.

Gerbes AL, Jüngst D, Xie Y, et al: Ascitic fluid analysis for the differentiation of malignancy-related and nonmalignant ascites: Proposal of a diagnostic sequence. Cancer 68:1808, 1991.
Ascites fluid cholesterol level >45 mg/dL (1.15 mmol/L) detected 49 of 50 patients with peritoneal cancer.

Gitt S, Haddad F, Leverson S: Tuberculous peritonitis: An overlooked diagnosis. Hosp Pract 27:224, 1992.
Important condition to keep in mind.

Hoefs JC, Jonas GM: Diagnostic paracentesis. In La Mont JT (ed): Adv Intern Med 37:391, 1992.
Guidelines for determining the cause of ascites.

Kajani MA, Yoo YK, Alexander JA, et al: Serum-ascites albumin gradients in nonalcoholic liver disease. Dig Dis Sci 35:33, 1990.
Serum ascites albumin gradient <1.1 g/dL (11 g/L) may occur in patients with nonmalignant ascites associated with nonalcoholic liver disease.

Runyon BA, Antillon MR: Ascitic fluid pH and lactate: Insensitive and nonspecific tests in detecting ascitic fluid infection. Hepatology 13:929, 1991.
Neutrophil count >0.25 × 10^3 cells/μL (0.25 × 10^9 cells/L) is the most sensitive test for spontaneous bacterial peritonitis.

Runyon BA, Montano AA, Akriviadis EA, et al: The serum-ascites albumin gradient is superior to the exudate-transudate concept in the differential diagnosis of ascites. Ann Intern Med 117:215, 1992.
Albumin gradient correctly differentiated ascites due to portal hypertension from that with a different cause 91.7% of the time.

Williams JW Jr, Simel DL: Does this patient have ascites? How to divine fluid in the abdomen. JAMA 267:2645, 1992.
Gives clinical guidelines for deciding whether a patient has ascites.

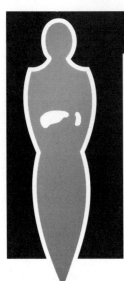

CHAPTER 6

DISEASES OF THE LIVER

Jaundice and Liver Function Tests
Acute Viral Hepatitis
Fatty Liver and Alcoholic Hepatitis
Acute Nonviral, Nonalcoholic Hepatitis
Chronic Persistent and Chronic Active Hepatitis
Cirrhosis
Cholestasis and Obstructive Liver Disease

Jaundice and Liver Function Tests

1.   In patients with jaundice use clinical findings, liver function tests, and other procedures to diagnose liver disease and to help decide whether it is due to hepatocellular or infiltrative disease or to extrahepatic obstruction.

The Patient Care Committee of the American Gastroenterological Association recommends the following workup of patients with jaundice.

In patients with probable hepatocellular or infiltrative liver disease categorize the disease as either probably benign or possibly malignant. Observe patients with probably benign disease and consider performing liver biopsy and ultrasonography. Study patients with possibly malignant tumors, using ultrasonography or computed tomography (CT).

In patients with possible extrahepatic obstruction consider using ultrasonography or CT with or without biopsy. If the results are equivocal or negative, consider using endoscopic retrograde cholangiopancreatography (ERCP) or percutaneous transhepatic cholangiography.

In patients with probable extrahepatic obstruction, consider using ERCP or percutaneous transhepatic cholangiography.

2.   Interpret liver function tests in the context of clinical findings.

The composition of liver function tests (often referred to as *LFTs*) varies from one health care facility to another. One possible combination of serum tests for acute liver disease follows:

1. Aspartate aminotransferase (AST, SGOT)
2. Alanine aminotransferase (ALT, SGPT)
3. Alkaline phosphatase (ALP)
4. Bilirubin, total and conjugated
5. Gamma-glutamyl transferase (GGT)

For chronic or severe liver disease consider using two additional tests: (1) prothrombin time (PT) and (2) albumin and globulin determinations.

Serum GGT is a sensitive test for liver disease of any variety. The sensitivity of routine liver function tests for excluding liver disease can be increased by measuring serum GGT; however, the increased sensitivity is accompanied by decreased specificity.

In addition to clinical findings and abnormal serum test results, increased urinary bilirubin and urobilinogen determinations may serve as clues to the presence of liver disease. Negative test results are not reliable because these analytes are destroyed in urine that is not promptly analyzed.

Liver function tests are easier to understand and interpret if they are viewed according to the pathophysiological derangements that cause the test results to become abnormal. Thus five pathophysiological questions are useful to ask.

a. Is liver disease present or not? Measure all liver function tests.

If all test results are normal, it is unlikely that there is significant liver disease.

b. Is there liver cell injury, and what is its severity? Measure serum transaminase—AST (SGOT) and ALT (SGPT)—levels.

Both AST and ALT are liver cell enzymes that are released into the blood after injury to the liver cell membranes, and significantly increased values are characteristic of acute hepatitis. Increased serum transaminase values correlate poorly with abnormal liver cell morphology by light microscopy. Remember that ALT usually is higher than AST in patients with viral hepatitis and that the reverse is true in patients with alcoholic hepatitis. ALT has been used as a surrogate test for viral hepatitis.

c. Is there cholestasis? Measure serum ALP and total and conjugated bilirubin.

Serum ALP and bilirubin are good tests to detect intrahepatic or extrahepatic obstruction (cholestasis). ALP usually is more sensitive than bilirubin. Serum GGT is another good test for cholestasis. GGT is particularly useful when the patient has an increased serum ALP value and it is unclear whether the increased ALP is originating in liver or bone. GGT is high in liver disease but not in bone disease. Also GGT values can be useful in diagnosing liver disease in adolescents and pregnant women when the ALP cannot be used to assess the liver because it is high as a result of bone growth and the placenta, respectively. Serum bile acid values are always increased in patients with cholestasis, but they are normal in patients with hereditary hyperbilirubinemias such as Gilbert's disease. Cholesterol is also increased in patients with cholestasis. Cholestasis is characteristic of metastatic infiltrates in the liver and of granulomatous infiltrates (tuberculosis, histoplasmosis, sarcoidosis) and hepatic abscess(es).

d. Are the metabolic functions of the liver compromised? Measure plasma PT and serum albumin.

Determination of decreased synthesis of proteins, especially serum albumin and the plasma coagulation factors, is a sensitive test for metabolic derangement of the liver. Measurement of serum albumin by protein electrophoresis is more accurate than dye-binding methods such as using bromcresol green because bromcresol green reacts with alpha and beta globulins, resulting in overestimation of albumin when these globulins are high (e.g., with nephrotic syndrome). Determining plasma PT is a good test to assess plasma coagulation factors that are synthesized by the liver. In patients with hepatocellular damage a low serum albumin level suggests decreased protein synthesis, and a significantly prolonged PT indicates a poor prognosis.

e. Is the disease process acute or chronic? Measure serum globulins.

Most acute liver diseases do not cause a significant increase of serum globulins, but chronic liver diseases commonly show a polyclonal increase of gamma globulins (>3 g/dL [>30 g/L]). Measurement of gamma globulins by protein electrophoresis is especially useful to assess whether the liver disease is acute or chronic. For example, with chronic hepatitis and cirrhosis, polyclonal gammapathy or diffuse hypergammaglobulinemia are common findings.

3. If one or more test results are abnormal, liver disease may be present. Analyze the pattern of abnormalities for clues about the type of liver disease. Consider drug-related liver disease.

The best method for diagnosing liver disease is microscopic examination of a liver biopsy. Serum tests provide indirect information about hepatic pathophysiology. Although there is a great deal of overlap, four major patterns of liver function test results can occur:

• Acute hepatitis pattern: significantly increased serum transaminase values with varying abnormalities of other liver function tests
• Cirrhosis pattern: decreased albumin, polyclonal gammapathy or diffuse hypergammaglobulinemia, often with beta-gamma bridging, and prolonged PT with varying abnormalities of other liver function tests
• Chronic hepatitis pattern: combinations of the first two patterns
• Obstructive liver disease pattern: increased ALP and bilirubin, with varying abnormalities of other liver function test results

Drug-related liver disease can take the form of acute hepatitis, chronic hepatitis, cirrhosis, and obstructive liver disease and therefore can show any of the above patterns. Drugs that can induce jaundice follow*:

Hepatocellular injury

Acetaminophen
Acetohexamide (Dymelor)
Bleomycin (Blenoxane)
Carbenicillin (Geocillin)
Chlorambucil (Leukeran)
Clindamycin (Cleocin)
Colchicine
Cyclophosphamide (Cytoxan)
Emetine
Ketoconazole (Nizoral)
Methimazole (Tapazole)
Methotrexate (Folex, Rheumatrex)
Methyldopa (Aldomet)
Mithramycin (Mithracin)
Mitomycin (Mutamycin)
Monoamine oxidase inhibitors
Niacin (Nicobid)
Phenazopyridine (Pyridium)
Propylthiouracil
Pyrazinamide
Quinidine (Quinaglute, Quinidex)
Salicylates
Sulfasalazine (Azulfidine)
Tamoxifen (Nolvadex)

Cholestatic injury

Aminosalicylic acid
Amitriptyline (Elavil, Endep)
Androgens
Azathioprine (Imuran)
Benzodiazepines
Busulfan (Myleran)
Captopril (Capoten)
Carbamazepine (Tegretol)
Carisoprodol (Soma)
Chloramphenicol (Chloromycetin)
Chlordiazepoxide (Librium)
Chlorpropamide (Diabinese)
Chlorthalidone (Hygroton)
Diazepam (Valium)
Disopyramide (Norpace)
Disulfiram (Antabuse)
Erythromycin estolate (Ilosone)
Erythromycin ethylsuccinate (E.E.S.)
Estrogens
Ethambutol (Myambutol)
Flurazepam (Dalmane)
Griseofulvin (Fulvicin, Grifulvin, Grisactin)
Mercaptopurine (Purinethol)
Nifedipine (Adalat, Procardia)
Oral contraceptives
Oxacillin (Bactocill, Prostaphlin)
Penicillamine (Cuprimine, Depen)
Phenobarbital
Phenothiazines
Progestins
Propoxyphene (Darvon)
Thiabendazole (Mintezol)
Thiazides
Tolazamide (Tolinase)
Tolbutamide (Orinase)
Trimethoprim
Troleandomycin (Tao)
Verapamil (Calan, Isoptin)
Warfarin (Coumadin, Panwarfin)

Both hepatocellular and cholestatic injury

Allopurinol (Zyloprim)
Cimetidine (Tagamet)
Dantrolene (Dantrium)
Dapsone
Gold sodium thiomalate (Myochrysine)
Haloperidol (Haldol)
Hydralazine (Apresoline)
Inhalation anesthetics
Isoniazid (INH, Laniazid, Nydrazid)
Nitrofurantoin (Furadantin, Macrodantin)
Nonsteroidal anti-inflammatory drugs
Phenytoin (Dilantin)
Rifampin (Rifadin, Rimactane)
Sulfonamides
Tetracyclines
Tricylic antidepressants

*Source: McKnight JT, Jones JE: Jaundice. Am Fam Physician 45(3):1142, March 1992. Published by the American Academy of Family Physicians.

Remember that there are tissue sources other than the liver for increased serum transaminase and ALP values. High transaminase values can originate in heart, pancreas, and skeletal muscle, and high ALP values can originate in bone, intestines, and placenta.

4. If the liver function test results are all normal, the liver is probably normal—the level of confidence is higher if serum GGT values are also normal.

Normal results for liver function tests are good evidence against liver disease, and if serum GGT values are also normal, the probability of liver disease is very low indeed, perhaps only 1% to 2%. Still, a liver disorder occasionally is present with normal liver function test results—a common example is fatty liver. Excretion tests (e.g., sulfobromphthalein [Bromsulphalein]) are obsolete.

5. In patients with persistently increased liver enzyme values who are otherwise well (discovered during blood donation or routine health checks), perform a thorough evaluation and consider a liver biopsy.

In studies of this clinical situation the most common abnormality was fatty liver. Other disorders in decreasing order of frequency included non-cirrhotic alcoholic liver disease; chronic active (viral) hepatitis; chronic persistent hepatitis; cirrhosis; hemochromatosis; granulomatous liver disease; and autoimmune liver disease. Drug-related hepatitis was rare. Several hematological, biochemical, and serological tests may further aid the diagnosis: mean red cell volume (MCV); serum iron, transferrin, ferritin, ceruloplasmin, and α_1-antitrypsin levels; smooth muscle, antimitochondrial, and antinuclear antibodies; immunoglobulins; and markers for hepatitis A, B, and C. Ultrasonography should be done to exclude infiltrative liver disease and extrahepatic abnormalities. Ultrasound and isotope scans, CT, or magnetic resonance imaging (MRI) techniques are of little value in differentiating the major forms of parenchymal liver disease. Liver biopsy is essential for the evaluation of a patient with persistently (>6 months) increased enzymes. Asymptomatic individuals with threefold to eightfold increased transaminase values frequently have chronic active hepatitis and often cirrhosis.

6. If you intend to perform a percutaneous liver biopsy (mortality rate, 0.01%), remember to exclude a bleeding disorder and other contraindications.

A negative history of unusual bleeding after surgery, previous biopsies, or dental work plus normal or only mildly abnormal tests for coagulation exclude a significant bleeding disorder. Minimal acceptable guidelines include a PT no more than 4 seconds greater than midrange normal, an activated partial thromboplastin time (APTT) no more than 9 seconds greater than midrange normal, a platelet count $>50 \times 10^3/\mu L$ ($50 \times 10^9/L$), and a normal bleeding time. Aspirin and other nonsteroidal anti-inflammatory agents can prolong the bleeding time and, ideally, should be omitted for approximately 1-2 weeks before the test. Correction of any coagulation abnormality should be undertaken before biopsy. Other relative contraindications to biopsy include lack of patient cooperation, ascites, and right lower lobe pneumonia.

7.   In patients with liver disease with clinical findings of hepatic failure (hepatorenal syndrome, hepatic encephalopathy), request determinations of serum urea nitrogen, creatinine, and urine sodium together with arterial blood ammonia.

Ordinary liver function tests may not be useful to monitor hepatic failure (e.g., the serum transaminase level may be low in a patient with massive hepatic necrosis because the hepatic cell transaminase content has been exhausted). Rising serum urea nitrogen and creatinine values and falling urinary volume and sodium excretion characterize the renal failure of the hepatorenal syndrome as intrarenal shunting deprives the renal cortex of blood. Because these findings do not differentiate the hepatorenal syndrome from prerenal azotemia, patients should be initially treated as though they had prerenal azotemia. Although blood ammonia, short-chain fatty acids, false neurotransmitters, and amino acids have been implicated as the cause of hepatic encephalopathy, determination of arterial blood ammonia is the only widely available test to diagnose this syndrome.

BIBLIOGRAPHY

Frank BB, Members of the Patient Care Committee of the American Gastroenterological Association: Clinical evaluation of jaundice: A guideline of the Patient Care Committee of the American Gastroenterological Association. JAMA 262:3031, 1989.
Recommendations for the workup of patients with jaundice.
Hay JE, Czaja AJ, Rakela J, et al: The nature of unexplained chronic aminotransferase elevations of a mild to moderate degree in asymptomatic patients. Hepatology 9:193, 1989.
Asymptomatic patients with mildly to moderately increased aminotransferase values frequently have chronic active hepatitis and often cirrhosis.
Kassirer JP, Kopelman RI: Case 13—A picture is worth a thousand words. In Learning Clinical Reasoning. Baltimore, Williams & Wilkins, 1991, p 97.
Discusses clinical reasoning in a patient with alcoholic liver disease and the hepatorenal syndrome.
Kothur R, Marsh F Jr, Posner G: Liver function tests in nonparenteral cocaine users. Arch Intern Med 151:1126, 1991.
Minimally increased liver enzymes are common in nonparenteral cocaine users without evidence of severe hepatotoxicity.
Kumar S, Rex DK: Failure of physicians to recognize acetaminophen hepatotoxicity in chronic alcoholics. Arch Intern Med 151:1189, 1991.
High index of suspicion is necessary to detect acetaminophen-related hepatitis in alcoholics.
McKnight JT, Jones JE: Jaundice. Am Fam Physician 45:1139, 1992.
Good discussion of the differential diagnosis and management of jaundice.
McVay PA, Toy P: Lack of increased bleeding after liver biopsy in patients with mild hemostatic abnormalities. Am J Clin Pathol 94:747, 1990.
Mildly abnormal platelet count, PT, and APTT do not increase the risk of bleeding after liver biopsy.

Sherman KE: Alanine aminotransferase in clinical practice. Arch Intern Med 151:260, 1991.

Reviews the biochemistry and clinical relevance of alanine aminotransferase in patient care.

Speicher CE, Widish JR, Gaudot FJ, et al: An evaluation of the overestimation of serum albumin by bromcresol green. Am J Clin Pathol 69:347, 1978.

Bromcresol green reacts with alpha and beta globulins. This can cause overestimation of albumin when these globulins are high (e.g., with nephrotic syndrome).

Van Ness MM, Diehl AM: Is liver biopsy useful in the evaluation of patients with chronically elevated liver enzymes? Ann Intern Med 111:473, 1989.

The higher the liver enzyme values (AST, ALT, GGT), the more accurate is the noninvasive diagnosis, but liver biopsy ensures maximal diagnostic accuracy.

What's up with the enzymes? Lancet 335:140, 1990. Editorial.

Outlines the most common diagnoses in patients with increased liver enzymes and encourages performance of a liver biopsy.

Acute Viral Hepatitis

1. For patients with clinical findings and liver function test results of acute viral hepatitis, request serological tests for hepatitis A, B, and C; namely, anti-hepatitis A IgM antibody, hepatitis B surface antigen, anti-hepatitis B core IgM antibody, and anti-hepatitis C antibody. Reserve anti-hepatitis D antibody and hepatitis B e antigen testing for patients who are positive for hepatitis B. Another cause of viral hepatitis, for which there is no test, is hepatitis E. In certain individuals screening for viral hepatitis is appropriate.

The Centers for Disease Control (CDC) recommends prenatal screening for hepatitis B, and the American Academy of Pediatrics recommends hepatitis B vaccine for all normal newborns. Moreover, there is a growing trend to screen health care workers for immunity to common infectious diseases, including viral hepatitis, and to immunize those workers who are at risk. In the United States, effective in early 1992, the Occupational Safety and Health Administration (OSHA) required employers to make available the hepatitis B vaccine and vaccination series to all employees who have occupational exposure. The first hepatitis A vaccine was recently licensed in Europe, and a vaccine may be available in the United States by 1994.

The following clues about different varieties of viral hepatitis are helpful. Hepatitis A has fecal and oral transmission, a 20- to 37-day incubation period, and up to a 45% prevalence in some groups in the United States, whereas hepatitis B has percutaneous or venereal transmission, a 60- to 110-day incubation period, and up to a 5% to 15% prevalence in some groups in the United States. The transmission of hepatitis C resembles that of hepatitis B, whereas the transmission of hepatitis E resembles that of hepatitis A. Hepatitis C causes most cases of posttransfusion hepatitis.

Testing for hepatitis D should not be done unless it has been determined the patient has hepatitis B and a deteriorating clinical condition caused by hepatitis. One other hepatitis A test is for anti-hepatitis A IgG antibody. Its presence indicates a hepatitis A infection in the remote past. Several other tests for hepatitis B are available—those for anti-hepatitis B surface antibody, anti-hepatitis B core IgG antibody, hepatitis B e antigen, and anti-hepatitis B e antibody. These other tests for hepatitis B are useful only after it has been determined that a patient has hepatitis B since they can help to answer three questions: (1) when was the infection resolved; (2) what is the risk that this patient may infect others; and (3) when did the infection become chronic? A second-generation antibody test for hepatitis C has recently been approved, which has a sensitivity of approximately 54% in patients with acute hepatitis C.

The serum AST (SGOT) and ALT (SGPT) values are usually increased from 600 to 5000 U/L or more, but <500 U/L may occur in mild illness. Usually the ALT exceeds the AST. The magnitude of the transaminase increase is not well correlated with the severity of liver damage. Serum bilirubin is commonly increased from 5 to 20 mg/dL (85 to 342 μmol/L); values >30 mg/dL (513 μmol/L) suggest severe disease or hemolysis. ALP is slightly increased but may be markedly increased in the presence of severe cholestasis. Serum gamma globulins may be slightly increased: concentrations >3 g/dL (30 g/L) suggest chronic disease. Decreased serum albumin and a prolonged PT reflect impairment of liver protein synthesis and parallel the severity of the disease. A PT >20 seconds suggests the development of acute hepatic insufficiency.

2.   Evaluate the serological test results.

VIRAL SEROLOGICAL TESTS IN ACUTE HEPATITIS

TYPE OF HEPATITIS	DIAGNOSTIC SEROLOGICAL TESTS RESULTS
A	Anti-hepatitis A IgM antibody *positive*
	Hepatitis B surface antigen *positive**
	Anti-hepatitis B core IgM antibody *negative*
	or
	Hepatitis B surface antigen *positive*
	Anti-hepatitis B core IgM antibody *positive*
	or
	Hepatitis B surface antigen *negative*
B	Anti-hepatitis B core IgM antibody *positive*
	Anti-hepatitis C antibody *positive*
C	(confirm with supplemental assay)
D	Anti-hepatitis D antibody *positive*

*Vaccination causes a positive test for hepatitis B surface antibody but does not cause a positive test for hepatitis B surface antigen.

The serological profile for acute hepatitis B follows:

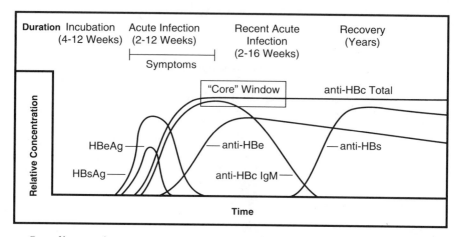

Serodiagnostic assessment of acute viral hepatitis. (Source: Abbott Diagnostics Educational Services, Abbott Laboratories, Abbott Park, Ill, January 1990.) Key: HBsAg = hepatitis B surface antigen; HBeAg = hepatitis B e antigen; anti-HBe = antibody to hepatitis B e antigen; anti-HBc IgM = antibody (IgM) to core antigen; anti-HBc total = total antibody (IgG and IgM) to core antigen; anti-HBs = antibody to hepatitis B surface antigen.

If hepatitis B becomes chronic, hepatitis B surface antigen persists and antibody to hepatitis B surface antigen does not develop. Hepatitis B may be complicated by hepatitis D. A hepatitis D infection can occur as a coinfection with hepatitis B or can be superimposed on a preexisting hepatitis B infection.

In an individual with hepatitis B, hepatitis B surface antigen initially appears approximately 4 to 12 weeks after exposure, followed by anti-hepatitis B core IgM antibody a little later, and anti-hepatitis B surface IgG antibody still later. There is a time period when hepatitis B surface antigen disappears and anti-hepatitis B surface IgG antibody has not yet appeared during which anti-hepatitis B core IgM antibody may be the only positive diagnostic test result (the "core" window). During the first 2 weeks of symptoms, hepatitis B surface antigen is more sensitive than the test for anti-hepatitis B core IgM antibody, but this is reversed 2 weeks after the onset of symptoms. The test for anti-hepatitis B core IgM antibody is better than the hepatitis B surface antigen test for detecting hepatitis B in the asymptomatic patient. There may be times when hepatitis B surface antigen and anti-hepatitis B core IgM antibody are present simultaneously or anti-hepatitis B core IgM antibody and anti-hepatitis B surface antibody IgG are present simultaneously. Almost all patients with acute hepatitis B have titers of anti-hepatitis B core IgM antibody at the time of initial examination, whereas chronic carriers of the virus may have only low titers or no detectable anti-hepatitis B core IgM antibody at all.

Posttransfusion non-A, non-B hepatitis is nearly always due to hepatitis C. Diagnosis is established by a positive anti-hepatitis C antibody test. In patients with clinical findings of hepatitis C and a negative anti-hepatitis C antibody test, repeat the test at 3 and 6 months.

Hepatitis D is diagnosed by the presence of anti-hepatitis D antibody. The usual clinical situation is that of a patient with chronic, asymptomatic, or acute hepatitis B who suddenly becomes markedly worse clinically. In some of these patients the level of hepatitis B surface antigenemia drops precipitously. However, even in these patients, anti-hepatitis B core positivity remains. A characteristic biphasic aminotransferase elevation may result from the sequential infection of hepatitis B followed by hepatitis D.

Hepatitis E is a diagnosis of exclusion since there is no available test. ALT may be used as a surrogate test.

3. If hepatitis B surface antigen or anti-hepatitis B core IgM antibody or both are present, diagnose acute hepatitis B and request testing for hepatitis B e antigen and anti-hepatitis B e antibody. If anti-hepatitis A IgM antibody is present, diagnose hepatitis A. If anti-hepatitis C antibody is present, consider a supplemental assay for specificity. The presence of anti-hepatitis C antibody indicates acute, chronic, or resolved hepatitis C infection.

The presence of hepatitis B e antigen indicates patients who are very infectious and much more likely to infect others than patients who are simply hepatitis B surface antigen positive without e antigen. If anti-hepatitis B e antibody is present, the hepatitis is beginning to resolve. If hepatitis C is suspected and the test for anti-hepatitis C antibody is negative, the test should be repeated at 3 and 6 months. First-generation tests for anti-hepatitis C antibody have produced not only false-negative results but also false-positive results. Second-generation tests for anti-hepatitis C antibody are about 54% sensitive. If possible, patients with a positive anti-hepatitis C antibody should have the diagnosis confirmed with a supplemental assay (e.g., a recombinant immunoblot assay in a reference laboratory). Patients with a confirmed positive test should be evaluated to determine whether they have acute, chronic, or resolved hepatitis C.

4. If diagnostic test results for hepatitis A, hepatitis B, hepatitis C, and hepatitis D are negative, consider other causes of an acute viral hepatitis-like syndrome.

Other causes of an acute viral hepatitis-like syndrome that should be considered include acute cholangitis, ischemic liver injury, drug-related hepatitis, syphilis, acute exacerbation of underlying chronic hepatitis, and several miscellaneous viral infections.

Hepatitis E

Hepatitis E may occur sporadically but is probably rare in the United States. Since there are no specific serological tests for hepatitis E, the diagnosis relies on clinical findings and surrogate test results such as increased ALT. Like hepatitis A, hepatitis E does not progress to chronic disease.

Epstein-Barr Hepatitis

Consider Epstein-Barr hepatitis (often part of the infectious mononucleosis syndrome) with these findings: nausea and vomiting, jaundice, and increased serum transaminase values. The presence of heterophil antibodies (positive Monospot test) or a rise in titer of specific antibodies to Epstein-Barr virus confirms the diagnosis.

Cytomegalovirus Hepatitis

Consider cytomegalovirus hepatitis (sometimes as part of an infectious mononucleosis syndrome without adenopathy or tonsillopharyngeal involvement) in patients with clinical and laboratory findings of mild acute hepatitis. Infection can be demonstrated by inoculation of appropriate tissue culture with urine or an increase in complement-fixation or indirect hemagglutination titers after an attack.

Herpes Virus Hepatitis

Consider hepatitis caused by herpes simplex or varicella virus in patients with clinical and laboratory findings of acute hepatitis, often accompanied by typical skin lesions in immunocompromised patients. Presence of herpetic skin lesions demonstrable by a Tzanck test does not necessarily mean that the hepatitis is caused by a herpes virus.

Paramyxovirus Hepatitis

Consider paramyxovirus hepatitis in patients with severe hepatitis of unknown cause in which the liver biopsy shows replacement of liver cells by syncytial giant cells.

5.   After diagnosing acute viral hepatitis, begin therapy and monitor the patient's progress, using chemical and serological (immunological) test results.

For acute hepatitis A there is no carrier state or possibility of chronic hepatitis, so serological monitoring of these patients is not necessary.

For acute hepatitis B serological monitoring is mandatory. Anti-hepatitis B core IgG antibody appears before hepatitis B surface IgG antibody and persists throughout life. It is the best single marker of exposure to hepatitis B virus. To determine when the infection has resolved, test for hepatitis B surface IgG antibody monthly. If by 6 months after the acute episode the patient is no longer hepatitis B surface antigen positive and is anti-hepatitis B surface IgG antibody positive, the patient has eliminated the virus, and a full and complete recovery has occurred. Such a patient will have no chronic sequelae and can no longer infect others. After 1 to 23 months anti-hepatitis B surface antibody may be lost, but anti-hepatitis B core antibody always persists. For patients who are hepatitis B e antigen positive, test for anti-hepatitis B e antibody monthly because the appearance of anti-hepatitis B e antibody indicates when the patient is less infectious to others. In patients who do not develop anti-hepatitis B surface IgG antibody, the finding of two positive hepatitis B surface antigen results 6 months or more apart indicates chronic hepatitis (approximately 10% of acute hepatitis B patients develop chronic hepatitis). If there is no clinical and laboratory evidence of hepatitis, the patient is termed a *chronic carrier* (more often in men than women). If laboratory or biopsy evidence of hepatitis is present, the diagnosis is termed *chronic persistent hepatitis* or *chronic active hepatitis*, depending on the histological findings. Patients with chronic active hepatitis may develop cirrhosis and hepatoma.

The ALT value may be used to follow the course of acute viral hepatitis because it is often the last test to return to normal. This test is especially helpful in following patients with hepatitis C in whom 50% to 70% persistently have enzyme abnormalities after 6 months duration (i.e., they develop chronic hepatitis).

6.   In patients with acute viral hepatitis in addition to abnormal liver function tests, the following abnormal blood test results may occur:

↓ **Hemoglobin and hematocrit,** mild and transient; rarely, aplastic anemia.

↑ **Platelets** in fulminant disease.

↓ **Glucose,** often mild and insignificant; profound hypoglycemia can occur in fulminant hepatitis.

↑ **Lactate dehydrogenase** from hepatocellular damage.

↑ **Lymphocytes** and atypical lymphocytes; mild leukocytosis may occur.

↑ **Uric acid** related to hepatocellular damage.

↑ **Amylase** with concurrent pancreatitis.

↓ **Cholesterol** from decreased liver synthesis; degree parallels severity of hepatitis.

BIBLIOGRAPHY

Abbott Laboratories Diagnostics Division: Enzyme immunoassay for the qualitative detection of antibody to hepatitis C virus (anti-HCV) in human serum or plasma. Abbott Laboratories, Abbott Park, Ill, April 1992. Package Insert.
Technical and clinical information about a second-generation test for anti-hepatitis C antibody.
Arvan DA: Acute viral hepatitis. In Panzer RJ, Black ER, Griner PF (eds): Diagnostic Strategies for Common Medical Problems. Philadelphia, American College of Physicians, 1991, p 141.
Suggests strategies for the differential diagnosis of acute hepatitis.
Barnes HV: Viral hepatitis. In Spivak JL, Barnes HV (eds): Manual of Clinical Problems in Internal Medicine, 4th ed. Boston, Little, Brown & Co, 1990, p 272.
Good discussion of diagnosis and management with annotated key references.

Brodell RT, Helms SE, Devine M: Office dermatologic testing: The Tzanck preparation. Am Fam Physician 44:857, 1991.
Describes how to do a Tzanck preparation.

Consensus on HCV Testing and Treatment, 1992. Advanced Therapeutic Communications, 400 Plaza Drive, Secaucus, NJ 07094.
Summarizes consensus statements and algorithms of the National Hepatitis Detection and Treatment Program for hepatitis C.

Eng TR, Borges ML, Harlin VK, et al: Screening for hepatitis B during pregnancy: Awareness of current recommendations among Washington hospitals. West J Med 155:613, 1991.
CDC recommends prenatal HBsAg screening of all women or, for women who do not have a history of prenatal care, screening at the time of delivery.

Ergun GA, Miskovitz PF: Viral hepatitis: The new ABS's. Postgrad Med 88:69, 1990.
Reviews the different kinds of viral hepatitis, including clinical and laboratory features.

Harrison PM, Lau JYN, Williams R: Hepatology. Postgrad Med J 67:719, 1991.
Reviews the diagnosis and management of viral hepatitis.

Hepatitis A: A vaccine at last. Lancet 339:1198, 1992. Editorial.
Reports the availability of a hepatitis A vaccine in Europe.

Hoofnagle JH, Di Bisceglie AM: Serologic diagnosis of acute and chronic hepatitis. Semin Liver Dis 11:73, 1991.
Reviews the serological diagnosis of viral hepatitis.

Katkov WN, Ault MJ, Dubin SB: Absence of hepatitis B surface antigenemia after vaccination. Arch Pathol Lab Med 113:1290, 1989.
Positive hepatitis B surface antigen should not be attributed to vaccination.

Phillips MJ, Blendis LM, Poucell S, et al: Syncytial giant-cell hepatitis: Sporadic hepatitis with distinctive pathological features, a severe clinical course, and paramyxoviral features. N Engl J Med 324:455, 1991.
Describes 10 cases of a new form of hepatitis that occurred in Toronto.

Tedder RS, Gilson RCJ, Briggs M, et al: Hepatitis C virus: Evidence for sexual transmission. BMJ 302:1299, 1991.
Provides strong evidence that hepatitis C can be transmitted through both sexual contact and blood transfusions.

Fatty Liver and Alcoholic Hepatitis

1. In patients with clinical findings and liver function test results of fatty liver or alcoholic hepatitis, to accurately diagnose the lesion, consider a needle biopsy of the liver.

Alcohol abuse causes three main pathological lesions: fatty liver, alcoholic hepatitis, and cirrhosis. Patients may have clinical features particular to each of these lesions or mixed clinical findings caused by combinations of these pathological lesions. Often the patient can be treated without a liver biopsy; however, if the clinical findings are severe enough to require an accurate diagnosis, a biopsy is appropriate.

In fatty liver the AST value may be normal to modestly increased, up to 400 U/L (ratio of AST to ALT is often $\geq 2:1$). Increased serum bilirubin values to 5 mg/dL (85 μmol/L) may occur with mildly increased ALP. Occasionally intense cholestasis develops. Serum albumin and globulin values are abnormal in approximately 25% of patients, and serum GGT is usually increased. Mild anemia and leukocytosis may occur. An increased GGT level, by itself, may not warrant a liver biopsy. Occasionally severe fatty liver may be the only significant finding in sudden unexpected death.

In patients with alcoholic hepatitis there are fever and leukocytosis that may exceed 30 to 40 × 10^3 cells/μL (30 to 40 × 10^9 cells/L). Regarding the liver, the AST may be increased to 600 U/L, and AST is usually higher than ALT. Frequently, the AST is more than twice as high as ALT. A high AST:ALT ratio may also occur in nonhepatic disease such as acute myocardial infarction, skeletal muscle necrosis, hemolysis, renal necrosis, and cerebral necrosis. Serum bilirubin and ALP levels may increase moderately, and a small percentage of patients develops a cholestatic picture, with high bilirubin (up to 30 mg/dL [513 μmol/L]) and high ALP levels as the predominant abnormalities. Prolongation of the PT, hypoalbuminemia, and hyperglobulinemia may be present.

2.   Evaluate the tests.

The best method for the diagnosis of fatty liver and alcoholic hepatitis is microscopic examination of a liver biopsy.

3.   If a liver biopsy shows fatty change of the large droplet variety, it is consistent with the fatty liver of alcohol abuse.

Large-droplet fatty change is not specific for alcohol abuse but may be seen in other conditions such as obesity, protein-calorie malnutrition (e.g., kwashiorkor, jejunoileal bypass), and/or diabetes mellitus. The lesion may also be caused by corticosteroids, methotrexate, and perhexilene. Alcoholic fatty liver is reversible if the patient stops drinking.

4.   If a liver biopsy shows hepatocellular necrosis with infiltration by polymorphonuclear leukocytes, the findings are consistent with alcoholic hepatitis.

The essential feature of alcoholic hepatitis is hepatocellular necrosis and infiltration by polymorphonuclear leukocytes. Alcoholic hyalin may be present or absent. Fibrosis may be present within the lobule and around the central vein where it can cause obstruction of blood flow and portal hypertension. Patients with alcoholic hepatitis may develop the hepatorenal syndrome—rising serum urea nitrogen and creatinine levels indicate a poor prognosis, and these patients may develop cirrhosis. Amiodarone toxicity can simulate alcoholic hepatitis.

BIBLIOGRAPHY

Ireland A, Hartley L, Ryley N, et al: Raised gamma-glutamyltransferase activity and the need for liver biopsy. BMJ 302:388, 1991.
   Isolated increase in GGT by itself may not be enough to warrant a liver biopsy.
Lieber CS, Guadagnini KS: The spectrum of alcoholic liver disease. Hosp Pract 25:51, 1990.
   Good discussion of the pathophysiology of alcoholic liver disease, including fatty liver, early fibrosis, alcoholic hepatitis, and cirrhosis.

Zakim D, Boyer TD: Hepatology: A Textbook of Liver Disease, 2nd ed. Philadelphia, WB
Saunders Co, 1990.
Good discussion of fatty liver and alcoholic hepatitis.

Acute Nonviral, Nonalcoholic Hepatitis

**In patients with clinical findings and liver function test results of acute
hepatitis in whom acute viral hepatitis and alcoholic hepatitis have been
excluded, consider hepatitis caused by drugs, toxins, heart failure, hepatic
vein occlusion, and Reye's syndrome.**

All of these kinds of hepatitis may be confused with acute viral hepatitis
because of similar clinical and laboratory findings such as an increased serum
transaminase level. Since there are few specific diagnostic tests, diagnosis
often depends on a careful analysis of the history, physical examination,
laboratory findings, and results of other studies.

DRUG-RELATED HEPATITIS

Consider drug-related hepatitis in patients with these findings: clinical and
chemical evidence of acute hepatitis and onset of hepatitis 2 to 6 weeks after
starting drug therapy (but may occur as early as the first day or not until 6
months later). The hepatitis may progress even after drug withdrawal, and
failure to withdraw the offending drug can cause death. Almost any drug
can occasionally cause unpredictable hepatitis. Older patients and women
appear more susceptible. Acetaminophen can cause hepatitis, especially in
alcoholics—acetylcysteine treatment is safe and effective even in later stages
of poisoning.

See the preceeding discussion of jaundice and liver function tests for
drugs that can induce jaundice.

Examples of different types of drug-related liver disease follow:

TISSUE REACTION	EXAMPLES	TISSUE REACTION	EXAMPLES
Microvesicular fat	Tetracycline	Macrovesicular fat	Methotrexate
	Salicylates		Perhexiline
Cholestasis	Chlorpromazine		Ethanol
(with or without hepatocellular injury)	Sex steroids, including oral contraceptives	Centrilobular necrosis	Acetaminophen
			Halothane
		Massive necrosis	Halothane
Hepatitis, acute to chronic	Isoniazid		Acetaminophen
	Oxyphenisatin		Alpha-methyldopa
	Alpha-methyldopa	Fibrosis-cirrhosis	Methotrexate
	Nitrofurantoin		Cinchophen
	Phenytoin		Amiodarone
	Cinchophen	Veno-occlusive disease	Cytotoxic drugs

Tissue Reaction	Examples	Tissue Reaction	Examples
Granuloma formation	Sulfonamides Alpha-methyl-dopa Quinidine Phenylbutazone Hydralazine Allopurinol	Hepatic or portal vein thrombosis Focal nodular hyperplasia	Estrogens, including oral contraceptives ?C-17 alkylated steroids, including oral contraceptives
Adenoma	Oral contraceptives		
Hepatocellular carcinoma	?Anabolic steroids, oral contraceptives		

*Source: Cotran RS, Kumar V, Robbins SL: The liver and biliary tract. In Robbins Pathologic Basis of Disease, 4th ed. Philadelphia, WB Saunders, 1989, p 963.

Toxic Hepatitis

Consider toxic hepatitis in patients with severe acute hepatitis who were exposed to poisoning such as carbon tetrachloride or the wild mushroom *Amanita phalloides*. The mortality rate is high.

Heart-Failure Hepatitis

Consider heart-failure hepatitis in patients with increased serum transaminase values up to thousands of units per liter and sometimes jaundice. These patients may have marked hypotension, shock, or severe acute congestive heart failure.

Hepatic Vein—Occlusion Hepatitis

Consider hepatic vein—occlusion hepatitis (Budd-Chiari syndrome) in patients with these findings: acute abdominal pain, tender hepatomegaly, ascites, and liver function test results consistent with acute hepatitis. Causes include polycythemia vera, pregnancy, the postpartum state, the use of oral contraceptives, paroxysmal nocturnal hemoglobinuria, and intra-abdominal cancers, particularly hepatocellular carcinoma.

Reye's Syndrome

Consider Reye's syndrome in children with these findings: sudden onset of intractable vomiting a few days after a viral illness, history of aspirin ingestion, cloudy sensorium, seizures, coma, enlarged liver, hypoglycemia, and abnormal liver function tests. Liver biopsy reveals fatty change of the small-droplet variety, with little or no inflammation. Small-droplet fatty change may also occur in patients with acute fatty liver of pregnancy, Jamaican vomiting sickness, drug (tetracycline and valproic acid) hepatotoxicity, and occasionally ethanol ingestion.

BIBILIOGRAPHY

Cohen JA, Kaplan MM: Left-sided heart failure presenting as hepatitis. Gastroenterology 74:583, 1978.
Discusses several cases of heart-failure hepatitis that presented as a viral—hepatitis-like syndrome.

Keays R, Harrison PM, Wendon JA, et al: Intravenous acetylcysteine in paracetamol induced fulminant hepatic failure: A prospective controlled trial. BMJ 303:1026, 1991.
Acetylcysteine therapy is effective even in late stages of poisoning.

Kothur R, Marsh F Jr, Posner G: Liver function tests in nonparenteral cocaine users. Arch Intern Med 151:1126, 1991.
Minimally increased liver enzymes are common in nonparenteral cocaine users, without evidence of severe hepatotoxicity.

Kumar S, Rex DK: Failure of physicians to recognize acetaminophen hepatotoxicity in chronic alcoholics. Arch Intern Med 151:1189, 1991.
High index of suspicion is necessary to detect acetaminophen-related hepatitis in alcoholics.

Zakim D, Boyer TD: Hepatology: A Textbook of Liver Disease, 2nd ed. Philadelphia, WB Saunders Co, 1990.
Good discussion of nonviral, nonalcoholic liver disease.

Chronic Persistent and Chronic Active Hepatitis

1. For patients with clinical findings and liver function test results of chronic hepatitis, request serological tests for viral hepatitis (namely, hepatitis B surface antigen and anti-hepatitis C antibody). To diagnose the lesion accurately, consider performing a needle biopsy of the liver.

Chronic hepatitis is caused by viruses, drugs, unusual metabolic diseases such as α_1-antitrypsin deficiency and Wilson's disease, alcoholic liver disease, and unknown factors. Primary biliary cirrhosis and primary sclerosing cholangitis may be confused with chronic hepatitis.

When chronic hepatitis follows acute hepatitis, persistence longer than 6 months can be used to make the diagnosis. Sometimes, however, the disease begins insidiously, or the problem may arise when an apparently healthy person is found to have a high serum transaminase value by laboratory screening or a positive serological test for hepatitis is discovered when an individual attempts to donate blood. In these latter instances, a polyclonal gammopathy or diffuse hypergammaglobulinemia on serum protein electrophoresis may be a clue that the patient has chronic hepatitis.

In a patient with chronic persistent hepatitis serum transaminase values may vary from normal to moderately increased (40 to 200 U/L), and the values may fluctuate. Serum ALP and bilirubin levels may be normal to slightly increased, and serum albumin values and the plasma PT are usually normal. Moderately increased gamma globulins up to approximately 2 g/dL (20 g/L) may be seen. Antinuclear antibodies (ANAs) are usually absent, and the lupus erythematosus (LE) cell preparation is negative.

In patients with chronic active hepatitis serum transaminase values >400 U/L are common, with possible increases to much higher levels, usually occurring during exacerbations of the disease. Serum ALP may be increased, and bilirubin levels of 3 to 10 mg/dL (51 to 171 μmol/L) or more commonly occur. Decreased serum albumin values and a prolonged PT may occur, and the degree of abnormality parallels the severity of the disease process. Serum globulins are commonly increased and may reach the 3 to 7 g/dl (30 to 70 g/L) range. Positive ANAs are frequently found, and the LE cell preparation is positive in 10% to 20% of patients.

2.   Evaluate the tests.

The best method for the diagnosis of chronic hepatitis and the differentiation of chronic persistent hepatitis from chronic active hepatitis is microscopic examination of a liver biopsy.

With the exception of α_1-antitrypsin deficiency, the cause of chronic active hepatitis cannot be determined from the histology. Periodic acid-Schiff (PAS) reaction-positive material in hepatocytes after diastase treatment is characteristic of α_1-antitrypsin deficiency. Copper stains for Wilson's disease are often unreliable.

VIRAL SEROLOGICAL TESTS IN CHRONIC HEPATITIS

TYPE OF HEPATITIS	DIAGNOSTIC SEROLOGICAL TEST RESULTS
B	Hepatitis B surface antigen *positive*
C	Anti-hepatitis C antibody *positive* (confirm with supplemental assay)
D	Hepatitis B surface antigen *positive* Anti-hepatitis D antibody *positive*

3.   If a liver biopsy shows chronic active hepatitis, determine its cause so that appropriate therapy may be chosen. If serological test results are positive for hepatitis B, request tests for anti-hepatitis B core IgM antibody, hepatitis B e antigen, and anti-hepatitis D antibody if appropriate. If anti-hepatitis C antibody is present, consider a supplemental assay for specificity.

Approximately 20% of cases of chronic active hepatitis are associated with and probably caused by hepatitis B with or without superimposed hepatitis D infection. In contrast to patients with acute hepatitis B who have high titers of anti-hepatitis B core IgM antibody at the time of initial examination, chronic carriers of the virus have low titers or no detectable anti-hepatitis B core IgM antibody. However, chronic carriers with the antibody are more likely to have active liver disease, hepatitis B e antigen positivity, and detectable viremia (hepatitis B virus DNA positive by DNA-DNA hybridization). Chronic active hepatitis may also be due to hepatitis C, so a history of transfusion is important. As stated previously, approximately 50% to 70% of cases of hepatitis C become chronic. A second-generation test for anti-hepatitis C is available and is positive in approximately 86% of cases of chronic hepatitis C. If chronic hepatitis C is suspected and the test for anti-hepatitis C antibody is positive, consider a supplemental assay for specificity (e.g., a recombinant immunoblot assay performed in a reference laboratory). Hepatitis A and hepatitis E do not cause chronic hepatitis. In any case of chronic hepatitis, but particularly when considering non-A, non-B hepatitis, one should exclude alcoholic liver disease, autoimmune liver disease, gall-stones, hemochromatosis, Wilson's disease, α_1-antitrypsin deficiency, and drug-related hepatitis.

Drugs that can cause chronic active hepatitis include amiodarone, dan-trolene, isoniazid, methyldopa, nitrofurantoin, oxyphenisatin, perhexilene maleate, phenytoin, propylthiouracil, and sulfonamides. Long-term use of acetaminophen, aspirin, and ethanol may occasionally cause the syndrome. Patients with Wilson's disease and α_1-antitrypsin deficiency may be seen initially with chronic active hepatitis. In many patients the cause is unknown. A number of these patients (usually young women) with no known cause will exhibit clinical features and serological findings of autoimmune chronic active hepatitis (formerly lupoid hepatitis) such as positive ANAs, a positive LE cell preparation, double-stranded DNA antibody, smooth muscle anti-body, and a polyclonal hypergammaglobulinemia with the IgG fraction pre-dominating.

Patients with chronic active hepatitis may develop cirrhosis. Hepatocel-lular carcinoma is another possible complication. Serum α-fetoprotein and ultrasonography are the most sensitive studies for early detection of the cancer. An increased serum α-fetoprotein concentration up to approximately 200 ng/mL (200 µg/L) is a sensitive but not very specific marker for he-patocellular carcinoma. Values >1000 ng/mL (1000 µg/L) or progressively increasing concentrations are highly suggestive of the cancer.

4.   If the liver biopsy shows chronic persistent hepatitis, reassure the patient and continue observation.

For chronic persistent hepatitis related to hepatitis B, regular monitoring (approximately every 6 months) is mandatory to determine whether hepatitis B and e antigens persist or whether these antigens are replaced by anti-hepatitis B and e antibodies, in which case the patient is cured. Approxi-mately 15% of patients with chronic hepatitis B develop antibodies and are cured each year.

5.   In patients with chronic active hepatitis, in addition to abnormal liver function tests, the following abnormal blood test results may occur:

↓ **Hemoglobin and hematocrit.**

↓ **Platelets.**

↓ **Leukocytes.**

↓ **Glucose** related to destruction of hepatic tissue.

BIBLIOGRAPHY

Abbott Laboratories Diagnostics Division: Enzyme immunoassay for the qualitative detec-tion of antibody to hepatitis C virus (anti-HCV) in human serum or plasma. Abbott Laboratories, Abbott Park, Ill, April 1992. Package Insert.
Technical and clinical information about a second-generation test for anti-hepatitis C antibody.

Alter HJ, Purcell RH, Shih JW, et al: Detection of antibody to hepatitis C virus in pro-spectively followed transfusion recipients with acute and chronic non-A, non-B hep-atitis. N Engl J Med 321:1494, 1989.

Hepatitis C is the predominant agent of transfusion-associated non-A, non-B hepatitis.

Babb RR: Chronic liver disease: The scope of causes and treatments. Postgrad Med 91:89, 1992.

Discusses the differential diagnosis of chronic liver disease.

Harrison PM, Lau JYN. Williams R: Hepatology. Postgrad Med J 67:719, 1991.

Reviews the diagnosis and management of viral hepatitis.

Hoofnagle JH, Di Bisceglie AM: Serologic diagnosis of acute and chronic hepatitis. Semin Liver Dis 11:73, 1991.

Reviews the serological diagnosis of viral hepatitis.

Sánchez-Tapias JM, Barrera JM, Costa J, et al: Hepatitis C virus infection in patients with nonalcoholic chronic liver disease. Ann Intern Med 112:921, 1990.

Testing for anti-hepatitis C antibody may be helpful in the differential diagnosis between viral and autoimmune chronic liver disease.

Summary of a workshop on screening for hepatocellular carcinoma. MMWR 39:619, 1990.

Suggests serum α-fetoprotein and ultrasonography to detect hepatocellular carcinoma.

Williams ALB, Hoofnagle JH: Ratio of serum aspartate to alanine aminotransferase in chronic hepatitis: Relationship to cirrhosis. Gastroenterology 95:734, 1988.

AST:ALT ratio >1 in patients with nonalcoholic chronic liver disease suggests that cirrhosis is present or developing.

Yarze JC, Martin P, Muñoz SJ, et al: Wilson's disease: Current status. Am J Med 92:643, 1992.

Discusses pathophysiology, diagnosis, and management of Wilson's disease.

Cirrhosis

1.   In patients with clinical findings and liver function test results of cirrhosis, to accurately diagnose the lesion, consider a needle biopsy of the liver.

In patients with cirrhosis the liver function test results vary according to the rate of hepatocellular destruction and the amount of tissue replaced by fibrosis. Thus AST and ALT activities may be normal or increased. In patients with alcoholic cirrhosis AST values can increase to 200 to 300 U/L. The increase of ALT is typically less. ALP may be normal to increased, up to three times the upper normal limit, and the bilirubin is normal to increased, up to 20 to 40 mg/dL (342 to 684 μmol/L) in decompensated alcoholic cirrhosis. Albumin is typically decreased, the globulins increased, and the PT prolonged.

2.   Evaluate the tests.

Percutaneous liver biopsy is the procedure of choice to diagnose cirrhosis accurately. In 10% to 20% of cases of presumed alcoholic cirrhosis another disease is found on biopsy. Whereas a needle biopsy is usually diagnostic for micronodular cirrhosis, a single needle biopsy can miss the morphological diagnosis of macronodular cirrhosis, and three separate biopsies may be necessary to exclude macronodular cirrhosis because the needle can puncture the center of a large macronodule in which the histology does not show cirrhosis.

3.   If the liver biopsy shows cirrhosis, determine its cause so that appropriate therapy can be chosen.

The most common causes of cirrhosis in the Western world are alcoholic cirrhosis, cryptogenic cirrhosis, postnecrotic cirrhosis, biliary cirrhosis (primary and secondary), and pigment cirrhosis (in hemochromatosis). Cirrhosis associated with Wilson's disease, α_1-antitrypsin deficiency, and other forms of cirrhosis is rare.

4.   In patients with cirrhosis the following additional abnormal blood test results may occur:

↓ **Hemoglobin and hematocrit** related to chronic disease, gastrointestinal bleeding, and/or hypersplenism.

↑ **Erythrocyte sedimentation rate.**

↓ **Glucose.**

↑ **Creatinine** caused by the hepatorenal syndrome.

↓ or ↑ **Uric acid.**

↓ **Potassium,** frequently in patients with ascites and edema.

↓ **Phosphorous,** particularly after glucose administration.

↓ **Leukocytes** related to hypersplenism.

↓ **Platelets** related to hypersplenism and/or disseminated intravascular coagulation.

↓ **Urea nitrogen** caused by decreased synthesis of urea.

↑ **Urea nitrogen** due to gastrointestinal hemorrhage or the hepatorenal syndrome.

↓ **Sodium,** especially in patients with ascites.

↓ **Calcium.**

↓ **Magnesium.**

↑ **Amylase,** which correlates with high incidence of patients with pancreatic disease.

↑ **α-Fetoprotein** as a marker for hepatoma: >200 ng/ml (200 μg/L), sensitive but not specific; >1000 ng/ml (1000 μg/L), highly suggestive.

BIBLIOGRAPHY

Castilla A, Prieto J, Fausto N: Transforming growth factors beta-1 and alpha in chronic liver disease: Effects of interferon alfa therapy. N Engl J Med 324:933, 1991; and Schiff ER: Hepatic fibrosis: New therapeutic approaches. N Engl J Med 324:987, 1991. *New information on the pathogenesis of cirrhosis.*

Colombo M, De Franchis R, Del Ninno E, et al: Hepatocellular carcinoma in Italian patients with cirrhosis. N Engl J Med 325:675, 1991. *Cirrhotic patients should be carefully followed for the development of hepatoma.*

Czaja AJ, Wolf AM, Baggenstoss AH: Clinical assessment of cirrhosis in severe chronic active liver disease: Specificity and sensitivity of physical and laboratory findings. Mayo Clin Proc 55:360, 1980. *Three separate needle biopsies may be required to exclude macronodular cirrhosis.*

Melato M, Laurino L, Mucli E, et al: Relationship between cirrhosis, liver cancer, and hepatic metastases: An autopsy study. Cancer 64:455, 1989.
Most neoplasms in cirrhotic livers are primary.

Cholestasis and Obstructive Liver Disease

1. For patients with clinical findings and liver function test results of obstructive liver disease consider appropriate radiographic and other studies and liver biopsy. See the discussion of jaundice and liver function tests for the workup of patients with jaundice.

Cholestasis refers to disorders that impair bile formation or bile flow. It is sometimes referred to as *obstructive liver disease,* which may be either intrahepatic or extrahepatic. Intrahepatic obstructive processes may be due to hepatocellular disease (e.g., acute viral hepatitis, drug-induced hepatitis); hepatocellular and cholestatic disease (e.g., acute cholestatic viral hepatitis, chronic active hepatitis, cirrhosis, drug-related cholestatic hepatitis); and cholestatic disease (drug-related cholestasis [e.g., chlorpromazine, sex steroids], infiltrative neoplastic or granulomatous hepatic disease, and primary biliary cirrhosis). Extrahepatic obstruction is usually due to mechanical obstruction (e.g., common duct stone and perampullary carcinoma). Some causes of cholestatic jaundice follow*:

Alcoholic hepatitis	Postoperative cholestasis
Amyloidosis	Sarcoidosis
Benign recurrent cholestasis	Sclerosing cholangitis
Biliary cirrhosis	Shock
Cholestasis of pregnancy	Sickle cell disease
Chronic active hepatitis	Total parenteral nutrition
Congestive heart failure	Toxic chemicals (e.g., paraquat)
Drugs†	Transplant rejection
Hepatic cirrhosis	Viral hepatitis
Mechanical obstruction	

---

*Source: McKnight JT, Jones JE: Jaundice. Am Fam Physician 45(3):1143, March 1992. Published by the American Academy of Family Physician.

†See the preceding discussion of jaundice and liver function tests for drugs that can cause jaundice.

By strict definition, cholestasis does not include prehepatic jaundice (hemolysis) or the hereditary hyperbilirubinemias such as Gilbert's disease, the Crigler-Najjar syndrome, the Dubin-Johnson syndrome, and Rotor's syndrome. Cholestasis is characterized by increased serum bile acids, and in all the hereditary hyperbilirubinemias, bile acids are typically normal.

Increased ALP and GGT levels are valuable in identifying cholestasic disorders but are not very useful in determining the cause of the cholestasis or whether the obstruction is intrahepatic or hepatic. Moreover, in this regard even liver biopsy has limitations. Radiographic and endoscopic studies are often necessary to diagnose the nature and location of the obstruction.

Appropriate procedures to consider include ultrasonography, CT, ERCP, and percutaneous transhepatic cholangiography.

2. Interpret test results in the context of clinical findings.

If the liver function test results show a cholestatic pattern, determine whether the biliary obstruction is intrahepatic or extrahepatic (i.e., medical versus surgical obstruction). Serum bile acid values may be helpful in excluding prehepatic jaundice. Determine the exact cause of either medical or surgical obstruction so that appropriate therapy can be chosen.

BIBLIOGRAPHY

Arvan DA: Obstructive jaundice. In Panzer RJ, Black ER, Griner PF (eds): Diagnostic Strategies for Common Medical Problems. Philadelphia, American College of Physicians, 1991, p 131.
Recommends strategies for the differential diagnosis of obstructive jaundice.

Hadjis NS, Blenkharn JI, Hatzis G, et al: Patterns of serum alkaline phosphatase activity in unilateral hepatic duct obstruction: A clinical and experimental study. Surgery 107:193, 1990.
Increased serum alkaline phosphatase may be the only abnormality in patients with unilateral hepatic duct obstruction.

Panzer RJ: Hepatic metastases. In Panzer RJ, Black ER, Griner PF (eds): Diagnostic Strategies for Common Medical Problems. Philadelphia, American College of Physicians, 1991, p 152.
Recommends strategies for the diagnosis of hepatic metastases.

Rocklin MS, Senagore AJ, Talbott TM: Role of carcinoembryonic antigen and liver function tests in the detection of recurrent colorectal carcinoma. Dis Colon Rectum 34:794, 1991.
Carcinoembryonic antigen measurements are sufficient to monitor patients for possible metastatic colorectal cancer. Liver function tests are unnecessary.

Sartin JS, Walker RC: Granulomatous hepatitis: A retrospective review of 88 cases at the Mayo Clinic. Mayo Clin Proc 66:914, 1991.
Discusses differential diagnosis of granulomatous hepatitis.

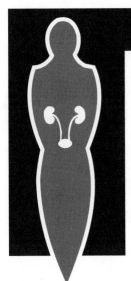

CHAPTER 7

URINARY TRACT DISEASES

The Urinalysis
Glucosuria
Proteinuria
Hematuria and Colored Urine
Urinary Tract Infection in Women
Acute Renal Failure

The Urinalysis

1. Screen asymptomatic persons at high risk for urinary tract disease, using a reagent strip (dipstick) that includes the nitrite test and leukocyte esterase test. In asymptomatic individuals, if all reagent strip test results are negative, omit microscopic examination of the sediment.

Performance of a screening urinalysis is controversial. Because a urine reagent strip is such an economical and effective way to detect urinary tract disease and because urinary tract disorders are so prevalent, many physicians perform reagent strip screening. Use of reagent strips is particularly well suited for screening asymptomatic high-risk populations (e.g., diabetics, pregnant women, preschool children, persons more than age 60).

In the routine health care setting urinalysis may be compromised by a poorly collected specimen, delays in testing, lack of standardization of procedures, and lack of proficiency by the examiner. Microscopic examination of the sediment is particularly vulnerable to these poor practices. To obtain medically reliable information, emphasis must be placed on proper collection of a fresh specimen, which is quickly tested by a competent examiner, using standardized and controlled techniques.

The traditional macroscopic examination consists of a description of the urine, including its color and specific gravity. The usual reagent strip provides a semiquantitative estimation of pH, glucose, protein, hemoglobin, ketones, bilirubin, and urobilinogen. Recently two new reagent strip tests have been added: the nitrite test and the leukocyte esterase test.

Each of these new tests is designed to detect the presence of urinary tract infections (UTIs). Many gram-negative bacteria reduce nitrates to nitrites, and polymorphonuclear leukocytes in urine release leukocyte esterase.

The microscopic examination is done by centrifuging 10 mL of urine at 2000 rpm for 5 minutes at approximately $450 \times g$ and resuspending the sediment in 1 mL of urine. Under high power, red blood cells (RBCs), white blood cells (WBCs), and renal epithelial cells are counted in 10 representative fields. Bacteria and yeast are noted. Crystals are reported if their number is unusually large or they are abnormal. If casts are present, they are identified, and the number of casts per low-power field in 10 fields is reported. With the introduction of the nitrite and leukocyte esterase tests to detect bacteria and WBCs in the urine, there have been a number of studies to determine whether it is necessary to perform a labor-intensive microscopic examination of the urinary sediment if all reagent strip tests are completely negative.

A study of the results of a nine-parameter reagent strip test examination of 1385 urine specimens gave the following results: all positive protein tests confirmed by the sulfosalicylic acid test; 81.9% sensitivity for pyuria (five WBCs, per high-power field); 94.5% sensitivity for blood; 25.9% sensitivity for bacteria; and 1139 (82.2%) of specimens positive for one or more elements. Only 28 (3.8%) of the 730 specimens with negative reagent strip tests had positive microscopic findings. The reagent strip had a 98.1% sensitivity for bacteria in specimens that had positive cultures.

A practical approach appears advisable—application of urine reagent strip technology is an effective test to detect covert pyuria, hematuria, and proteinuria as a part of a routine physical examination. The test is inexpensive and can detect diseases that cause serious morbidity. A negative result is also useful as baseline information. A urine reagent strip test may even be useful to detect sexually transmitted disease in men. Pregnant women should have regular urinalyses with urine cultures if pyuria is noted. Clearly the microscopic examination is the most time-consuming and costly part of the urinalysis, and it can be omitted in the context of screening for urinary tract disorders if all the reagent strip test results are negative.

2.   In patients with clinical findings of urinary tract disease obtain a complete urinalysis—reagent strip and microscopic examination of the sediment—regardless of the reagent strip results. Consider obtaining a culture.

Because a reagent strip is not 100% sensitive for abnormal findings in the microscopic sediment and because the results of both reagent strip test and microscopic examination are clinically useful, it is prudent to perform both reagent strip tests and microscopic examination of the sediment in patients who are symptomatic. If there are clinical findings of UTI, obtaining a urine culture may be appropriate.

3. Interpret urinalysis test results in the context of clinical findings.

Positive test results, either macroscopic or microscopic, should always be explored. The presence of glucose, protein, or hemoglobin in the urine may be a clue to serious disease or may represent a benign finding that, once explained, can be disregarded. RBCs, WBCs, epithelial cells, bacteria, casts, and other findings in the urinary sediment may constitute key information in diagnosing a urinary tract disorder. The problems that follow discuss the workup of glucosuria, proteinuria, and hemoglobinuria and the use of urinalysis in the diagnosis of UTI in women.

BIBLIOGRAPHY

Abyad A: Screening for asymptomatic bacteriuria in pregnancy: Urinalysis vs urine culture. J Fam Pract 33:471, 1991.
Suggests complete urinalysis at first prenatal visit with cultures if five or more leukocytes per high-power field.

Akin BV, Hubbell FA, Frye EB, et al: Efficacy of routine admission urinalysis. Am J Med 82:719, 1987.
Concludes that routine hospital admission urinalysis is not very useful.

Cramer AD, Chogyoji M, Saxena S, et al: Macroscopic screening urinalysis. Laboratory Medicine 20:623, 1989.
A study of 1385 urine specimens that supports omission of the microscopic sediment exam if all reagent test results are negative.

Is routine urinalysis worthwhile? Lancet 1:747, 1988. Editorial.
Concludes that the high prevalence of urinary abnormalities justifies routine urinalysis both in the ambulatory care and hospital settings.

Kiel DP, Moskowitz MA: The urinalysis: A critical appraisal. Med Clin North Am 71:607, 1987.
Good review of the technical and medical aspects of urinalysis.

Lachs MS, Nachamkin I, Edelstein PH, et al: Spectrum bias in the evaluation of diagnostic tests: Lessons from the rapid dipstick test for urinary tract infection. Ann Intern Med 117:135, 1992.
Sensitivity and specificity of the leukocyte esterase and nitrite reagent strip test for UTI may differ among different patient groups.

Pappas PG: Laboratory in the diagnosis and management of urinary tract infections. Med Clin North Am 75:313, 1991.
Good discussions of urinalysis, urine culture, noninvasive methods of UTI localization, and office diagnosis of UTIs.

Sadof MD, Woods ER, Emans J: Dipstick leukocyte esterase activity in first-catch urine specimens: A useful screening test for detecting sexually transmitted disease in the adolescent male. JAMA 258:1932, 1987; and Shafer MA, Schachter J, Moscicki AB, et al: Urinary leukocyte esterase screening test for asymptomatic chlamydial and gonococcal infections in males. JAMA 262:2562, 1989.
Urine reagent strip leukocyte esterase testing can detect sexually transmitted disease in the male.

U.S. Preventive Services Task Force, Washington, DC: Screening for asymptomatic bacteriuria, hematuria, and proteinuria. Am Fam Physician 42:389, 1990.
Recommends screening for bacteriuria in diabetics, pregnant women, and possibly preschool children using leukocyte esterase and nitrite tests—cultures also suggested in pregnancy. Screening for bacteriuria, hematuria, and proteinuria may also be wise in persons over age 60.

Glucosuria

1.   In patients with glucosuria assess the clinical findings, perform a complete urinalysis, including microscopic examination of the urinary sediment, and measure serum glucose, creatinine, and urea nitrogen.

Glucosuria usually occurs when the serum glucose concentration is greater than 180 to 200 mg/dL (9.99 to 11.10 mmol/L), but glucose may appear in the urine at lower serum glucose values, varying in individuals. The serum glucose concentration at which glucose appears in the urine is termed the *renal threshold* for glucose. Glucosuria should be distinguished from other conditions involving sugars in the urine such as lactosuria and galactosuria. In addition to the serum glucose concentration, other factors that affect the appearance of glucose in the urine include glomerular blood flow, tubular reabsorption rate, and urinary flow. Follow-up studies are necessary to determine whether the glucosuria is caused by hyperglycemia or renal tubular dysfunction. Glucosuria in the absence of hyperglycemia is called *renal glucosuria.*

Glucosuria may occur as an isolated finding, or it may be accompanied by other abnormal findings. A complete urinalysis can provide clues to a variety of disorders such as diabetic nephropathy and UTI. A serum glucose measurement can help determine whether glucosuria is an overflow phenomenon or related to a renal disorder, and serum urea nitrogen and creatinine measurements are useful to assess renal function.

2.   Evaluate the tests.

Reduction methods (copper reduction test) for measuring urinary glucose are obsolete. A reagent strip method using glucose oxidase currently is the most commonly used technique. Large doses of ascorbic acid (vitamin C) can cause a false-negative urinary glucose test result using the glucose oxidase method. Ascorbic acid does not affect reduction methods, but other drugs can give false-positive results or unusual colors with the copper reduction test, especially the cephalosporins (e.g., cephalexin [Keflex]) and radiocontrast agents. Reduction methods are useful to detect nonglucose meliturias, which can occur in infants. In the presence of other sugars such as lactose and galactose, the reduction test is positive, and the glucose oxidase test is negative.

3.   If the serum glucose concentration is increased in a patient with glucosuria, conclude that the urinary glucose is an overflow phenomenon, and determine whether the increased serum glucose is due to diabetes mellitus or some other cause for hyperglycemia.

Serum glucose may be increased in a patient with diabetes mellitus, during stress, and with a variety of diseases such as pancreatitis, central nervous system lesions, and disorders secondary to drugs (e.g., corticosteroids).

4. If the serum glucose concentration is normal in a patient with glucosuria, consider renal tubular dysfunction (i.e., renal glucosuria).

Glucosuria without hyperglycemia is usually caused by renal tubular dysfunction, which may be inherited (uncommon) or acquired. In patients with renal tubular dysfunction glucose is not the only substance with impaired tubular reabsorption. For example, in patients with Fanconi's syndrome the reabsorption of water, amino acids, sodium, bicarbonate, and phosphate is also impaired. Other examples of conditions associated with tubular dysfunction include galactosemia, cystinosis, lead poisoning, and myeloma.

BIBLIOGRAPHY

Freeman JA, Beeler MF: Laboratory Medicine/Urinalysis and Medical Microscopy, 2nd ed. Philadelphia, Lea & Febiger, 1983.
  Good general reference on urinalysis and glucosuria.
Kiel DP, Moskowitz MA: The urinalysis: A critical appraisal. Med Clin North Am 71:607, 1987.
  Discusses differential diagnosis of glucosuria.

Proteinuria

1. In patients with proteinuria assess the clinical findings, request a complete urinalysis, including microscopic examination of the urinary sediment, and measure serum creatinine and urea nitrogen. Consider testing diabetics and hypertensive patients for microalbuminuria with a special method.

Proteinuria is a common and easily detected sign of renal disease. In the past normal urine was believed free of protein. It now is known that healthy individuals excrete a small amount of protein, which is undetectable by routine methods. Normally the composition of urinary protein is approximately 40% albumin, 40% tissue proteins from renal and other urogenital tissues, 15% immunoglobulins, and 5% other plasma proteins. Proteinuria may be caused by (1) an overflow of increased plasma proteins, (2) increased glomerular permeability, (3) tubular proteinuria, and (4) altered renal hemodynamics.

Proteinuria may occur as an isolated finding during a urinalysis or together with other abnormal findings. A urinalysis can provide clues to a variety of disorders such as fatty casts, oval fat bodies, and doubly refractile fat globules for the nephrotic syndrome; RBC casts for glomerulonephritis; and glucosuria for diabetes mellitus. When these other findings are present, they corroborate the significance of the proteinuria. Serum creatinine and urea nitrogen measurements are useful to evaluate renal function.

Many diabetologists and nephrologists believe that the early detection and reversal of microalbuminuria in diabetics may delay or prevent frank diabetic nephropathy. There is a growing interest in detecting and reversing microalbuminuria in hypertensive patients. The usual reagent strip test is not sensitive enough to screen for microalbuminuria.

Digital rectal examination of the prostate does not cause proteinuria.

2.   Evaluate the tests.

Urinary protein can be measured by reagent strip, turbidimetric, chemical, and immunological methods. With reagent strip test methods, false-positive results can occur with highly concentrated urine, highly alkaline (pH >7) urine, and contamination of the urine with bacteria, blood, quaternary ammonium compounds, and chlorhexidine. False-negative results can occur with urinary immunoglobulin light chains (Bence Jones protein) and highly dilute urine. With turbidimetric methods, false-positive results can occur if the urine contains tolbutamide, radiocontrast agents, or high levels of cephalosporin, penicillin, or sulfonamide derivatives.

The usual reagent strip test can detect 200 to 300 mg/L of albumin and is less sensitive to globulins, Bence Jones protein, and mucoprotein. To quantify microalbuminuria, a special method is necessary: a detection limit of at least 5 mg/L and a range of 5 to 200 mg/L are preferred, and normal values are less than 20 mg/L. Available methods include radioimmunoassay, radial immunodiffusion, enzyme-linked immunosorbent assay (ELISA), and immunoturbidimetry. The collection method must be standardized.

3.   If proteinuria is present, documented, and confirmed, measure serum creatinine, urea nitrogen, and a 24-hour protein excretion (alternatively, measure urinary protein and creatinine in a random urine specimen and calculate the protein:creatinine ratio to estimate protein excretion). Consider the possibility of transient and orthostatic proteinuria.

Spot urinary measurements of protein and creatinine reliably detect significant proteinuria. This method avoids the cumbersome, inconvenient, and often unreliable collection of a 24-hour urine sample. The protein:creatinine ratio can distinguish healthy individuals from those with renal disease and can differentiate nephrotic range proteinuria from that seen with other renal diseases. The protein:creatinine ratio in healthy individuals seldom exceeds 200 mg of protein per gram of creatinine. For patients with nephrotic range proteinuria (>4 g/day), the ratio exceeds 3000 mg per gram.

Transient proteinuria may be associated with strenuous exercise, emotional stress, extreme cold, epinephrine administration, congestive heart failure, and seizures. Transient proteinuria can be documented by several protein free urinalyses after the precipitating cause has passed. The mechanism of proteinuria is believed related to hemodynamic changes. The patient should be reassured, and no further workup is indicated.

Orthostatic proteinuria is characterized by the presence of proteinuria with the patient in the erect position and the absence of proteinuria as shown by a negative reagent strip test result or one <50 mg/L with the patient in the recumbent position. The true mechanism is unknown but probably is increased glomerular permeability. The proteinuria usually does not exceed 2 g/day. Long-term follow-up studies over several decades have shown excellent prognosis, with normal renal function.

**4.   If proteinuria is persistent and nonorthostatic, perform a more exten-
sive evaluation. Other useful laboratory tests include complement studies,
serum albumin, serum total protein, serum and urinary immunoelectrophoresis, and radiological evaluation.**

The spectrum of lesions in isolated proteinuria is wide. In patients with
fixed proteinuria <2 g/day without hematuria, systemic disease, or impaired
renal function, renal biopsy usually is not performed unless a change in
clinical status occurs or the patient requests a biopsy. Nephrotoxic agents
such as gold salts and nonsteroidal anti-inflammatory drugs are an important
cause of proteinuria to consider.

BIBLIOGRAPHY

Cembrowski GS: Testing for microalbuminuria: Promises and pitfalls. Laboratory Medi-
cine 21:491, 1990.
Suggests strategies for monitoring microalbuminuria in diabetic patients.
Kaplan NM: Microalbuminuria: A risk factor for vascular and renal complications of
hypertension. Am J Med 92(suppl 4B):4B-8S, 1992.
In hypertensive patients testing for microalbuminuria should be routinely performed.
McKenna MJ, Arias C, Feldkamp CS, et al: Microalbuminuria in clinical practice. Arch
Intern Med 151:1745, 1991.
Concludes that testing for microalbuminuria is useful for early detection of diabetic nephropathy.
Roe TF, Costin G, Kaufman FR, et al: Blood glucose control and albuminuria in type 1
diabetes mellitus. J Pediatr 119:178, 1991.
*Maintenance of hemoglobin A1$_c$ values at 9% or less significantly decreases the risk of diabetic
nephropathy.*
Schwab SJ, Christensen RL, Dougherty K, et al: Quantitation of proteinuria by the use of
protein-to-creatinine ratios in single urine samples. Arch Intern Med 147:943, 1987.
Suggests the use of single urine samples as a reliable way to quantitate proteinuria.
Waller KV, Ward KM, Mahan JD, et al: Current concepts in proteinuria. Clin Chem 35:755,
1989.
Good review of glomerular, tubular, and mixed proteinuria.

Hematuria and Colored Urine

**1.   In patients with hematuria, myoglobinuria, or colored urine, assess
the clinical findings, request a complete urinalysis, and measure serum
creatinine, urea nitrogen, creatine kinase, and haptoglobin. Obtain a carefully drawn serum specimen for visual inspection.**

Hematuria may be either gross (red, red-brown, or brown-black urine)
or microscopic (more than two RBCs per high-power field). It may be caused
by a disorder of hemostasis or therapeutic anticoagulation, or it may originate in a lesion located anywhere in the urinary tract. When hematuria is
gross, it is important to determine that the color of the urine is really caused
by blood and not another colored substance such as myoglobin or porphyrins. The diagnosis of the cause of hematuria depends on clinical find-

ings, radiographs, urological procedures, and laboratory tests. It helps to know whether the hematuria is painful or painless and whether it is accompanied by other urinary abnormalities such as protein and formed elements in the urine.

In patients with hemoglobinuria RBCs may be present or absent in the urinary sediment. If RBCs are absent and the urinary reagent test for blood is positive, hemoglobinuria must be distinguished from myoglobinuria. If a carefully drawn serum specimen can be examined (avoiding hemolysis), it often is pink with hemoglobinemia but a normal color with myoglobinemia. Serum myoglobin is rapidly cleared by the kidneys, but serum hemoglobin is not. Additional useful tests are determinations of serum creatine kinase (CK), which often is markedly increased in patients with myoglobinuria secondary to muscle damage, and serum haptoglobin, which is low in patients with hemoglobinuria and normal in those with myoglobinuria.

Hematuria may be present as an isolated finding on urinalysis or appear together with other abnormal findings. A complete urinalysis can provide clues to a variety of disorders such as UTI and urinary calculi. Creatinine and urea nitrogen measurements are useful to assess renal function.

2. Evaluate the tests.

The usual reagent strip test relies on the peroxidase-like activity of RBCs and hemoglobin. Both hemoglobin and myoglobin give a positive test result. False-positive results can occur when urine from menstruating women is tested or when the urine is contaminated with residues of strongly oxidizing cleaning agents in the urine container or with povidone-iodine. False-negative readings can occur when the urine contains large quantities of ascorbic acid (vitamin C) or is preserved with formalin.

Currently available reagent strip tests are capable of detecting two or three RBCs per high-power field, with a sensitivity of 97%. Intact RBCs hemolyze on the reagent strip, and the liberated hemoglobin produces a colored dot. Scattered or compacted dots indicate intact RBCs, whereas a uniform green color indicates free hemoglobin, hemolyzed RBCs, or myoglobin.

3. In patients with documented gross or microscopic hematuria determine the source of the hemoglobin or bleeding.

Hemoglobinuria can be caused by hemolytic disorders, which may be either inherited or acquired. After a race, marathon runners may have hematuria. Myoglobinuria can be caused by rhabdomyolysis, which may occur with the following conditions: primary muscle injury, increased muscle energy consumption (strenuous exercise, status epilepticus), decreased muscle energy consumption (diabetic ketoacidosis), decreased muscle oxygenation, infections, and toxins.

The most common causes of hematuria originating in the urinary tract are cystitis, urethritis, and bleeding from the prostate; the most serious are bladder and kidney carcinoma, urinary calculi, and renal tuberculosis. Glomerulonephritis is an important cause of hematuria, in which the question of whether or not to perform a renal biopsy is often raised. Approximately

10% of patients with gross hematuria and 35% with microscopic hematuria have so-called "hematuria of unknown cause."

Cytological examination of the urine without endoscopic examination of the bladder may be a simple, cost-effective method for evaluating asymptomatic microhematuria in women. In patients with idiopathic hematuria renal biopsy makes no difference therapeutically or prognostically and is therefore unnecessary for routine management of asymptomatic hematuria.

If no pathological cause of hematuria is present, consider an entity known as *familial hematuria* in which hematuria is present in other family members and good renal function is maintained during long-term follow-up.

4. In patients with red or brown urine, if the reagent strip test for blood is negative, conclude that a substance other than hemoglobin or myoglobin is responsible for the colored urine.

Red, red-brown, or brown-black urine can result from either ingested substances or substances that originate in the body. Ingested substances include azodyes (phenazopyridine [pyridium]), phenolsulfonphthalein, *p*-aminosalicylic acid, anthraquinones, nitrofurantoin, metronidazole, sulfa compounds, chloroquine, methyldopa, levodopa, phenacetin, salicylates, methocarbamol, cresol, iron sorbitol citrate, and beets (individuals who can absorb betanin). Phenytoin is not a cause of red urine. Substances originating in the body include bilirubin, porphyrin, melanin (in melanoma), homogentisic acid (in alkaptonuria), and the red pigment produced by *Serratia marcescens* (in infection by that organism).

5. In patients with myoglobinuria (acute rhabdomyolysis) the following additional abnormal blood test results may occur:

↓ **Serum urea nitrogen: creatinine ratio** (<10:1) because creatine from injured muscles is rapidly converted into creatinine.

↑ **Uric acid** caused by conversion of muscle purines to uric acid. Renal failure may further increase uric acid.

↑ **Calcium** from muscle.

↓ **Calcium** (early) followed by increased calcium (later). Possible deposition of calcium in damaged muscle tissue.

↑ **Phosphorus,** probably from muscle. Renal failure may further increase phosphate.

BIBLIOGRAPHY

Britton JP, Dowell AC, Whelan P: Dipstick hematuria and bladder cancer in men over 60: Results of a community study. BMJ 299:1010, 1989.
  Discusses hematuria in men with bladder cancer.
Connelly JE: Microscopic hematuria. In Panzer RJ, Black ER, Griner PF (eds): Diagnostic Strategies for Common Medical Problems. Philadelphia, American College of Physicians, 1991, p 412.
  Recommends strategies for diagnosing the cause of microscopic hematuria.
Paola AS: Hematuria: Essentials of diagnosis. Hosp Pract 25:144, 1990.
  Describes differential diagnosis of hematuria.

Sutton JM: Evaluation of hematuria in adults. JAMA 263:2475, 1990.
Gives an approach to adults with hematuria.
What urine color tells you. Emergency Medicine 20:155, 1988.
Describes a way to determine the cause of different colored urines: brown or black, yellow or orange, colorless or milky, and blue or green.

Urinary Tract Infection in Women

1.   For women with clinical findings of a lower UTI, request a urinalysis. If the clinical findings suggest pyelonephritis (fever, rigors, nausea, vomiting, flank pain, costovertebral angle tenderness), obtain a urine Gram stain and culture and a urinalysis.

Patients with findings of lower UTI and possible subclinical pyelonephritis (pregnancy, underlying urinary tract disease, diabetes mellitus, immunosuppression, symptoms for more than 7 days, three or more UTIs in past year, past history of pyelonephritis, recent use of antibiotics, poor city neighborhood) should have a urine Gram stain and culture and a urinalysis.

For sexually active patients with possible chlamydial or gonococcal urethritis, request a urinalysis and obtain a Gram stain and culture of urethral (or cervical os) discharge. Urethritis in the sexual partner, a new sexual partner, or mucopurulent endocervical secretions are suggestive findings.

For women with findings of vaginitis, obtain a microscopic examination of any abnormal vaginal discharge and consider a culture.

Since the decision to treat a lower UTI is based on the presence of pyuria rather than bacteriuria, only a urinalysis is required when the clinical findings (e.g., dysuria, urgency, and frequency) are limited to the lower urinary tract.

Since false-negative results with the reagent strip nitrite test can occur when the urine has not been retained in the bladder long enough for gram-negative bacteria to reduce nitrates in the urine to nitrites, a first-morning urine specimen is best. Other causes of a false-negative nitrite test result are deficient dietary nitrate and a urinary ascorbic acid concentration >75 mg/dL (4.28 mmol/L). Other factors that can influence test results include hydration status (is patient forcing fluids?), urinary pH, antibiotics, and other drugs.

Women should be requested to clean manually the labia and area around the urethral meatus thoroughly with a mild soap and water solution, stroking away from the meatus of the urethra once it has been cleaned. In a squatting position, either over a bedpan or on a toilet seat, the female patient should separate the labia with one hand and begin voiding. During the void, preferably at the approximate midpoint, a collection bottle or cup held in the other hand should be inserted into the urine stream without halting the void. When an adequate sample has been collected, the cup should be withdrawn, and the patient should complete the urination into the toilet or bedpan.

Specimens for gonococcal culture should include cervical and urethral swabs, and the rectum may also be sampled. Maximal recovery of *Chlamydia* is achieved by culture of both cervix and urethra. These specimens should be collected with synthetic fiber swabs because wooden shafts and calcium alginate swabs are toxic to *Chlamydia* and to a lesser extent to gonococci. Chlamydial cultures require immediate inoculation of the specimen into a suitable transport medium such as 2SP. Specimens for gonococci taken in a physician's office should be cultured immediately and placed in an incubator at 95° F (35° C) in 5% to 10% carbon dioxide, and these cultures should be incubated overnight before being sent to a laboratory for analysis.

Microscopic examination using a drop of 10% potassium hydroxide to dissolve cellular material is useful to identify the pseudohyphae and budding forms of *Candida;* a gram stain is also helpful. A wet mount of fresh discharge with a drop of warm normal saline solution can be prepared to identify the motile flagellated *Trichomonas* and "clue" cells, which are bacilli within epithelial cells often present in patients with *Gardnerella vaginalis* (formerly *Haemophilus vaginitis*). Cultures are necessary to diagnose the rare cases of purulent vaginitis from gonorrhea.

After collection, the urine specimen should be promptly (within 20 minutes) cultured or refrigerated if culture is delayed. A Gram stain of mixed but unspun urine is a rapid test for the presence of WBCs and bacteria >100,000 per milliliter that may be useful in the office or clinic setting.

2.   Evaluate the tests.

The two most common pathogens in lower urinary tract bacterial infection or subclinical pyelonephritis in women are *Escherichia coli* and *Staphylococcus saprophyticus.*

Whenever mixed bacterial species are grown on culture, the likelihood of contamination is high. Moreover, *Staphylococcus epidermidis,* diphtheroids, and lactobacilli are commonly found in the distal urethra and rarely cause infection. If contamination is suspected and culture results are still important, the culture should be repeated.

3.   Interpret pyuria, Gram stains, and urine cultures in the context of the clinical findings.

Lower Urinary Tract Infection

In patients with findings of lower UTI the presence of pyuria justifies giving immediate therapy, whereas the absence of pyuria justifies withholding therapy. Pyuria is present in 90% to 95% of patients with lower UTI and colony counts >100,000 bacteria/mL of urine, in 70% of patients with lower UTI and colony counts of 100 to 100,000 bacteria/mL, and in only 1% of asymptomatic nonbacteriuric patients. If the patient has pyuria without bacteriuria (by examination of unstained sediment), consider the possibility of chlamydial urethritis, gonococcal urethritis, or urinary infection with gram-positive cocci. Lower UTI caused by yeasts (*Candida* species, *Torulopsis*) can also exhibit pyuria. Urinary tract yeast infections occur more commonly in diabetics.

PYELONEPHRITIS

In patients with findings of acute pyelonephritis or subclinical pyelonephritis, urinalysis typically shows pyuria with possible proteinuria, hematuria, and casts. A urine Gram stain and culture are necessary to isolate the responsible organism and identify the pattern of antibacterial sensitivities. Usually, but not always, the colony count will be greater than 100,000 bacteria per milliliter of urine.

CHLAMYDIAL URETHRITIS

Urethral infection with *Chlamydia trachomatis* accounts for 2% to 20% of cases of acute dysuria in women. The urinalysis shows pyuria without bacteriuria. Hematuria is very unusual, as is proteinuria. Routine urine culture will not isolate *C. trachomatis* and often is negative for other organisms. The sensitivity of a single culture for *Chlamydia* is approximately 80%. *C. trachomatis* can also be detected with a nucleic acid probe.

GONOCOCCAL URETHRITIS

Neisseria gonorrhoeae typically produces pyuria. Gram stain shows gram-negative intracellular diplococci, and culture on Thayer-Martin or New York City medium will isolate the organism. Positive Gram stains of cervical discharge are suggestive but not diagnostic of gonococci. These Gram stains should be interpreted with caution if vaginal epithelial cells are present because anaerobic gram-negative bacteria and coccobacillary bacteria can resemble gonococci. *N. gonorrhoeae* can also be detected with a nucleic acid probe.

OTHER URETHRAL INFECTIONS

Urethritis may also be caused by herpes simplex virus, *Trichomonas vaginalis,* and *Candida albicans.* Herpes simplex and *T. vaginalis* produce pyuria, but candidal infection may not.

VAGINITIS

Patients with vaginitis may have dysuria (plus frequency and urgency) as their chief complaint. Typically pyuria is absent except when trichomonal infection involves both the urethra and the vagina. Microscopic examination of the abnormal discharge may reveal budding yeast and pseudohyphae, trichomonads, and clue cells.

ASYMPTOMATIC WOMEN WITH BACTERIURIA

The value of identifying asymptomatic bacteriuria (>100,000 bacteria/mL) in asymptomatic, nonpregnant women is controversial. Asymptomatic bacteriuria apparently is correlated with an increased mortality rate in the elderly, but there is no evidence that treatment alters the rate. Asymptomatic bacteriuria in pregnant women must be treated since therapy reduces the occurrence of acute pyelonephritis and possibly low-birth-weight babies. Therefore pregnant women should have regular urinalyses in the prenatal period, with urine cultures if pyuria is noted.

SYMPTOMATIC WOMEN WITHOUT PYURIA

Many women with dysuria have no pyuria, have no recognized pathogen, and do not respond to antimicrobial treatment. These women should have a urinalysis and urine culture. In these women consider the possibility of urethral inflammation from physical or chemical agents or from trauma.

BIBLIOGRAPHY

Bickley LS: Acute vaginitis. In Panzer RJ, Black ER, Griner PF (eds): Diagnostic Strategies for Common Medical Problems. Philadelphia, American College of Physicians, 1991, p 249.
  Recommends diagnostic strategies for acute vaginitis.
Cook RL, Reid G, Pond DG, et al: Clue cells in bacterial vaginosis: Immunofluorescent identification of the adherent Gram-negative bacteria as *Gardnerella vaginalis*. J Infect Dis 160:490, 1989.
  Recent study of clue cells in bacterial vaginosis.
Johnson JR, Stamm WE: Urinary tract infections in women: Diagnosis and treatment. Ann Intern Med 111:906, 1989.
  Reviews recent developments in the diagnosis and management of these infections.
Komaroff AL: Acute dysuria in adult women. In Panzer RJ, Black ER, Griner PF (eds): Diagnostic Strategies for Common Medical Problems. Philadelphia, American College of Physicians, 1991, p 239.
  Recommends diagnostic strategies for acute dysuria in women.
Komaroff AL: Urinalysis and urine culture in women with dysuria. In Sox HC Jr (ed): Common Diagnostic Tests: Use and Interpretation, 2nd ed. Philadelphia, American College of Physicians, 1990, p 286.
  Good review of the use of urinalysis and urine culture for diagnosing dysuria in women.
Kunin CM: Detection, Prevention, and Management of Urinary Tract Infection, 4th ed. Philadelphia, Lea & Febiger, 1987.
  Good reference text for UTIs.
Pappas PG: Laboratory in the diagnosis and management of urinary tract infections. Med Clin North Am 75:313, 1991.
  Discusses the use of laboratory tests to diagnose UTIs.
Wright RA, Blum R: Infectious disease update: Diagnostic imperatives for urinary tract infection. Modern Medicine 58:46, 1990.
  Describes the use of the reagent strip, examination of the urinary sediment, and in-office culture kits.

Acute Renal Failure

1.   In patients with clinical findings of acute renal failure document azotemia by measuring serum urea nitrogen and creatinine.

Renal failure is characterized by high serum urea nitrogen and creatinine concentrations. If the renal failure occurs suddenly, over a period of days to weeks, it is acute. If it occurs slowly, over a period of months to years, it is chronic. Division of renal failure into acute and chronic varieties is helpful in arriving at the cause, for the differential diagnoses of acute and chronic renal failure differ.

Acute azotemia may be prerenal, intrarenal, or postrenal. Prerenal failure is characterized by azotemia secondary to inadequate perfusion of the kidneys and is reversible within 24 hours if the systemic cause of the renal hypoperfusion is corrected. Postrenal failure is characterized by azotemia resulting from mechanical obstruction distal to the kidneys; in this case renal function may be restored or improved if the obstruction is removed. Intrarenal azotemia is a diagnosis of exclusion. First, prerenal and postrenal causes of azotemia must be excluded; then the exact cause of the intrarenal disease must be determined. Causes of acute intrarenal azotemia include ischemic disorders, nephrotoxicities, diseases of glomerular and small blood vessels, and diseases of major renal blood vessels.

2.   If azotemia is present, request the following studies to help determine its cause: complete blood count (CBC); serum sodium, potassium, chloride, bicarbonate, calcium, magnesium, phosphorous, uric acid; and urinary volume, sediment, osmolality, sodium, urea nitrogen, and creatinine.

Prerenal and postrenal causes of acute renal failure must be vigorously excluded before the diagnosis can be assumed to be intrinsic renal disease, for which immediate specific treatment is only rarely available.

3.   Use clinical findings plus serum and urinary test results to diagnose postrenal and prerenal causes of acute renal failure. Intrinsic renal disease is a diagnosis of exclusion.

If the laboratory tests establish the presence of acute azotemia (a sudden increase of serum creatinine >2 mg/dL [177 μmol/L] and urea nitrogen >25 mg/dL [4.2 mmol/L]), the next step is to exclude a postrenal cause and prerenal cause. A postrenal cause can be excluded by ruling out obstructive uropathy; a prerenal cause can be excluded by clinical information, radiographic studies, and the use of urinary indices as shown on p. 167.

A postrenal cause for acute azotemia may be excluded by working up the patient for an enlarged prostate, palpable bladder, large residual urinary volume, hydronephrotic kidneys, ureteral obstruction, and a history of renal calculi. Usually no urinary sediment abnormalities are found with postrenal azotemia; however, the sediment may contain WBCs and RBCs in infected patients. Patients with urinary tract obstruction have urinary indices that are

Index	Prerenal	Acute Tubular Injury
Urinary osmolality, mOsm/kg water	>500	>350
Urinary sodium (Na), mEq/L	<20	>40
Urinary/plasma creatinine	>40	<20
Fractional sodium excretion*	<1	>1

Source: Grantham JJ: Acute renal failure. In Wyngaarden JB, Smith LH, Bennett JC (eds): Cecil Textbook of Medicine, 19th ed. Philadelphia, WB Saunders Co, 1992, p 531.

$$*\frac{Urine/serum\ (Na)}{Urine/serum\ (creatinine)} \times 100$$

indistinguishable from those of patients with prerenal failure (in patients with obstructions lasting more than 2 days in duration, the indices are similar to those seen with intrarenal tubular injury). If an obstruction is found and if it is relieved, a brisk diuresis ensues, which can be as high as 6 to 8 L per hour. Salt and water losses can be significant and, if not replaced, can result in shock. Hypokalemia can occur.

A prerenal cause for acute azotemia (i.e., volume depletion, congestive heart failure, or severe liver disease) can be excluded by the clinical context and by measuring serum and urine analytes and computing indices.

A rising serum creatinine level >2.5 mg/dL (221 μmol/L) strongly suggests established renal failure as opposed to prerenal azotemia. The urea nitrogen:creatinine ratio is usually about 10:1 in patients with renal parenchymal disease but is greater than 15:1 in patients with prerenal azotemia and urinary tract obstruction. Urinary sediment abnormalities, except for hyaline casts, are usually not found with prerenal azotemia. In intrarenal failure, urinary sediment findings may be helpful, e.g., hematuria, proteinuria, red cell casts, and granular casts suggest acute glomerulonephritis.

4. In patients with acute renal failure the following additional abnormal blood test results may occur:

Anemia.
Leukocytosis not necessarily related to infection.
Thrombocytopenia.
↑ Glucose.
↑ Uric acid.
↓ Sodium.

↑ Potassium.
↓ Bicarbonate with metabolic acidosis.
↓ Calcium.
↑ Magnesium.
↑ Phosphorus.
↑ Amylase.

BIBLIOGRAPHY

Martinez-Maldonado M, Kumjian DA: Acute renal failure due to urinary tract obstruction. Med Clin North Am 74:919, 1990.
    Reviews the causes of acute renal failure due to obstruction.
Simenhoff ML: Acute renal failure. In Conn RB: Current Diagnosis, 8th ed. Philadelphia, WB Saunders Co, 1991, p 1151.
    Describes a diagnostic approach to acute renal failure.

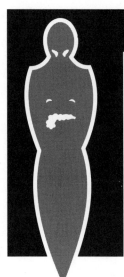

CHAPTER 8

ENDOCRINE AND METABOLIC DISEASES

Hypothyroidism and Hyperthyroidism
Hypocalcemia and Hypoparathyroidism
Hypercalcemia, Cancer, and Hyperparathyroidism
True Hypoglycemia and the Idiopathic
    Postprandial Syndrome
Diabetes Mellitus
Gestational Diabetes Mellitus
Adrenal Insufficiency

Hypothyroidism and Hyperthyroidism

1. For patients with clinical findings of hypothyroidism or hyperthyroidism or if you wish to screen for these disorders, request a serum free thyroxine index (FT₄I) and a serum sensitive thyrotropin assay (S-TSH). In 1990, the American Thyroid Association suggested using both tests.

Most authorities recommend against general wellness screening using thyroid function testing; however, some experts endorse selective wellness screening for thyroid dysfunction for individuals at increased risk.

Ordinarily restrict performance of thyroid tests to patients with clinical findings. Testing asymptomatic individuals for thyroid dysfunction is appropriate in high-risk populations such as newborns, individuals with a strong family history of thyroid disease, older patients, postpartum women 4 to 8 weeks after delivery, individuals with autoimmune diseases such as Addison's disease and type I diabetes mellitus, and persons with abnormal serum cholesterol values. A persistently increased serum creatine kinase concentration in patients with cardiovascular symptoms may be a clue to hypothyroidism.

2.   Evaluate the tests.

Reference ranges may vary in different laboratories.

REFERENCE RANGES

Test	Specimen	Conventional Units	International Units
Free thyroxine index (FT$_4$I)	Serum	4.2-13.0	4.2-13.0
Thyroxine (T$_4$), total	Serum	10-60 yr: 5-12 μg/dL >60 yr: M, 5.0-10.0 μg/dL F, 5.5-10.5 μg/dL	65-155 nmol/L 65-129 nmol/L 71-135 nmol/L
Triiodothyronine resin uptake test (T$_3$RU)	Serum	Adult: 24%-34%	24-34 arbitrary units (AU)
Triiodothyronine (T$_3$), total	Serum	100-200 ng/dL	1.54-3.08 nmol/L
Thyrotropin (TSH)	Serum	<10 μU/mL	<10 mU/L
Sensitive thyrotropin (S-TSH)*	Serum	0.4-5 μU/mL	0.4-5 mU/L

*Subclinical hypothyroidism has been recognized for 20 years and is characterized by patients who are clinically euthyroid and have normal or equivocal serum T$_4$ and T$_3$ concentrations and increased TSH. The old TSH test was effective for diagnosing hypothyroidism but not hyperthyroidism. With the new S-TSH test, a group of patients will be recognized who have subclinical hyperthyroidism (i.e., clinically euthyroid, normal, or equivocal serum T$_4$ and T$_3$ concentrations and a decreased S-TSH).

3.   To diagnose hypothyroidism, interpret test results in the context of clinical findings.

a.   Primary hypothyroidism in ambulatory patients is characterized by a low FT$_4$I and a high S-TSH. In a patient with early or mild primary hypothyroidism the FT$_4$I may be normal and the S-TSH high. In one with secondary hypothyroidism the FT$_4$I is low, and the S-TSH is normal or low.

The cause of primary hypothyroidism may be previous iodine 131 therapy, thyroidectomy, ingestion of antithyroid drugs, a familial disorder, Hashimoto's thyroiditis, or the postpartum state. Significantly increased titers of antithyroid microsomal antibodies indicate that the patient suffers from Hashimoto's thyroiditis or postpartum thyroid dysfunction.

Approximately 10% of hypothyroid patients have secondary hypothyroidism due to pituitary failure in which there is a low FT_4I and a low S-TSH. Additional endocrinological testing and radiographic studies may be used to establish the diagnosis. Drugs can decrease or increase T_4, T_3, and FT_4I values in euthyroid patients; however, the S-TSH is generally reliable as a true indicator of thyroid function (two exceptions are large doses of glucocorticoids and dopamine, which may decrease S-TSH values).

  b. **A useful approach for diagnosing hypothyroidism in sick patients is to consider patients with mild to moderate illness (uncomplicated patients) separately from those with severe illness (e.g., intensive care patients).**

Mild to Moderately Ill Patients

The criteria for diagnosing hypothyroidism in mild to moderately ill patients are the same as for uncomplicated ambulatory patients. In the absence of thyroid disease, the FT_4I and S-TSH are generally normal, but occasionally the FT_4I is high.

Severely Ill Patients With a Low FT_4I and a Normal S-TSH

The FT_4I may be low in severely ill patients such as intensive care patients, but the S-TSH is usually normal, and these patients are usually euthyroid. A simultaneously low FT_4I and a high S-TSH may indicate primary hypothyroidism. A pitfall is that the use of dopamine and corticosteroids in critically ill patients can suppress a high S-TSH into the normal range.

Severely Ill Patients With a Low FT_4I and a High S-TSH

A low FT_4I and a high S-TSH in patients recovering from a severe illness are compatible with either primary hypothyroidism or euthyroidism. Since unrecognized hypothyroidism has a prevalence of only 1% in the adult population, most patients with these findings are euthyroid. As the sick euthyroid patient recovers, the S-TSH decreases to normal in a few days or weeks. Previous treatment for Graves' disease, thyroid surgery, high titers of antithyroid microsomal antibodies, or physical findings of hypothyroidism favor diagnosis of primary hypothyroidism.

Severely Ill Patients With a Low FT_4I and a Low S-TSH

A severely ill patient with a low FT_4I and a low S-TSH presents a rare situation—consider secondary hypothyroidism. Look for signs of hypogonadism and hypoadrenalism and measure serum cortisol to detect an undiagnosed pituitary deficiency. Sometimes a measurable level of S-TSH is found in a patient with secondary hypothyroidism that results from an abnormal TSH with decreased biological activity. Provided the patient is not receiving dopamine or corticosteroids and in the absence of hypothalamic or pituitary disease, a normal S-TSH excludes primary thyroid disease.

c. **If you diagnose hypothyroidism and decide to treat the patient with thyroid replacement hormone, measure S-TSH to monitor therapy 2 to 6 months after the full replacement dose is achieved.**

The ideal dose of thyroid hormone will lower the S-TSH level into the normal but not the subnormal range. Excessive replacement therapy may cause osteoporosis and findings of hyperthyroidism. There is a risk of osteoporosis even when hyperthyroid findings are not apparent.

d. **In the hypothyroid patient the following additional abnormal blood test results may occur:**

Anemia, mild and typically normocytic, but may be macrocytic; sometimes pernicious anemia with Hashimoto's thyroiditis.

↑ **Erythrocyte sedimentation rate.**

↓ **Partial pressure of oxygen (Po$_2$)** with dyspnea secondary to pleural effusion.

↑ **Glucose.**

↓ **Glucose.**

Slightly high creatinine, urea nitrogen, and uric acid, which are related to lower glomerular filtration and which return to normal with replacement therapy; uric acid frequently high and may lead to attacks of gout.

↑ **Bicarbonate** related to increased CO$_2$.

↓ **Sodium** with or without the inappropriate antidiuretic hormone (ADH) syndrome; may also be caused by pseudohyponatremia associated with hyperlipidemia.

↑ **Calcium.**

↑ **Magnesium.**

↑ **Creatine kinase,** ↑ **aspartate aminotransferase, and high lactate dehydrogenase** caused by skeletal muscle myopathy.

↓ **Alkaline phosphatase** caused by low osteoblastic activity.

↑ **Albumin.**

↑ **Cholesterol** in hypothyroidism of thyroid (but not pituitary) origin.

↑ **Triglyceride.**

↓ **Ferritin,** presumably because of low protein turnover.

4. **To diagnose hyperthyroidism, interpret test results in the context of clinical findings.**

a. **Primary hyperthyroidism in uncomplicated patients is characterized by a low S-TSH and a high FT$_4$I. In patients with a normal FT$_4$I and a low S-TSH, request a serum T$_3$ determination to investigate the possibility of T$_3$ thyrotoxicosis.**

The serum FT$_4$I is increased in approximately 95% of ambulatory hyperthyroid patients; an occasional hyperthyroid patient may have a normal FT$_4$I and increased serum T$_3$ (T$_3$ thyrotoxicosis). The magnitude of elevation of T$_3$ provides a quantitative assessment of the severity of the thyrotoxic state. The serum S-TSH should be clearly subnormal, that is, <0.1 μU/mL (0.1 mU/L) to make the diagnosis of hyperthyroidism. The cause of hyperthyroidism may be Graves' disease (diffusely enlarged gland and exophthalmos), toxic adenoma, or toxic multinodular goiter (confirm by thyroid scan with radioactive iodine [do not administer to pregnant women or nursing mothers]). If one of these common causes is unclear, perform a radioactive iodine uptake examination—results are generally increased in patients with Graves' disease and decreased in ones with hyperthyroidism caused by subacute thyroiditis, "silent" (lymphocytic) thyroiditis, postpartum thyroid dysfunction, or thyrotoxicosis factitia. To diagnose thyrotoxicosis factitia, measure serum thyroglobulin, which is low with thyrotoxicosis factitia and high with any form of primary thyrotoxicosis.

> **b. Several other confusing combinations of test results may be found that are suggestive of hyperthyroidism.**

Patients With a Normal FT$_4$I, Normal T$_3$, and Low S-TSH

In the absence of medication that suppresses thyrotropin secretion, patients with a normal FT$_4$I, normal T$_3$ level, and low S-TSH probably have mild thyrotoxicosis with minimal hypersecretion of thyroid hormone. Their abnormal thyroid function may be further established using a T$_3$-suppression test or by demonstrating a lack of responsiveness of serum TSH to thyrotropin-releasing hormone (TRH).

Patients With High FT$_4$I, High T$_3$, and Normal or High S-TSH

Findings of high FT$_4$I, high T$_3$, and normal or high S-TSH are rare. Consider secondary hyperthyroidism caused by increased and autonomous thyrotropin secretion, generally from a pituitary tumor.

Patients With High Serum FT$_4$I and Normal S-TSH

Patients with high serum FT$_4$I and normal S-TSH are encountered infrequently and are usually euthyroid. Some may have familial dysalbuminemic hyperthyroxinemia. Others may have circulating anti-T$_4$ and/or anti-T$_3$ antibodies.

> **c. Hyperthyroid patients with a nonthyroidal illness may show confusing combinations of test results. It is useful to consider patients with mild to moderate illness separately from patients with severe illness. In puzzling situations consult an endocrinologist.**

Hyperthyroid Patients With a Nonthyroidal Illness	Tests Results
Mild illness	T$_4$ and T$_3$ are high. S-TSH should be less than 0.1 µU/mL (0.1 mU/L).
Moderate illness	T$_3$ may be normal, but the T$_4$ is generally high. S-TSH should be less than 0.1 µU/mL (0.1 mU/L).
Severe illness	T$_4$ and T$_3$ levels may be normal or low. S-TSH should be less than 0.1 µU/mL (0.1 mU/L).

Remember that with nonthyroidal illness or treatment with dopamine or large doses of corticosteroids, a low S-TSH may be found. Monitor serial serum S-TSH levels and/or perform TRH testing to clarify the diagnosis.

Recently screening of 651 elderly nursing home residents detected 11 patients (1.7% prevalence) with high FT_4I levels and normal S-TSH levels. These patients were clinically determined euthyroid.

d. In the hyperthyroid patient the following additional abnormal blood test results may occur:

Mild anemia, typically normocytic.

↑ **Erythrocyte sedimentation rate.**

Moderate neutropenia.

Idiopathic thrombocytopenic purpura in Graves' disease and Hashimoto's thyroiditis.

↓ **PO_2.**

↓ **Partial pressure of carbon dioxide (PCO_2)** with respiratory alkalosis.

↑ **Glucose** from accelerated glycogenolysis secondary to increased catecholamines.

↑ **Urea nitrogen and creatinine** associated with excessive protein catabolism.

↑ **Sodium** caused by hypercalcemic diabetes insipidus.

↓ **Potassium** and periodic paralysis.

↑ **Calcium** due to bone dissolution by osteoclasts.

↑ **Phosphorus** with increased bone dissolution and increased renal reabsorption.

↓ **Magnesium.**

↑ **Alkaline phosphatase** from stimulation of osteoclasts by thyroid hormones.

↓ **Amylase** in thyrotoxicosis.

↓ **Albumin** possibly related to rapid turnover.

↑ **Bilirubin** caused by hemolysis or ↓ **Bilirubin** related to decreased RBC mass and low albumin.

↓ **Cholesterol and** ↓ **triglycerides.**

BIBLIOGRAPHY

Bayer MF: Effective laboratory evaluation of thyroid status. Med Clin North Am 75:1, 1991.
  Reviews the use of laboratory tests for diagnosing and managing thyroid disease.
Drinka PJ, Nolten WE, Voeks S, et al: Misleading elevation of the free thyroxine index in nursing home residents. Arch Pathol Lab Med 115:1208, 1991; and Oxley DK: Screening for hyperthyroidism. Arch Pathol Lab Med 115:1201, 1991.
  Interesting example of false-positive thyroid function tests in the elderly.
Greenspan SL, Greenspan FS, Resnick NM, et al: Skeletal integrity in premenopausal and postmenopausal women receiving long-term L-thyroxine therapy. Am J Med 91:5, 1991.
  If the FT_4I is maintained in the physiological range, the changes in bone density are minimal.
Hay ID, Bayer MF, Kaplan MM, et al: American Thyroid Association assessment of current free thyroid hormone and thyrotropin measurements and guidelines for future clinical assays. Clin Chem 37:2002, 1991.
  Guidelines from the American Thyroid Association for choosing appropriate tests for free thyroid hormone and sensitive TSH assays.
Hayward RSA, Steinberg EP, Ford DE, et al: Preventive care guidelines: 1991. Ann Intern Med 114:758, 1991.
  Recommendations about wellness screening using thyroid function testing.

Helfand M, Crapo LM: Testing for suspected thyroid disease. In Sox HC Jr (ed): Common
   Diagnostic Tests: Use and Interpretation, 2nd ed. Philadelphia, American College of
   Physicians, 1990, p 148.
   Reviews the use of thyroid function tests to diagnose thyroid dysfunction.
Kassirer JP, Kopelman RI: Case 5—A hit after a miss. In Learning Clinical Reasoning.
   Baltimore, Md, Williams & Wilkins, 1991, p 63.
   *Discusses clinical reasoning in the diagnosis and management of a patient with hypothyroidism
   in which hypercholesterolemia is the initial clue.*
LeMar HJ Jr, West SG, Garrett CR, et al: Covert hypothyroidism presenting as a cardio-
   vascular event. Am J Med 91:549, 1991.
   *Increased creatine kinase concentration may be a clue to hypothyroidism in patients with cardio-
   vascular findings.*
Sawin CT: Thyroid dysfunction in older persons. In Siperstein MD (ed): Adv Intern Med
   37:223, 1991.
   Discusses the problem of undiagnosed or misdiagnosed thyroid disease in the elderly.
Sundbeck G, Jagenburg R, Johansson P-M, et al: Clinical significance of low serum thy-
   rotropin concentration by chemiluminometric assay in 85-year-old women and men.
   Arch Intern Med 151:549, 1991.
   *Approximately 2% of elderly asymptomatic persons have low TSH levels with new sensitive assays,
   but the majority of these patients are not hyperthyroid.*
Surks MI, Chopra IJ, Mariash CN, et al: American Thyroid Association Guidelines for
   use of laboratory tests in thyroid disorders. JAMA 263:1529, 1990.
   *Recommendations by The American Thyroid Association for using tests to diagnose thyroid dys-
   function, which constitute the basis for most of the guidelines in this problem.*
Symposium on sensitive TSH assays: Introduction, Parts I, II, and III. Mayo Clin Proc
   63:1026, 1988.
   Excellent review of the role of sensitive TSH assays in patient care.
Wynne AG, Gharib H, Scheithauer BW, et al: Hyperthyroidism due to inappropriate
   secretion of thyrotropin in 10 patients. Am J Med 92:15, 1992.
   Reports 10 cases of secondary hyperthyroidism from the Mayo Clinic.

Hypocalcemia and Hypoparathyroidism

**1.   For patients with clinical findings of hypocalcemia or for an individual
with a low serum calcium concentration, request at least three measurements of serum calcium together with a complete blood count (CBC), serum
albumin and globulin determinations by electrophoresis, and determinations of phosphorus, magnesium, alkaline phosphatase, urea nitrogen, creatinine, and electrolyte levels. In certain circumstances measurement of
serum ionized calcium may be helpful.**

Remember that certain drugs such as anticonvulsants, corticosteroids,
diuretics, and laxatives may be associated with a low serum calcium concentration.

Measurements of calcium, albumin, phosphorus, and magnesium are useful to verify the presence of hypocalcemia and to attempt to determine its
cause. Serum urea nitrogen, creatinine, and electrolyte determinations help
assess renal function, and a CBC and an alkaline phosphatase determination
may provide valuable clues about the presence of malignancy.

See the discussion of hypercalcemia, which follows this section, for specimen collection and handling issues.

2.   Evaluate the tests.

See the discussion of hypercalcemia, which follows this section, for testing issues.

3.   If hypocalcemia is documented by at least three serum calcium measurements and drugs are not the cause, consider the differential diagnosis as follows.

Prior thyroid surgery is a common cause of a low serum calcium value secondary to hypoparathyroidism. If hypoparathyroidism is suspected, low ionized calcium and low parathyroid hormone values can confirm the diagnosis. Idiopathic hypoparathyroidism may also occur. In addition to a deficiency of parathyroid hormone, a low serum calcium level may be caused by failure of the kidneys to respond to normal amounts of parathyroid hormone, a condition known as *pseudohypoparathyroidism*. In a patient with either hypoparathyroidism or pseudohypoparathyroidism the serum phosphorus level is high. Both hypomagnesemia and hypermagnesemia can impair parathyroid hormone secretion, causing hypocalcemia. Renal failure is perhaps the most common of all causes of hypocalcemia: the serum urea nitrogen, creatinine, and phosphorus levels are all increased. In patients with intestinal malabsorption defective absorption of both calcium and vitamin D can occur, resulting in hypocalcemia. Miscellaneous causes of hypocalcemia include acute pancreatitis, osteoblastic metastatic bone disease, excessive transfusion with citrated blood, and rhabdomyolysis-induced renal failure. After parathyroid surgery hypocalcemia may be caused by the hungry bone syndrome in which remineralization of the skeleton causes hypocalcemia and hypophosphatemia, often with tetany, requiring vigorous, prolonged calcium and vitamin D therapy.

4.   If hypocalcemia can be explained as an effect of drug therapy, improper specimen collection and handling, or laboratory error, conclude that the patient does not have a pathological cause.

Hypocalcemia may be the result of a methodology problem, or it may be related to a low serum albumin level. Certain drugs such as phenytoin and other anticonvulsant medications have been implicated as a cause of vitamin D deficiency and borderline-low serum calcium values. It is important to identify these causes of hypocalcemia so that a needless search for some underlying disease or disorder can be averted.

5.   In patients with hypoparathyroidism the following abnormal blood test results may occur:

↑   **Creatine kinase** associated with myopathy.

BIBLIOGRAPHY

Barnes HV: Hypoparathyroidism. In Spivak JL, Barnes HV: Manual of Clinical Problems
   in Internal Medicine, 4th ed. Boston, Little Brown & Co, 1990, p 199.
   Discussion of differential diagnosis with annotated key references.
Brasier AR, Nussbaum SR: Hungry bone syndrome: Clinical and biochemical predictors
   of its occurrence after parathyroid surgery. Am J Med 84:654, 1988.
   After parathyroid surgery remineralization of the skeleton may cause hypocalcemia.
Riancho JA, Arjona R, Valle R, et al: The clinical spectrum of hypocalcemia associated
   with bone metastases. J Intern Med 226:449, 1989.
   Osteoblastic metastatic bone disease, particularly from prostate cancer, may cause hypocalcemia.

Hypercalcemia, Cancer, and Hyperparathyroidism

1.   For patients with clinical findings of hyperparathyroidism or for an individual with hypercalcemia, request at least three measurements of serum total calcium together with a CBC, serum albumin and globulin determinations by electrophoresis, determinations of phosphorus, magnesium, alkaline phosphatase, urea nitrogen, creatinine, and electrolyte levels, thyroid function tests, and a 24-hour urinary calcium determination. In certain circumstances measurement of serum ionized calcium may be helpful. Review the drug history for a possible hypercalcemic effect.

Before undertaking the differential diagnosis of hypercalcemia, artifactual causes of hypercalcemia should be excluded. If the serum calcium is truly high, the cause should be determined, keeping in mind that cancer and hyperparathyroidism are among the more common causes.

The laboratory studies should be part of a thorough workup that includes a careful history and physical examination, chest roentgenography, renal ultrasonography, and skeletal survey radiographs. Drugs such as vitamin D or antacids together with milk can cause hypercalcemia (milk-alkali syndrome).

In the past patients with hyperparathyroidism usually were seen with clinical features of the disease before hypercalcemia was detected. With the advent of laboratory screening, the current typical presentation of patients with hyperparathyroidism is unexplained hypercalcemia. Although some experts believe that screening for hypercalcemia is valuable, others argue that there is no advantage in treating asymptomatic hyperparathyroidism and that screening with serum calcium measurements should be omitted.

Other causes of hypercalcemia that must be differentiated from hyperparathyroidism are shown in the table on the next page.

Common causes for hypercalcemia are cancer and hyperparathyroidism. Most hospitalized patients with hypercalcemia will have cancer, but most ambulatory patients will have hyperparathyroidism, with only a few having cancer. Additional conditions associated with hypercalcemia include adrenal insufficiency; acromegaly; vitamin A intoxication; pheochromocytoma; the

INCREASED GASTROINTESTINAL ABSORPTION OF CALCIUM	INCREASED RESORPTION OF BONE	INCREASED RENAL RESORPTION
Sarcoidosis	Cancer of bone*	Thiazide diuretics
Other granuloma-tous diseases		
Milk-alkali syndrome	Ectopic PTH syndrome	Familial hypocal-ciuric hypercal-cemia
Hypervitaminosis D	Hyperthyroidism	
	Paget's disease of bone	
	Immobilization	

*These are usually the osteolytic metastases of carcinoma of the breast, lung, and prostate or are multiple myeloma, acute leukemias, certain lymphomas, and Hodgkin's disease. Sometimes bone involvement is absent, and the hypercalcemia is induced by a parathyroid hormone–related humoral mediator.

watery diarrhea, hypokalemia, achlorhydria syndrome; lithium therapy; and postrenal transplant.

Diurnal variation of serum calcium concentrations, although slight, makes a morning sample desirable. Remember that posture affects serum calcium levels. Since serum calcium is bound to albumin and since albumin is higher in ambulatory than in recumbent patients, calcium levels are higher in ambulatory patients than in recumbent patients. Prolonged application of a tourniquet or muscular exercise of the limb chosen for venipuncture can artifactually increase the serum calcium concentration. Serum or heparinized plasma is a satisfactory sample, but do not allow prolonged contact with red blood cells since with time the cells become permeable to calcium. Using a cork stopper on the patient's sample can increase the calcium concentration because cork contains calcium.

Serum inorganic phosphorus concentration may be difficult to interpret unless the specimen is collected in the morning after an overnight fast (with no intravenous fluids). Under these conditions the reference range for adults is 3 to 4.5 mg/dL (0.97 to 1.45 mmol/L). The concentration is slightly higher before puberty and after gonadal failure.

Total calcium concentration in serum includes three forms: a protein-bound fraction (40%); a chelated fraction (10%); and an ionized, physiologically active fraction (50%). Serum measurements of total calcium are sometimes misleading, especially among patients in intensive care units, in neonates, in patients undergoing liver and cardiac transplant surgery, and in patients with renal disease. In these patients determining serum ionized calcium concentrations may be helpful. Blood samples should be collected anaerobically and without venous stasis. If use of an anticoagulated specimen is necessary, use the smallest amount of heparin possible because heparin binds calcium and will cause a decrease in the ionized calcium concentration.

Ionized calcium should not be measured in specimens containing citrate or ethylenediaminetetraacetic acid (EDTA).

2. Evaluate the tests and the results.

The accuracy and precision of present calcium methods is not good enough to distinguish normocalcemia sharply from borderline hypercalcemia. Remember the effect of altered serum albumin values.

REFERENCE RANGE

Test	Specimen	Conventional Units	International Units
Calcium, ionized (iCa)	Serum, plasma, or whole blood (with heparin)	4.65-5.28 mg/dL	1.16-1.32 mmol/L

Serum total calcium measurements >12 mg/dL (2.99 mmol/L) are associated with toxicity (e.g., hypercalcemic coma), and medical therapy is indicated. Make certain that serum calcium is measured by an accurate and precise method. The reference method is atomic absorption. In addition, patients with mild hyperparathyroidism may have intermittent elevations. Thus repeat measurements of serum calcium should be obtained. In questionable cases it may be useful to space the samples over several weeks or months.

The reference range for serum total calcium should be corrected for serum albumin concentration according to the ratio of 0.5 mg/dL (0.12 mmol/L) of serum calcium for every 1 g/dL (10 g/L) of serum albumin above or below the middle of the reference range. With an increase or decrease in albumin, other cations bound to albumin (e.g., magnesium and zinc) also will increase or decrease.

Serum concentrations of phosphorus, alkaline phosphatase, urea nitrogen, creatinine, electrolytes, and magnesium outside the reference range favor a pathological cause for an increased calcium value. Hypercalcemia may be caused by hyperlipoproteinemia or hyperproteinemia.

3. If hypercalcemia is documented by at least three serum calcium measurements and if drugs are not the cause, consider the differential diagnosis for hypercalcemia. If hyperparathyroidism is a serious consideration, measure immunoreactive parathyroid hormone.

Primary hyperparathyroidism can be diagnosed best by showing persistent hypercalcemia with an increased serum parathyroid hormone concentration. Patients with hypercalcemia from other causes such as malignancies and sarcoidosis have low-normal or decreased parathyroid hormone values. Recently the agent responsible for the humoral hypercalcemia of cancer was isolated: parathyroid hormone–related protein (PTHRP). In general, plasma PTHRP concentrations are not increased in patients with primary hyperparathyroidism, and plasma parathyroid hormone concentrations are not increased in the humoral hypercalcemia of cancer.

Severe hypercalcemia (>14 mg/dL [>3.49 mmol/L]) favors nonparathyroid causes, usually cancer. Milder serum calcium elevations are typically seen in patients with hyperparathyroidism; however, nonparathyroid causes may be responsible. A diagnostic rule of thumb is that hypercalcemia that lasts more than a year without signs of primary cancer (or another identifiable cause) is caused by parathyroid disease.

The ratio of serum chloride to phosphorus is helpful in differentiating hyperparathyroidism from other causes. In hyperparathyroid patients chloride values are high (mean, >107 mEq/L [>107 mmol/L]), and the chloride:phosphorus ratios range from 32 to 80, with 96% of values higher than 33. In patients with hypercalcemia from other causes the chloride values are lower (mean, 98 mEq/L [98 mmol/L]), the phosphorus measurement is higher (mean, 4.5 mg/dL [1.45 mmol/L]), and the chloride:phosphorus ratios range from 18 to 32, with 92% of values lower than 30.

If hypercalcemia is accompanied by an increased alkaline phosphatase level, the differential diagnosis includes hyperparathyroidism, hyperthyroidism, osteoblastic bone lesions, and malignancy. Alkaline phosphatase is not increased in multiple myeloma patients. A serum alkaline phosphatase value greater than twice the upper reference limit is unlikely to indicate uncomplicated primary hyperparathyroidism. A decreased serum alkaline phosphatase value may occur with hypervitaminosis D related to an increased phosphorus concentration.

Increased serum urea nitrogen and creatinine concentrations suggest the nephropathy of mild hyperparathyroidism.

Serum potassium values may be low in patients with hypercalcemia (32%), and potassium concentration varies inversely with calcium. Because patients with cancer have higher calcium values, these cancer patients have a higher prevalence of hypokalemia (52%).

A low urinary calcium concentration (usually <60 mg/24 hour [<1.50 mmol/24 hour]) is the diagnostic hallmark of familial hypocalciuric hypercalcemia, an autosomal dominant syndrome. The serum magnesium concentration may be increased. If a low urinary calcium value is found, this diagnosis should be considered, and family members should be screened for hypercalcemia.

4. If additional calcium measurements are normal and the increased calcium concentration can be explained on the basis of drug therapy, improper specimen collection and handling, or laboratory error, conclude that the patient does not have a pathological cause of hypercalcemia.

5. In patients with hypercalcemia the following abnormal blood test results may occur:

↓ **Hemoglobin or hematocrit** and a ↑ **erythrocyte sedimentation rate** suggest a nonparathyroid cause, particularly malignancy, although these findings may occur in primary hyperparathyroidism.

Leukopenia is frequent in hyperparathyroidism.

↓ **Pco₂ and bicarbonate** because parathyroid hormone increases urinary bicarbonate excretion.

↑ **Urea nitrogen, creatinine, and uric acid** secondary to nephropathy. Uric acid may be high in malignancy because of high cell turnover and proliferation.

↑ **Chloride** secondary to low bicarbonate.

↑ **Chloride metabolic acidosis** favors primary hyperparathyroidism.

↓ **Serum magnesium** may occur in hyperparathyroidism.

↑ **Phosphorus** without renal failure suggests a nonparathyroid cause.

↓ **Phosphorus** (when dietary phosphorus is adequate and patient is not taking oral phosphate-binding agents) favors primary hyperparathyroidism but can occur in malignancy.

↑ **Serum transaminase and alkaline phosphatase** with granulomatous hepatitis (e.g., sarcoidosis).

↑ **Alkaline phosphatase** often in malignancy and unlikely in primary hyperparathyroidism in the absence of osteitis fibrosa cystica. The Regan isoenzyme may occur in patients with carcinoma. Polyclonal hypergammaglobulinemia favors sarcoidosis but has been seen in primary hyperparathyroidism.

↑ **Lactate dehydrogenase** caused by high malignant cell turnover and proliferation.

BIBLIOGRAPHY

Arvan DA: Hypercalcemia. In Panzer RJ, Black ER, Griner PF (eds): Diagnostic Strategies for Common Medical Problems. Philadelphia, American College of Physicians, 1991, p 355.
   Recommends strategies for the differential diagnosis of hypercalcemia.
Barnes HV: Hypercalcemia and primary hyperparathyroidism. In Spivak JL, Barnes HV: Manual of Clinical Problems in Internal Medicine, 4th ed. Boston, Little, Brown & Co, 1990, pp 52, 216.
   Discusses diagnosis and management, with annotated key references.
Burtis WJ, Brady TG, Orloff JJ, et al: Immunochemical characterization of circulating parathyroid hormone–related protein in patients with humoral hypercalcemia of cancer. N Engl J Med 322:1106, 1990; and Bilezikian JP: Parathyroid hormone–related peptide in sickness and health. N Engl J Med 322:1151, 1990.
   Article and editorial describing the use of parathyroid hormone–related protein in differentiating the hypercalcemia of cancer from primary hyperparathyroidism.

Consensus Development Conference Panel: Diagnosis and management of asymptomatic primary hyperparathyroidism: Consensus Development Conference statement. Ann Intern Med 114:593, 1991.
Establishes guidelines for diagnosing and treating asymptomatic patients with hyperparathyroidism.
Gökçe C, Gökçe O, Baydinc C, et al: Use of random urine samples to estimate total urinary calcium and phosphate excretion. Arch Intern Med 151:1587, 1991.
Estimates of daily excretion of urinary calcium and phosphorus can be obtained by measuring random urinary calcium, phosphorus, and creatinine concentrations.
Gray TA, Paterson CR: The clinical value of ionized calcium assays. Ann Clin Biochem 25:210, 1988.
Reviews the use of ionized calcium measurements in patient care.
Heath H III: Primary hyperparathyroidism: Recent advances in pathogenesis, diagnosis, and management. In Siperstein MD (ed): Adv Intern Med 37:275, 1991.
Review of primary hyperparathyroidism from the Mayo Clinic.
Kassirer JP, Kopelman RI: Case 44—Watch and wait, or operate? In Learning Clinical Reasoning. Baltimore, Williams & Wilkins, 1991, p 222.
Discusses clinical reasoning in a patient with asymptomatic hyperparathyroidism.
Mallette LE, Beck P, Vandepol C: Malignancy hypercalcemia: Evaluation of parathyroid function and response to treatment. Am J Med Sci 302:205, 1991.
Discusses intact and midregion PTH assays for the evaluation of parathyroid function in patients with malignancy-associated hypercalcemia.
Nikkilä MT, Saaristo JJ, Koivula TA: Clinical and biochemical features in primary hyperparathyroidism. Surgery 105:148, 1989.
Discusses biochemical findings in 61 surgical cases.
Ratcliffe WA, Hutchesson ACJ, Bundred NJ, et al: Role of assays for parathyroid hormone—related protein in investigation of hypercalcemia. Lancet 339:164, 1992.
Discusses the usefulness of parathyroid hormone—related protein to discover malignancy in cases of hypercalcemia.

True Hypoglycemia and the Idiopathic Postprandial Syndrome

1. In patients with clinical findings of hypoglycemia measure serum glucose. Draw an additional 10 to 20 mL of blood for studies determined by clues from the clinical findings.

The only unequivocal diagnostic test for true hypoglycemia is documentation of a low serum glucose concentration during the time the patient experiences spontaneously developed symptoms. The true hypoglycemia syndrome refers to the presence of adrenergic or neuroglycopenic signs and symptoms in the presence of a low serum glucose concentration—generally <40 mg/dL (2.22 mmol/L)—in which the signs and symptoms can be relieved by the administration of glucose (Whipple's triad). In the idiopathic postprandial syndrome the serum glucose concentration is typically normal.

HYPOGLYCEMIC SIGNS AND SYMPTOMS

Adrenergic symptoms of hypoglycemia are induced by epinephrine secretion and consist of sweating, tremor, tachycardia, anxiety, and hunger. Neuroglycopenic findings are caused by low central nervous system glucose and consist of dizziness, headache, clouded vision, blunted mental acuity, confusion, abnormal behavior, convulsions, and coma. Persistent, very low central nervous system glucose values can cause features of decortication or decerebration and focal abnormalities, particularly hemiplegia. Without glucose administration, these defects may become permanent. Interestingly, the peripheral nervous system is seldom affected by hypoglycemia.

IDIOPATHIC POSTPRANDIAL SYNDROME

Idiopathic postprandial syndrome is a term applied to the adrenergic signs and symptoms (often reduced by glucose administration), for which the cause frequently is unclear, that occur in many individuals 2 to 5 hours after a meal. Generally, if serum glucose is measured, these individuals do not have hypoglycemia.

In the workup of a patient with hypoglycemia a detailed history is essential and should include information about every medication (prescription and nonprescription) and alcohol ingestion. For patients who have underlying disease, the results of the history and physical examination should determine the direction of the investigation. The following tests may be useful: serum glucose, insulin, calcium, phosphorus, uric acid, lipids, creatinine, liver function, insulin antibodies, and serum and urinary corticosteroids.

Be alert for artifactual hypoglycemia, which can occur in patients with leukemia, polycythemia, and hemolytic anemia with excessive nucleated red blood cells. Serum should be separated promptly from blood cells, or blood should be preserved with fluoride because blood cells metabolize glucose and decrease the serum glucose concentration.

2. Evaluate the serum glucose result.

A low serum glucose concentration is generally one that is <40 mg/dL (2.22 mmol/L). Normally, at glucose concentrations of 40 mg/dL (2.22 mmol/L) or less, little or no insulin is released. Vitamin C ingestion can depress values measured with the glucose oxidase method. The methodological considerations are the same as for diagnosing diabetes, which is discussed in the next section.

Serum glucose concentrations do not always correlate with an individual's signs and symptoms. Symptoms of hypoglycemia usually occur at serum glucose values <40 mg/dL (2.22 mmol/L), but some persons show no findings with values as low as 30 mg/dL (1.67 mmol/L). Other persons may show findings at values up to 100 mg/dL (5.55 mmol/L) when the serum glucose rapidly falls from a previously high concentration. Adrenergic signs and symptoms apparently are related to a rapidly falling glucose concentration. If glucose falls rapidly but central nervous system levels remain adequate, adrenergic findings can occur in the absence of neuroglycopenic findings. If the glucose concentration falls slowly to very low levels, neuroglycopenic findings can occur in the absence of adrenergic findings.

3.   If a patient has adrenergic signs and symptoms and a normal serum glucose concentration in the postprandial state, consider the idiopathic postprandial syndrome. Never use the 5-hour oral glucose tolerance test to diagnose the idiopathic postprandial syndrome.

In healthy individuals ingestion of a meal provokes a rise in serum glucose and a brisk insulin release, followed by a falling serum glucose concentration and a decrease in insulin. Frequently the falling glucose value drops below baseline, even below 40 mg/dL (2.22 mmol/L), but these persons usually have no symptoms. Insulin is the primary hypoglycemic hormone. Other hormones that affect serum glucose (i.e., cortisol, growth hormone, glucagon, catecholamines) tend to increase the serum concentration.

Patients in the postprandial state with clinical findings suggestive of hypoglycemia usually do not have a low serum glucose concentration. The 5-hour oral glucose tolerance test produces so many false-positive results it has become completely discredited. If the patient has adrenergic signs and symptoms and the serum glucose concentration is normal, the diagnosis is the idiopathic postprandial syndrome. Treatment is controversial; however, a high-protein, low-carbohydrate diet frequently is prescribed for patients with the idiopathic postprandial syndrome and may relieve symptoms.

4.   If a patient has a low serum glucose concentration in the postprandial state, consider the following.

ALIMENTARY HYPOGLYCEMIA

Alimentary hypoglycemia is the most common cause of postprandial hypoglycemia. After certain procedures such as gastrectomy, gastrojejunostomy, pyloroplasty, or vagotomy, patients may have rapid postprandial gastric emptying with rapid absorption of glucose and excessive release of insulin. Since blood glucose values tend to fall faster than insulin values, hypoglycemia may ensue.

OTHER CAUSES OF POSTPRANDIAL HYPOGLYCEMIA

In certain children with fructose intolerance or galactosemia, ingestion of fructose or galactose causes hypoglycemia. Rarely leucine causes hypoglycemia in susceptible infants. In Jamaica extreme hypoglycemia after ingestion of unripe ackee fruit is called the *toxic hypoglycemic syndrome*. True postprandial hypoglycemia of unknown cause or idiopathic hypoglycemia in which the patient has adrenergic signs and symptoms relieved by glucose administration is rare.

5.   If a patient has a low serum glucose concentration in the fasting state, consider the following causes:

- **Hyperinsulinism:** too much insulin in a diabetic patient; islet cell hyperplasia or tumor; factitious administration of insulin or sulfonylureas.
- **Drugs:** alcohol; salicylates in children; propranolol; disopyramide; sulfamethoxazole-trimethoprim in a patient with renal failure; pentamidine and quinine when used to treat cerebral malaria; chlorpropamide (may stimulate beta cells, producing hyperinsulinemia); miscellaneous drugs (see the references for a review article on this subject).
- **Acquired liver disease:** hepatic congestion; severe hepatitis; cirrhosis; Reye's syndrome; secondary to uremia or sepsis.
- **Renal failure:** low gluconeogenic substrate and/or glucagon deficiency.
- **Hormone deficiencies:** hypopituitarism; adrenal insufficiency.
- **Extrapancreatic tumors:** large mesenchymal tumors; carcinomas of liver, gastrointestinal tract, and adrenal gland.
- **Substrate deficiency:** severe malnutrition; late pregnancy.
- **Enzyme defects:** glucose-6-phosphatase; pyruvate carboxylase.
- **Insulin antibodies.**
- **Miscellaneous disorders:** diffuse carcinomatosis; rampant leukemia.

6.   To diagnose hyperinsulinism secondary to an insulinoma or insulin administration, proceed as follows.

Hypoglycemia in a diabetic who is taking insulin or a sulfonylurea is perhaps the most common cause of fasting hypoglycemia. The diagnosis is obvious.

Hypoglycemia secondary to islet cell hyperplasia or tumor can be provoked by fasting. Start with a 6- to 8-hour overnight fast, but remember that a 48- to 64-hour fast may be required (exercise such as walking up and down stairs for an hour can help provoke hypoglycemia). Thirty-five percent will become hypoglycemic in 12 hours, 75% in 24 hours, and more than 90% in 48 hours. When hypoglycemia occurs (glucose level <60 mg/dL [<3.34 mmol/L]), measurement of serum insulin and C peptide in simultaneous samples will show inappropriately increased values in most patients with an insulinoma.

Factitious hypoglycemia caused by insulin administration may be diagnosed by measuring serum insulin and C peptide. In patients with factitious hypoglycemia the serum insulin level is increased and the C peptide level is decreased because insulin is administered directly instead of being produced in the islet beta cells where proinsulin normally gives rise to increased serum levels of both insulin and C peptide. Insulin antibodies may also be present. Patients with factitious hypoglycemia are often suicidal, and a psychiatrist should be consulted before confronting these patients with the evidence.

7.   In patients with hypoglycemia the following abnormal blood test results may occur:

↓ **Potassium and ↓ phosphorus** caused by intracellular shifts after administration of glucose and insulin.

BIBLIOGRAPHY

Boyle PJ, Schwartz NS, Shah SD, et al: Plasma glucose concentrations at the onset of hypoglycemic symptoms in patients with poorly controlled diabetes and in nondiabetics. N Engl J Med 318:1487, 1988.
Poorly controlled diabetics may have symptoms of hypoglycemia at plasma levels that are normal or even above normal.

Nelson RL: Drug-induced hypoglycemias. In Service FJ (ed): Hypoglycemic Disorders: Pathogenesis, Diagnosis, and Treatment. Boston, GK Hall, 1983, p 97.
Many drugs have been implicated as a cause of hypoglycemia.

Service FJ: Hypoglycemias. West J Med 154:442, 1991.
Authoritative and comprehensive review of the diagnosis and management of hypoglycemia.

Snorgaard O, Binder C: Monitoring of blood glucose concentration in subjects with hypoglycemia symptoms during everyday life. BMJ 300:16, 1990.
Functional hypoglycemia more likely is due to something other than low blood sugar.

Toxic hypoglycemic syndrome: Jamaica, 1989-1991. MMWR 41:53, 1992.
In Jamaica extreme hypoglycemia can follow ingestion of unripe ackee fruit.

Diabetes Mellitus

1. In patients with obvious features of diabetes mellitus such as rapid weight loss, polyuria, polydipsia, and ketonuria, immediately measure serum glucose—fasting or nonfasting. A value >200 mg/dL (11.10 mmol/L) is diagnostic of diabetes.

The importance of obtaining a good blood sample for analysis cannot be overemphasized. Blood cells rapidly metabolize glucose at room temperature, but this metabolic loss of glucose can be prevented by promptly (within ½ hour) separating the serum from the blood cells or by using collection tubes containing fluoride. In the usual hospital setting serum glucose measurements are clinically acceptable; however, if the patient has a leukocytosis or a delay (>90 minutes) is anticipated, the specimens should be collected in a tube containing fluoride.

2. In patients with findings of subclinical diabetes such as unusual infections, worsening vision, or periodontal disease, measure the fasting serum glucose concentration (morning sample after a 10- to 16-hour fast). Routine screening of asymptomatic persons is not indicated. A value >140 mg/dL (7.77 mmol/L) is diagnostic. Do not test patients who are acutely ill.

Most authorities recommend against general wellness screening for diabetes mellitus using fasting serum glucose values; however, some endorse selective wellness screening for diabetes for individuals at increased risk.

A fasting serum glucose level >140 mg/dL (7.77 mmol/L) supports the diagnosis of diabetes and makes an oral glucose tolerance test unnecessary. A second fasting glucose level >140 mg/dL (7.77 mmol/L) is required to actually make the diagnosis. However, a fasting serum glucose level <140 mg/dL (7.77 mmol/L) but >115 mg/dL (6.38 mmol/L) does not exclude diabetes because it is not as sensitive a test for diabetes as is the oral glucose tolerance test. A fasting serum glucose level <115 mg/dL (6.38 mmol/L) excludes diabetes. Acute illness can affect serum glucose levels and cause misleading results. The sensitivity of fasting glucose to detect diabetes decreases with advancing age (50 to 79 years).

3.   If the fasting serum glucose is 115 to 140 mg/dL (6.38 to 7.77 mmol/ L), perform an early morning (before breakfast) oral glucose tolerance test. Do not test patients who are acutely ill.

Alternative methods to determine glucose tolerance such as measurement of a postprandial or random serum glucose concentration or performance of a glucose tolerance test regardless of the time of the last meal (except for pregnant women) are not recommended as definitive procedures.

The oral glucose tolerance test may be compromised if the protocol is not closely followed and the results correctly interpreted. Perform the oral glucose tolerance test in the morning after the person has fasted at least 10 hours but not more than 16 hours. The individual should not be ill or taking a medication known to affect the blood sugar and should have had normal physical activity and carbohydrate intake >150 g/day for at least 3 days before the test. The individual should remain seated and should not eat, smoke, or drink coffee, tea, or alcohol during the test. First, draw a fasting blood glucose sample, and afterward give 75 g of glucose orally (challenge dose for children is 1.75 g/kg of ideal body weight up to 75 g). The oral glucose solution should be ingested in less than 5 minutes, and the clock starts running when the patient begins to drink. Then draw blood samples every 30 minutes for 2 hours.

The following drugs and chemical agents are known to affect glucose tolerance:
- **Diuretics and antihypertensive agents:** chlorthalidone, clonidine, diazoxide, furosemide, thiazides.
- **Hormonally active agents:** corticotropin, glucagon, glucocorticoids, oral contraceptives, somatotropin, thyroid hormones.
- **Psychoactive agents:** chlorprothixene, haloperidol, lithium carbonate, phenothiazines, tricyclic antidepressants.
- **Catecholamines and other neurologically active agents:** epinephrine, isoproterenol, levodopa, norepinephrine, phenytoin.
- **Analgesic, antipyretic, and anti-inflammatory agents.**
- **Antineoplastic agents:** alloxan, L-asparaginase, streptozocin.
- **Miscellaneous agents:** encainide, isoniazid, nicotinic acid.

4.   Evaluate the tests and the results.

Use a laboratory with an accurately standardized glucose method. Enzymatic methods for measuring serum glucose such as hexokinase or glucose oxidase are best because they give the most accurate results. Reduction methods using substances such as ferricyanide and neocuproine are obsolete and tend to overestimate the serum glucose concentration because of non-glucose-reducing substances in the blood. In patients with uremia serious errors can occur using reduction methods because of overestimation of serum glucose up to 40 mg/dL (2.22 mmol/L) as a result of in-creased uric acid and creatinine levels. Patients taking vitamin C have er-roneously low glucose values when measured with the glucose oxidase method.

Try to measure the fasting serum glucose before doing the glucose tol-erance test. If the fasting serum glucose concentration is >140 mg/dL (>7.77 mmol/L), the diagnosis of diabetes is supported, and a glucose tolerance test is unnecessary. If the fasting serum glucose concentration is <115 mg/dL (<6.38 mmol/L), the diagnosis of diabetes is excluded. If the fasting serum glucose level is 115 to 140 mg/dL (6.38 to 7.77 mmol/L), proceed with the oral glucose tolerance test.

DIAGNOSTIC ORAL GLUCOSE TOLERANCE TEST

TIME	FINDINGS
Fasting	<140 mg/dL (<7.77 mmol/L)
½ hr	Both 2-hr sample and at least one
1 hr	other sample must be >200 mg/
1½ hr	dL (>11.10 mmol/L)
2 hr	

IMPAIRED ORAL GLUCOSE TOLERANCE TEST

TIME	FINDINGS
Fasting	<140 mg/dL (<7.77 mmol/L)
½ hr	2-hr sample must be 140-200 mg/dL
1 hr	(7.77-11.10 mmol/L) and at least
1½ hr	one other sample must be >200
2 hr	mg/dL (>11.10 mmol/L)

5.   If the diagnosis of diabetes is supported by an increased fasting serum glucose concentration or a positive oral glucose tolerance test, confirm the diagnosis by obtaining one or more additional positive results such as another increased fasting serum glucose concentration or another positive glucose tolerance test result.

In light of the many factors other than diabetes that increase fasting serum glucose and impair glucose tolerance, it is imperative that an increased fast-ing serum glucose concentration or a positive glucose tolerance test be dem-onstrated on more than one occasion before a clinical diagnosis of diabetes is made.

6.   If the diagnosis of impaired glucose tolerance is supported by the oral glucose tolerance test, reexamine the patient yearly.

Individuals with impaired glucose tolerance may develop overt diabetes (at the rate of 1% to 5% per year), revert to normal glucose tolerance, or

OSU FACULTY
STAFF & STAFF
HEALTH PLAN

DIABETES MELLITUS TYPE I (Insulin Dependent) and TYPE II (Insulin Requiring) INITIAL and ONGOING EVALUATION AND CARE
ANNUAL FLOW SHEET AND CARE GUIDELINES

Elements of Care	Initial	1	2	3	4	5	6	7	8	9	10	11	12	As Needed	Compli-cations
						MONTHS									
Comprehensive Evaluation*	☐	(may require frequent contact until stable)											☐		☐
Routine Examination, stable patients may only require examination every 6 months				☐			☐			☐			☐	☐	
Nutrition Evaluation and Teaching	☐												☐	☐	
Eye Examination (visual acuity, intra-ocular pressure, ophthalmic exam through dilated pupil in darkened room)	☐												☐		☐
Foot Examination	☐			☐			☐			☐			☐		☐
Dental Examination	☐						☐						☐		☐
Gynecologic Exam	☐												☐		☐
Pre-conception Counseling and Obstetrical Care	☐													☐	
Home Glucose Monitoring *Continuously 2-8 times per day. Record mean glucose at each visit.*	☐			☐			☐			☐			☐		
Fasting Plasma Glucose	☐			☐			☐			☐			☐		
HbA1c	☐												☐		
Fast Lipid Profile (tot chol, HDL, trigly)	☐												☐	☐	
Lytes, H&H, WBC, BUN, Creat	☐												☐		
UA per multistick, protein, ketones, leukocytes, etc.	☐												☐		
EKG	☐														
24 hour urine, albumin & creatinine clearance (5 years after diagnosis, then annually)	☐												☐	☐	

☐ Date
☐ Result
*According to ADA guidelines, annual visit to diabetes specialist is encouraged

Source: OSU Health Plan: Clinical Notes, vol 1, no 3, Spring 1991.

2/4/91

OSU FACULTY STAFF & STAFF HEALTH PLAN

DIABETES MELLITUS TYPE II (Non-Insulin Requiring) INITIAL and ONGOING EVALUATION AND CARE
ANNUAL FLOW SHEET AND CARE GUIDELINES

Elements of Care	Initial	1	2	3	4	5	6	7	8	9	10	11	12	As Needed	Compli-cations
						MONTHS									
Comprehensive Evaluation*		(may require frequent contact until stable)													
Routine Examination															
Nutrition Evaluation and Teaching															
Eye Examination (visual acuity, intra-ocular pressure, ophthalmic exam through dilated pupil in darkened room)															
Foot Examination															
Dental Examination															
Gynecologic Exam															
Pre-conception Counseling and Obstetrical Care															
Fasting Plasma Glucose															
HbA1c															
Fast Lipid Profile (tot chol, HDL, trigly)															
Lytes, H&H, WBC, BUN, Creat															
UA per multistick															
EKG (in adults)															
24 hour urine albumin & creatinine clearance															

☐ Date
☐ Result

*According to ADA guidelines, annual visit to diabetes specialist is encouraged

Source: OSU Health Plan: Clinical Notes, vol 1, no 3, Spring 1991.

2/4/91

189

remain in the intermediate range. Persons with impaired glucose tolerance rarely have clinically significant microvascular disease.

7.   If the diagnosis of diabetes is confirmed, begin therapy and monitor the patient to include the detection of the six most common complications: uncontrolled diabetes; retinopathy; nephropathy; cardiovascular disease; peripheral vascular disease and neuropathy leading to amputations; and adverse outcomes of pregnancy. For an example of guidelines for following these patients, see the schedules developed for The Ohio State University Health Plan on pp. 188-189.

As indicated in the schedules, regular monitoring of serum glucose and hemoglobin A_{1C} (Hb A_{1C}) provides far better identification of patients with poor glycemic control, leading to appropriate changes in therapy. In a recent study diabetics with mean annual Hb A_{1C} values below 1.1 times the upper limit of normal did not develop retinopathy or microalbuminuria. Patients taking insulin should monitor their glucose at home at regular intervals. Patients should be monitored for microalbuminuria and frank proteinuria (see the discussion of proteinuria in the chapter on urinary tract diseases).

8.   In diabetic patients the following abnormal blood test results may occur:

↑ **Platelets.**

↑ **Urea nitrogen, creatinine, and uric acid** with renal failure.

↑ **Creatinine** due to high glucose and acetone interference with the test.

↓ **Uric acid** caused by hyperuricosuria.

↓ **Sodium** caused by hyperglycemia.

↑ **Potassium** related to metabolic acidosis.

↓ **Total carbon dioxide** from ketoacidosis.

↑ **Calcium** from hyperalbuminemia with dehydration.

↓ **Calcium,** ↓ **potassium,** ↓ **sodium, and** ↓ **chloride** from osmotic diuresis caused by hyperglycemia.

↑ **Phosphorus** caused by glucose intolerance with hyperglycemia.

↑ **Creatine kinase, lactate dehydrogenase, and transaminase levels** caused by effects on skeletal muscle and fatty liver.

↑ **Alkaline phosphatase.**

↑ **Protein and high albumin** caused by dehydration.

↓ **Albumin.**

↑ **Cholesterol and** ↑ **triglyceride** caused by disturbed carbohydrate metabolism.

BIBLIOGRAPHY

Blunt BA, Barrett-Connor E, Wingard DL: Evaluation of fasting plasma glucose as screening test for NIDDM in older adults. Diabetes Care 14:989, 1991.
    Sensitivity of fasting glucose for diabetes decreases in older persons.
Chase HP, Jackson WE, Hoops SL, et al: Glucose control and the renal and retinal complications of insulin-dependent diabetes. JAMA 261:1155, 1989.
    Mean annual Hb A_{1C} values <1.1 times the upper limit of normal prevent diabetic retinopathy and microalbuminuria.

Hayward RSA, Steinberg EP, Ford DE, et al: Preventive care guidelines: 1991. Ann Intern Med 114:758, 1991.

Authoritative recommendations about wellness screening for diabetes mellitus using fasting serum glucose.

Israngkun PP, Speicher CE: Glucose: Review of methods. Chicago, American Society of Clinical Pathologists, Core chemistry no. PTS 91-3 (PTS-53), 1991.

Extensively reviews methodology for measuring glucose.

Larsen ML, Horder M, Mogensen EF: Effect of long-term monitoring of glycosylated hemoglobin levels in insulin-dependent diabetes mellitus. N Engl J Med 323:1021, 1990.

Discussion of the role of glycosylated hemoglobin levels in the management of diabetes.

Ohio State Faculty: Diabetes mellitus. Columbus, Ohio, The Ohio State University Health Plan Clinical Notes, vol 1, no 3, Spring 1991.

Medical practice guidelines for diabetes mellitus.

Position Statement: Office guide to diagnosis and classification of diabetes mellitus and other categories of glucose intolerance. Diabetes Care 14(suppl 2):3, 1991.

Recommendations of the American Diabetes Association for the diagnosis of diabetes mellitus.

Roe TF, Costin G, Kaufman FR, et al: Blood glucose control and albuminuria in type I diabetes mellitus. J Pediatr 119:178, 1991; and Travis LB: Prevention of renal disease in insulin-dependent diabetes mellitus: A "responsibility" for the pediatrician? J Pediatr 119:273, 1991.

Showed that patients with good diabetes control (glycosylated hemoglobin <9%) had less albuminuria.

Sazama K, Robertson EA, Chesler RA: Is antiglycolysis required for routine glucose analysis? Clin Chem 25:2038, 1979.

Use tubes with fluoride for patients with leukocytosis or when delays longer than 90 minutes are anticipated.

Singer DE, Coley CM, Samet JH, et al: Tests of glycemia in diabetes mellitus: Their use in establishing a diagnosis and in treatment. In Sox HC Jr (ed): Common Diagnostic Tests: Use and Interpretation, 2nd ed. Philadelphia, American College of Physicians, 1990, p 121.

Recommendations by the American College of Physicians for using tests to diagnose and manage diabetes mellitus.

Speicher CE: The bottom line: Can portable blood glucose monitoring improve the outcomes of diabetic patients? Am J Clin Pathol 95:112, 1991.

Discussion of the role of portable blood glucose monitoring in the management of diabetes.

Gestational Diabetes Mellitus

1. Screen all pregnant women for gestational diabetes mellitus between the twenty-fourth and twenty-eighth weeks of pregnancy with a 50 g oral glucose load without regard to the time of the last meal or the time of day, and measure serum glucose at 1 hour. If a pregnant woman has a history of diabetes, screen her in the same manner at the time of the initial visit.

Twenty-four to 28 weeks of pregnancy is the optimal time for screening for gestational diabetes mellitus since at this time its frequency peaks and there is still sufficient time for appropriate therapy. The specimen collection and handling and methodological considerations are the same as for diagnosing diabetes in nonpregnant individuals.

Recognition and treatment of gestational diabetes prevents both maternal mortality and morbidity (hypertension, hydramnios, cesarean section) and perinatal mortality and morbidity (intrauterine death, macrosomia, birth trauma, neonatal hypoglycemia, hyperbilirubinemia, hypocalcemia, polycythemia).

2.   If the 1-hour serum glucose level is more than 140 mg/dL (7.77 mmol/L), perform the 100 g pregnancy oral glucose tolerance test.

Perform the oral glucose tolerance test the same way as in screening for diabetes in the nonpregnant individual with these exceptions: give 100 g of glucose orally instead of 75 g, and draw blood samples every hour for 3 hours instead of every 30 minutes for 2 hours. The specimen collection concerns are the same as for diabetes mellitus as discussed in the preceding section.

3.   Evaluate the tests and the results.

The methodological considerations are the same as for diabetes mellitus.

DIAGNOSTIC ORAL GLUCOSE TOLERANCE TEST IN PREGNANCY

TIME	FINDINGS*
Fasting	>105 mg/dL (>5.83 mmol/L)
1 hr	>190 mg/dL (>10.55 mmol/L)
2 hr	>165 mg/dL (>9.16 mmol/L)
3 hr	>145 mg/dL (>8.05 mmol/L)

*Any two or more values exceeding these concentrations are diagnostic.

Because glucose methodology has changed, some advocate revising these criteria levels to fasting, >95 mg/dL (>5.27 mmol/L); 1 hour, >180 mg/dL (>9.99 mmol/L); 2 hours, >155 mg/dL (>8.60 mmol/L); and 3 hours, >140 mg/dL (>7.77 mmol/L).

4.   If the oral glucose tolerance test is diagnostic, the patient has gestational diabetes mellitus. Reexamine the patient after the pregnancy, using the strategy for the nonpregnant adult.

After pregnancy terminates, the woman must be reexamined to determine whether she has normal, diabetic, or impaired glucose tolerance. In the majority of patients with gestational diabetes mellitus glucose tolerance returns to normal postpartum, and the individual can be classified as having a previous abnormality of glucose tolerance. Approximately 40% of women with gestational diabetes mellitus will become diabetic within 15 years after delivery, and the risk increases with obesity. Once a woman has had the condition, a 90% probability exists for recurrence with future pregnancies.

5.   If the oral glucose tolerance test is not diagnostic of gestational diabetes mellitus but one value is increased, some authorities recommend repeating the test in 3 to 4 weeks.

Up to a third of women having one increased value on the oral glucose tolerance test will have a diabetic glucose tolerance test on repeat testing. These women are at increased risk for fetal macrosomia and preeclampsia or eclampsia.

BIBLIOGRAPHY

Corcoy R, Cabero L, de Leiva A: Gestational diabetes: What are the implications? Postgrad Med 91:393, 1992.
  Discusses gestational diabetes and the merits of screening tests for all pregnant women.
Cousins L, Baxi L, Chez R, et al: Screening recommendations for gestational diabetes mellitus. Am J Obstet Gynecol 165:493, 1991.
  Ninety-six percent of maternal-fetal medicine subspecialists and 84% of fellows of the American College of Obstetricians and Gynecologists use these guidelines in their practice.
Do gestational diabetes criteria need revision? Emergency Medicine 24:266, 1992.
  Because glucose measurements have changed from reduction methods to enzymatic methods, the criteria need downward revision.
Lindsay MK, Graves W, Klein L: The relationship of one abnormal glucose tolerance test value and pregnancy complications. Obstet Gynecol 73:103, 1989.
  Pregnant women with one abnormal value in the oral GGT are at increased risk for fetal macrosomia and preeclampsia/eclampsia.
Neiger R, Coustan DR: The role of repeat glucose tolerance tests in the diagnosis of gestational diabetes. Am J Obstet Gynecol 165:787, 1991.
  Suggest repeating the oral glucose tolerance test if one value is abnormal.
Position Statement: Gestational diabetes mellitus. Diabetes Care 14(suppl 2):5, 1991.
  Recommendations of the American Diabetes Association for the screening, diagnosis, and management of gestational diabetes mellitus.

Adrenal Insufficiency

1.   In patients with clinical findings of adrenal insufficiency, if the findings are severe, draw a blood sample for serum cortisol and adrenocorticotropic hormone (ACTH) levels before treating them with glucocorticoids. If the findings are early or mild, perform a cosyntropin test (rapid ACTH test).

To perform the rapid ACTH test, draw a baseline blood sample for a serum cortisol determination and give cosyntropin, 250 μg, intramuscularly or intravenously. Then draw additional blood samples for serum cortisol measurements at 30 minutes and 60 minutes.

2.   Evaluate the tests.

Reference ranges may vary among different laboratories.

REFERENCE RANGES

Test	Specimen	Conventional Units	International Units
Cortisol	Serum or plasma (with heparin)	0800 hr: 5-23 μg/dL 1600 hr: 3-15 μg/dL 2000 hr: ≤50% of concentration at 0800 hr	138-635 nmol/L 82-413 nmol/L ≤50% of concentration at 0800 hr
Adrenocorticotropic hormone (ACTH)	Plasma (with heparin)	0800 hr: 8-79 pg/mL 1800 hr: 7-30 pg/mL	8-79 ng/L 7-30 ng/L
Rapid ACTH test	(See below)		

3. Interpret test results in the context of clinical findings.

In severe cases a low serum cortisol level in the presence of an increased ACTH level indicates primary adrenal insufficiency, whereas a low cortisol level with a low or inappropriately "normal" level of ACTH indicates secondary adrenal insufficiency.

In early or mild cases, using the rapid ACTH test, a peak serum cortisol level ≥20 μg/dL (550 nmol/L) is a good indicator of normal adrenal function. It is reassuring also to see a rise in the serum cortisol level of ≥7 μg/dL (193 nmol/L) above the baseline level.

If the cortisol response to cosyntropin stimulation is low or subnormal, additional testing is necessary to diagnose primary versus secondary adrenal insufficiency, and an endocrinologist should be consulted.

4. In patients with adrenal insufficiency the following abnormal blood test results may occur:

↓ **Hemoglobin and hematocrit** with low reticulocytes.

↓ **Leukocytes.**

↑ **Eosinophils.**

↑ **Lymphocytes.**

↓ **Blood pH** with high potassium level and metabolic acidosis.

↓ **Glucose** and increased glucose tolerance with a flat curve.

↑ **Urea nitrogen and creatinine** related to dehydration and hypotension with prerenal impairment of renal function.

↓ **Sodium.**

↑ **Potassium.**

↓ **Chloride.**

↓ **Carbon dioxide.**

↑ **Calcium.**

↓ **Phosphorus.**

↑ **Magnesium.**

↑ **Protein** due to dehydration and hemoconcentration.

BIBLIOGRAPHY

Bravo EL: Acute adrenal insufficiency; and Gomez MT, Chrousos GP: Chronic adrenal insufficiency. In Conn RB: Current Diagnosis, 8th ed. Philadelphia, WB Saunders Co, 1991, pp 864, 865.
Discuss diagnostic strategies.
Grinspoon SK, Bilezikian JP: HIV disease and the endocrine system. N Engl J Med 327:1360, 1992.
The most important endocrine abnormality in HIV disease is adrenal insufficiency.

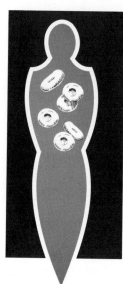

CHAPTER 9

HEMATOLOGICAL DISEASES

Classifying Blood Cell Disorders by a Complete
  Blood Count With Differential
Microcytic Anemia Without Reticulocytosis
Macrocytic Anemia Without Reticulocytosis
Normocytic Anemia Without Reticulocytosis
Anemia With Reticulocytosis
Classifying Bleeding Disorders by Laboratory Tests

Classifying Blood Cell Disorders by a Complete Blood Count With Differential

1.   For patients with clinical findings of a blood disorder or to screen for a blood disorder, request a complete blood count (CBC) with differential. If patients have abnormal findings, carefully review the peripheral blood smear.

Several authorities recommend against general wellness screening for iron deficiency anemia. Two of these authorities endorse selective screening for individuals at increased risk.

A Wright-stained peripheral blood smear can show helpful red blood cell (RBC), white blood cell (WBC), and platelet changes: sickling and targeting suggest sickle cell anemia (HbSS) or hemoglobin (Hb) S plus thalassemia minor; targeting and stippling suggest complications of thalassemia minor; marked targeting suggests Hb E, Hb C, or obstructive liver disease; RBC fragments and polychromatophilia suggest hemolysis; rouleaux suggest increased globulins and/or decreased albumin; and hypersegmented neutrophils with or without macrocytes suggest megaloblastic anemia. WBCs can be differentiated and the changes of the reactive disorders and leukemias noted. Any "left shift" (increased bands) can be noted. Unusual forms such as the bilobed neutrophils and eosinophils of the Pelger-Hüet anomaly or the large purple cytoplasmic granules of the Alder-Reilly anomaly may be present. The platelet count can be estimated, and abnormal forms such as small platelets, large platelets, or platelets with bizarre shapes and forms can be noted.

2.   Evaluate the tests.

A CBC performed on an automated hematology analyzer is widely available and provides hemoglobin and hematocrit values, RBC count, RBC indices, WBC values—and often the platelet count and an electronic WBC differential as well. The report from automated hematology analyzers such as the Coulter STKR (Coulter Electronics, Inc., Hialeah, Fla.) is expressed in a blood cell hemogram (modified for reproduction) as follows:

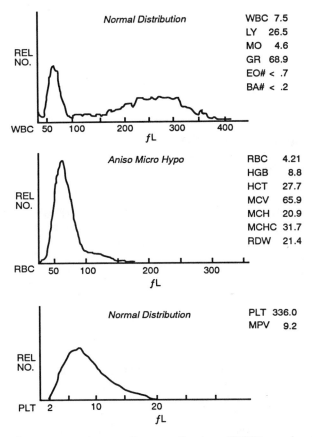

Source: Histogram printout from a Coulter STKR at the Ohio State University Hospitals Hematology Laboratory.

Key: WBC = white blood cell count; RBC = red blood cell count; PLT = platelets; Aniso = anisocytosis; Micro = microcytosis; Hypo = hypochromia; LY = % lymphocytes; MO = % monocytes; GR = % granulocytes; EO# = absolute number of eosinophils ($\times$ 10⁹/L); BA# = absolute number of basophils ($\times$ 10⁹/L); HGB = hemoglobin; HCT = hematocrit; MCV = mean corpuscular volume; MCH = mean corpuscular hemoglobulin; MCHC = mean corpuscular hemoglobin concentration; RDW = red cell distribution width; MPV = mean platelet volume; REL NO = relative number; fL = femtoliters.

In this hemogram the microcytic, hypochromic RBCs with anisocytosis (high RBC distribution width [RDW]) are consistent with iron deficiency anemia. Not only are the numerical results seen for the CBC, including WBC differential and RBC indices, but so are graphic displays of WBCs, RBCs and platelets. The RBC indices are calculated as follows:

$$\text{Mean corpuscular volume (MCV) (fL)} = \frac{\text{Hct (\%)} \times 10}{\text{RBC (in millions/}\mu\text{L)}} \ or \ \frac{\text{Hct (vol. fr.)} \times 1000}{\text{RBC (in millions/}\mu\text{L)}}$$

$$\text{Mean corpuscular hemoglobin (MCH) (pg)} = \frac{\text{Hb (g/dL)} \times 10}{\text{RBC (in millions/}\mu\text{L)}} \ or$$

$$\frac{\text{Hb (g/L)}}{\text{RBC (in millions/}\mu\text{L)}}$$

Mean corpuscular hemoglobin concentration (MCHC) (g/dL)
$$= \frac{\text{Hb (g/dL)} \times 100}{\text{Hct (\%)}} \ or \ \frac{\text{Hb (g/dL)}}{\text{Hct (vol. fr.)}}$$

The RDW is an estimate of RBC size variability (anisocytosis) and is calculated as follows:

$$\text{RDW} = \frac{\text{SD}}{\text{Mean}} \times 100 \ (13 \pm 1.5\%)$$

The deficiency anemias (iron, vitamin B_{12}, folic acid) tend to have higher RDWs (greater anisocytosis) than anemias caused by genetic defects (e.g., thalassemia) or primary bone marrow disorders.

3.   Interpret test results in the context of clinical findings.

CLASSIFYING RED BLOOD CELL DISORDERS

Anemia. In patients with anemia review the CBC with differential, determine the reticulocyte count, and examine the peripheral blood smear.

Pay attention to abnormal RBC indices, even when there is no anemia. A high MCV without anemia may be a clue to chronic alcoholism or an early vitamin B_{12} deficiency. Similarly, a low MCV without anemia may be a clue to heterozygous α- or β-thalassemia.

CRITERIA FOR ANEMIA IN MEN AND WOMEN

	WOMEN	MEN
Red blood cells	<4 × 10⁶ cells/μL (<4 × 10¹² cells/L)	<4.5 × 10⁶ cells/μL (<4.5 × 10¹² cells/L)
Hemoglobin	<12 g/dL (120 g/L)	<13.5 g/dL (135 g/L)
Hematocrit	<36% (0.36 volume fraction)	<40% (0.40 volume fraction)

Reticulocyte count. The reticulocyte count is a key value that should be determined as part of the initial workup of every anemic patient. Reticulocytes are 1- to 2-day-old young RBCs in the peripheral blood. They are macrocytic (MCV >100 fL) and contain aggregates of ribosomes that take up supravital stain (methylene blue). The reticulocyte count is expressed as the % reticulocytes per 500 or 1000 RBCs counted. The reference ranges for the reticulocyte count follow:

Test	Specimen	Conventional Units	International Units
% Reticulocytes	Peripheral blood smear	0.5%-1.5% of RBCs	0.005-0.015 (number fraction)
Absolute retic- ulocyte count	Peripheral blood smear	$<100 \times 10^3/\mu L$	$<100 \times 10^9/L$

Use the reticulocyte production index (RPI [normal = 1]) to correct for anemia for the longer presence of reticulocytes in the peripheral blood.

$$RPI = \% \text{ Reticulocytes} \times \frac{\text{Patient Hct}}{\text{Normal Hct}} \times \frac{1}{\text{Maturation time (days)}}$$

Maturation times (days) for Hct of 45%, 35%, 25%, and 15% are 1.0, 1.5, 2.0, and 2.5 respectively.

Characterize the anemia as having either a normal to low reticulocyte count or a high reticulocyte count. Classify anemia with a normal to low reticulocyte count according to whether the RBCs are microcytic, macrocytic, or normocytic. Examination of a peripheral blood smear may be helpful. Many patients with anemia do not require examination of the bone marrow. Classification of anemia according to RBC size and reticulocyte count has exceptions; nevertheless it provides a useful overall format for the differential diagnosis of anemia.

Anemia occurs secondary to decreased production of RBCs, increased loss, or a combination of the two. Classification of anemia according to RBC size and reticulocyte count is a useful first step toward finding a cause. For example, iron deficiency anemia, thalassemia minor, and anemia of chronic disease typically are seen as microcytic anemia with a normal to low reticulocyte count, whereas anemia caused by vitamin B_{12} or folate deficiency typically is seen as macrocytic anemia with a normal to low reticulocyte count. In contrast, anemia due to blood loss or hemolysis usually exhibits normocytic RBCs with a high reticulocyte count.

A bone marrow examination is not required in all patients with anemia. For example, a 65-year-old woman with microcytic anemia, a high RDW, and a low serum ferritin concentration has obvious iron deficiency anemia and does not require bone marrow aspiration to evaluate iron stores. Similarily, patients with obvious hemolytic anemias should be examined by other means and do not require bone marrow aspiration.

Polycythemia. Polycythemia is a condition in which the patient has an increased RBC volume, Hb concentration, Hct value, and RBC count. It may be primary (polycythemia vera) or secondary to another disorder such as chronic cardiac or pulmonary disease. See the references at the end of this section for a discussion of strategies for diagnosis.

CLASSIFYING WHITE BLOOD CELL DISORDERS

In patients with an abnormal WBC count, review the CBC with differential and examine the peripheral blood smear. Characterize the WBC count as normal, low, or high.

Leukopenia. When the WBC count is low, neutropenia (absolute neutrophilic granulocyte count [ANC] $<1.5 \times 10^3$ cells/μL [1.5×10^9 cells/L]) is a major concern. The ANC is calculated by multiplying the total WBC count by the percentage of bands and mature neutrophils (ANC = WBC × [% bands + % mature neutrophils] × 0.01). Susceptibility to infections in neutropenic patients is particularly related to the ANC. Once the ANC is documented as low, the cause should be determined. Drugs are an important common cause that should be ruled out by stopping medications and obtaining weekly WBC counts for 8 weeks. Patients with significant infections or who are still neutropenic after 8 weeks should be thoroughly examined.

Leukocytosis. When the WBC count is high, a major concern is whether the high count is due to a reactive process or to a leukemia. A reactive process with a WBC count exceeding 50×10^3 cells/μL (50×10^9 cells/L) is referred to as a *leukemoid reaction.*

A high WBC count may be due to neutrophila, eosinophila, basophilia, monocytosis, or lymphocytosis. Some causes follow:

- **Neutrophilia:** infections, leukemia, rheumatic and autoimmune disorders, neoplastic disorders, chemicals, trauma, endocrine and metabolic disorders, hematologic disorders, miscellaneous (e.g., drugs)
- **Eosinophilia:** infectious diseases, parasitic infections, allergic diseases, myeloproliferative and neoplastic diseases, cutaneous diseases, pulmonary diseases, connective tissue diseases, immunodeficiency diseases, gastrointestinal diseases, miscellaneous (e.g., long-term peritoneal dialysis)
- **Basophilia:** allergic reactions, chronic myeloid leukemia, myeloid metaplasia, polycythemia vera, ionizing radiation, hypothyroidism, chronic hemolytic anemia, post splenectomy
- **Monocytosis:** infections, neoplastic disorders, gastrointestinal disorders, sarcoidosis, drug reactions, recovering from marrow suppression
- **Lymphocytosis:** viral infections, lymphocytic leukemia, other infectious diseases, neoplastic disorders, other disorders (e.g., Graves disease)

Useful tests for differentiating a leukemoid reaction from chronic granulocytic leukemia follow:

TEST	LEUKEMOID REACTION	CHRONIC GRANULOCYTIC LEUKEMIA
WBC × 10³/μL (WBC × 10⁹/L)	<100	May be 30-500
%PMNs	Up to 95%	May be normal (60%-70%)
Immature granulocytes	To myelocyte	Usually includes occasional progranulocytes or blasts
Eosinophils, basophils	Normal or decreased	Slightly increased
Nucleated red blood cells	Occasional	Late; may be common
Bone marrow M:E ratio	6-8:1	≥15:1
LAP	>100	<10

Source: Kjeldsberg C, Beutler E, Bell C, et al (eds): Practical Diagnosis of Hematologic Disorders. Chicago, American Society of Clinical Pathologists, 1989, p 235.
PMN = polymorphonuclear leukocytes; M:E = myeloid:erythroid ratio; LAP = leukocyte alkaline phosphatase.

Infectious mononucleosis is a lymphocytic leukocytosis that may be confused with leukemia and other disorders. The presence of heterophil antibodies (Monospot test) in the context of the appropriate clinical and hematological findings is diagnostic for infectious mononucleosis. False-positive reactions are rare. Atypical lymphocytes usually account for more than 10% of the leukocytes in the peripheral blood smear.

Infectious conditions that may cause an infectious mononucleosis–like syndrome include streptococcal or gonococcal pharyngeal infection, cytomegalovirus infection, viral hepatitis, toxoplasmosis, human immunodeficiency virus (HIV) infection, and adenovirus infection.

In patients with infectious mononucleosis the following abnormal blood test results may occur:

Autoimmune hemolytic anemia caused by cold agglutinins against i antigens.
White blood cell count may be high, normal, or low; a relative and absolute neutropenia is present in 60% to 90% of patients.
Thrombocytopenia is common.
↑ **Uric acid** caused by accelerated lymphocyte nucleic acid turnover.
↑ **Transaminase levels (AST [SGOT] and ALT [SGPT])** in approximately 90% of patients.

↑ **Lactate dehydrogenase.**
↑ **Alkaline phosphatase (ALP).**
↓ **Serum albumin** related to decreased hepatic synthesis.
↑ **Serum globulins** caused by antibodies to Epstein-Barr virus and first IgM, then IgG.
↑ **Bilirubin,** usually mild and only occasionally 6 mg/dL (103 μmol/L) or greater; rarely bilirubin levels of 10.2 to 23 mg/dL (174 to 393 μmol/L) are encountered.

BIBLIOGRAPHY

Conley CL: Polycythemia vera. JAMA 263:2481, 1990; and Djulbegovic B, Hadley T, Joseph G: A new algorithm for the diagnosis of polycythemia. Am Fam Physician 44:113, 1991.
  Two articles that discuss polycythemia vera, including strategies for diagnosis.
Dale DC: A new look at an old laboratory test: The WBC count. J Gen Intern Med 6:264, 1991; and Chang R, Wong GY: Prognostic significance of marked leukocytosis in hospitalized patients. J Gen Intern Med 6:199, 1991.
  Discuss the WBC count and the prognostic significance of a neutrophilic leukocytosis >20 × 10³ cells/μL (20 × 10⁹ cells/L).
Griner PF: Infectious mononucleosis. In Panzer RJ, Black ER, Griner PF (eds): Diagnostic Strategies for Common Medical Problems. Philadelphia, American College of Physicians, 1991, p 196.
  Recommends strategies for the diagnosis of infectious mononucleosis.
Hayward RSA, Steinberg EP, Ford DE: Preventive care guidelines: 1991. Ann Intern Med 114:758, 1991.
  Authoritative recommendations for wellness screening for iron deficiency anemia.
Lambore S, McSherry J, Kraus AS: Acute and chronic symptoms of mononucleosis. J Fam Pract 33:33, 1991.
  Discusses the clinical findings of infectious mononucleosis.
Rice L: Anemia: Using a rational approach to diagnosis. Consultant 30:39, 1990.
  Believes that therapeutic trials are inappropriate.
Rotenberg Z, Harell D, Weinberger I, et al: Total lactate dehydrogenase and its isoenzymes in serum of patients with infectious mononucleosis. Clin Chem 37:116, 1991.
  Recommends lactate dehydrogenase studies for every patient with clinical suspicion of infectious mononucleosis.
Simel DL: Is the RDW-MCV classification of anemia useful? Clin Lab Haematol 9:349, 1987.
  Discusses the use of RDW and MCV for diagnosing microcytic anemia.
Welborn JL, Meyers FJ: A three-point approach to anemia. Postgrad Med 89:179, 1991.
  Gives a three-step approach to evaluate patients with anemia.

Microcytic Anemia Without Reticulocytosis

1. In patients with microcytic anemia (MCV <80 fL) and a normal to low reticulocyte count, causes include iron deficiency anemia, thalassemia minor, anemia of chronic disease, and sideroblastic anemia. Consider the following studies: examination of a peripheral blood smear, serum iron, total iron-binding capacity, percent saturation, ferritin, free erythrocyte protoporphyrin, and hemoglobin electrophoresis. A bone marrow examination occasionally is necessary.

Useful findings include the following: (1) in an otherwise healthy woman anemia is usually caused by iron deficiency (probability, 80% to 90%); (2) microcytic RBCs with little or no anemia are usually caused by thalassemia minor (probability >90%); and (3) in individuals with early or mild iron deficiency, anemia of chronic disease, and sideroblastic anemia, the RBCs may be normocytic instead of microcytic. Iron loss may be physiological (e.g., menstruation, pregnancy) or pathological (e.g., colon cancer). A complete gastrointestinal workup is necessary in men and postmenopausal women in whom iron deficiency has been discovered.

A practical approach in the absence of an obvious chronic disease is to determine initially whether the anemia is caused by iron deficiency. Determinations of the serum iron, total iron-binding capacity, and iron saturation are generally more easily available than that for serum ferritin, and if they are diagnostic, there is no need to measure serum ferritin. When the probability of uncomplicated anemia caused by iron deficiency is high on clinical grounds alone, the values for serum iron, total iron-binding capacity, and percent saturation are approximately equal to that for ferritin in confirming the diagnosis of iron deficiency anemia, but when the clinical probability is low, determining the ferritin value is the better test. Another approach to the diagnosis of iron deficiency anemia is a therapeutic trial: determine whether iron therapy produces reticulocytosis. Clues to the diagnosis of thalassemia minor are a normal RDW and a MCV <80 fL in patients with normal or borderline iron studies and no evidence of other causes of microcytosis. An MCV <70 fL is almost always due to iron deficiency or thalassemia.

Serum for iron studies should be drawn in the morning because of the diurnal variation (peak value, 7 to 10 A.M.) in iron values and the fact that reference ranges are for morning samples.

2. Evaluate the tests.

Reference ranges may vary among different laboratories.

REFERENCE RANGES

Test	Specimen	Conventional Units	International Units
Iron	Serum	M: 65-175 μg/dL	11.6-31.3 μmol/L
		F: 50-170 μg/dL	9.0-30.4 μmol/L
Total iron-binding capacity	Serum	250-450 μg/dL	44.8-80.6 μmol/L
Iron saturation	Serum	M: 20%-50%	0.20-0.50 (saturation fraction)
		F: 15%-50%	0.15-0.50
Ferritin	Serum	M: 20-250 ng/mL	20-250 μg/L
		F: 10-120 ng/mL	10-120 μg/L
Free erythrocyte protoporphyrin	Whole blood (EDTA or heparin)	30-80 μg/dL packed cells	0.534-1.424 μmol/dL packed cells
Hemoglobin electrophoresis	Whole blood (EDTA, citrate, or heparin)	Hb A >95% Hb A₂ 1.5%-3.5%	Hb A >0.95 (mass fraction) Hb A₂ 0.015-0.035 (mass fraction)

3. Interpret test results in the context of clinical findings.

The common anemias show characteristic patterns of test results.

COMMON ANEMIAS

TEST	IRON DEFICIENCY ANEMIA	ANEMIA OF CHRONIC DISEASE	THALASSEMIA MINOR	SIDEROBLASTIC ANEMIA
Peripheral blood smear	Normocytic to microcytic, hypochromic RBCs	Normocytic to microcytic, hypochromic RBCs	Normocytic to microcytic RBCs, target cells, basophilic stippling	Dimorphic; hypochromic, microcytic, and macrocytic RBCs with Pappenheimer bodies
RBC distribution width (RDW)	High (>16)	Usually normal	Normal	High
Iron	Low	Low	Normal to high	Normal to high
Total iron-binding capacity	High	Normal to low	Normal	Normal to low
Iron saturation	Low	Normal to low	Normal to high	High
Ferritin	Low	Normal to high	Normal to high	Normal to high
Free erythrocyte protoporphyrin	High	High	Normal	Normal to high
Hemoglobin electrophoresis	Normal	Normal	High Hb A$_2$ in β-thalassemia but normal in α-thalassemia	Normal
Bone marrow	Iron absent	Normal to high iron Low number of sideroblasts	Normal to high iron	High iron Ringed sideroblasts

IRON DEFICIENCY ANEMIA

Although iron deficiency anemia is typically a microcytic anemia, in mild cases of iron deficiency the RBCs may be normocytic. Initially there is a loss of stainable bone marrow iron and a decrease in the serum ferritin level, which is followed by a decrease in the serum iron level and an increase in the total iron-binding capacity. Then anemia occurs, with a decreasing MCV, increasing anisocytosis, poikilocytosis, and hypochromia, but no basophilic stippling. Indices are often normal until the Hb concentration falls below 10 g/dL (100 g/L). A decreasing RBC count and an increasing RDW are early changes. The fall in the erythrocyte count usually is less than the fall in Hb. Generally examination of the bone marrow is not required to establish a diagnosis of iron deficiency anemia. An exception is the clinical situation in which iron deficiency coexists with a chronic disease. A normal serum iron and iron-binding capacity does not exclude iron deficiency when the Hb concentration is greater than 9 g/dL (90 g/L) in women and 11 g/dL (110 g/L) in men.

ANEMIA OF THALASSEMIA MINOR

The anemia of thalassemia minor (α-or β-thalassemia minor) and Hb E is typically microcytic and, in contrast to iron deficiency anemia, is characterized by a normal or increased RBC count. For example, at a hemoglobin level of 9 g/dL (90 g/L), an iron-deficient patient typically has a RBC count of approximately 3×10^6 cells/μL (3×10^{12} cells/μL), whereas a patient with thalassemia minor has a count of approximately 5×10^6 cells/L (5×10^{12} cells/L). The variation in size is no more than normal, and the RDW is usually normal. There may be basophilic stippling. If the Hb value is greater than 10 g/dL (100 g/L) but the MCV is decreased, thalassemia is more likely than iron deficiency anemia. In the case of β-thalassemia minor, the diagnosis is established by demonstrating an increased concentration of Hb A_2 using Hb A_2 quantitation and Hb electrophoresis. Sometimes the diagnosis is more difficult; with α-thalassemia minor, Hb A_2 is not increased. With Hb E disease, however, the abnormal Hb is identified by Hb electrophoresis.

ANEMIA OF CHRONIC DISEASE

The anemia of chronic disease is typically normocytic. In approximately 25% of cases the anemia is microcytic, but the MCV rarely falls below 78 fL. Because this form of anemia is specifically related to acute or chronic inflammation rather than chronic disease, the term *anemia of inflammation* has been suggested for this disorder. In contrast to iron deficiency anemia, the serum iron level is low, total iron-binding capacity is normal or low, and the serum ferritin value is usually greater than 100 ng/mL (100 μg/L). Iron deficiency and anemia of chronic disease may occur together such as in patients with inflammatory bowel disease or rheumatic diseases treated with aspirin or other nonsteroidal anti-inflammatory drugs. With these conditions the iron saturation (iron and total iron-binding capacity) may be quite low, even without iron deficiency. If the saturation is greater than 30%, iron deficiency is excluded. A serum ferritin level <50 ng/mL (50 μg/L) in patients with these inflammatory conditions suggests iron deficiency because serum ferritin is an acute-phase reactant and usually is increased in these inflammatory states. In patients with rheumatoid arthritis a red cell MCV <80 fL and a serum ferritin concentration <50 ng/mL (50 μg/L) are 79% sensitive, but 100% specific for iron deficiency. A serum ferritin concentration <50 ng/mL (50 μg/L) is a good indicator of iron deficiency anemia in hospitalized geriatric patients. When serum ferritin values are borderline (i.e., 50 ng/mL [50 μg/L]), a bone marrow aspirate for iron stain can settle the question.

SIDEROBLASTIC ANEMIA

Sideroblastic anemia constitutes a group of refractory anemias with erythroid hyperplasia of the marrow. The cause may be either hereditary (sex-linked or autosomal recessive) or acquired. If acquired, it may be drug induced (e.g., lead, alcohol, isoniazid [INH]) or idiopathic (myelodysplastic syndromes). The peripheral blood smear exhibits hypochromic microcytic RBCs; but the picture is dimorphic, and macrocytes may prevail, making the MCV normal or high. There may be coarse basophilic stippling. Typically the serum iron and ferritin levels are normal to high, and the serum total iron-binding capacity is normal to low with a high saturation. Free erythrocyte porphyrin levels may be normal or high. The bone marrow contains increased iron stores and ringed sideroblasts. The Hb A_2 level is normal.

BIBLIOGRAPHY

Beutler E: The common anemias. JAMA 259:2433, 1988.
  Excellent discussion of thalassemia, iron deficiency anemia, and anemia of chronic disease.
Bick RL, Baker WF: Iron deficiency anemia. Laboratory Medicine 21:641, 1990.
  Good discussion of iron deficiency anemia and its differentiation from other microcytic anemias.
Brown RG: Determining the cause of anemia: General approach, with emphasis on microcytic hypochromic anemias. Postgrad Med 89:161, 1991.
  Recommends strategies for diagnosis.
Finch CA, Bellotti V, Stray S, et al: Plasma ferritin determination as a diagnostic tool. West J Med 145:657, 1986.
  Review of the use of plasma ferritin to diagnose iron deficiency and iron overload.
Griner P: Microcytic anemia. In Panzer RJ, Black ER, Griner PF (eds): Diagnostic Strategies for Common Medical Problems. Philadelphia, American College of Physicians, 1991, p 448.
  Suggests strategies for the differential diagnosis of microcytic anemia.
Guyatt GH, Oxman AD, Ali M, et al: Laboratory diagnosis of iron-deficiency anemia: An overview. J Gen Intern Med 7:145, 1992.
  Suggests serum ferritin radioimmunoassay as the most powerful test for iron deficiency anemia.
Joosten E, Hiele M, Ghoos Y, et al: Diagnosis of iron-deficiency anemia in a hospitalized geriatric population. Am J Med 90:653, 1991.
  Ferritin is best to diagnose iron deficiency anemia in hospitalized geriatric patients.
Schilling RF: Anemia of chronic disease: A misnomer. Ann Intern Med 115:572, 1991.
  Suggests the term anemia of inflammation *instead of* anemia of chronic disease.
Spivak JL: Anemia and chronic disease, iron deficiency, and sideroblastic anemia. In Spivak JL, Barnes HV (eds): Manual of Clinical Problems in Internal Medicine, 4th ed. Boston, Little, Brown & Co, 1990, pp 287, 331, 370.
  Good discussion of diagnosis and management with annotated key references.
Wallerstein RO Jr: Laboratory evaluation of anemia. West J Med 146:443, 1987.
  Good strategy for the laboratory evaluation of anemia using RBC size, reticulocyte count, and other selected studies.

Macrocytic Anemia Without Reticulocytosis

1.   In patients with macrocytic anemia (MCV >100 fL) and a normal to low reticulocyte count, causes include macrocytic megaloblastic anemia and macrocytic nonmegaloblastic anemia. Consider performing the following studies: examination of a peripheral blood smear and bone marrow aspirate; serum vitamin B_{12} and folate determinations; thyroid function tests; and liver function tests.

Useful findings include the following: (1) the higher the MCV, the greater is the probability of vitamin B_{12} or folate deficiency (MCV $\leq$95 fL equals 0.1% probability; MCV >130 fL equals almost 100% probability); and (2) an MCV of 100 to 110 fL is often due to other causes such as alcoholism, hypothyroidism, or liver disease. Patients with partially treated macrocytic anemia due to vitamin B_{12} or folate deficiency can show reticulocytosis.

The causes of macrocytic megaloblastic anemia include vitamin B_{12} or folate deficiency and drug-induced anemia. The causes of macrocytic nonmegaloblastic anemia include alcoholism, liver disease, hypothyroidism, aplastic anemia, sideroblastic anemia, and reticulocytosis.

2.   Evaluate the tests.

Reference ranges may vary among different laboratories.

REFERENCE RANGES

TEST	SPECIMEN	CONVENTIONAL UNITS	INTERNATIONAL UNITS
Peripheral blood smear	Presence of oval macrocytes, hypersegmented neutrophils (>5% neutrophils with five lobes or any neutrophil with six lobes), and giant platelets is consistent with megaloblastic anemia. Round macrocytes are consistent with other causes. Target cells occur with liver disease.		
Bone marrow	Presence of megaloblasts separates megaloblastic causes from nonmegaloblastic causes.		
Vitamin B_{12}	Serum	100-700 pg/mL	74-516 pmol/L
Folate	Serum erythrocytes (EDTA)	3-16 ng/mL 130-628 ng/mL packed cells	7-36 mmol/L 294-1422 nmol/L packed cells
Thyroid function		See Chapter 8	
Liver function		See Chapter 6	

3.   Interpret test results in the context of clinical findings.

MACROCYTIC MEGALOBLASTIC ANEMIA

In patients with macrocytic megaloblastic anemia there are not only macrocytic RBCs in the peripheral blood but also megaloblasts in the marrow. Causes include vitamin B_{12} deficiency, folate deficiency, antimetabolite drugs, and antifolate drugs. If drugs are excluded as a cause, the most likely diagnosis is either vitamin B_{12} deficiency or folate deficiency. The distinction between these two causes is very important for two reasons: (1) folate will not correct the neuropsychiatric abnormalities caused by vitamin B_{12} deficiency; and (2) a diagnosis of vitamin B_{12} deficiency commits the patient to parenteral therapy for life.

Vitamin B_{12} Deficiency. In addition to serum vitamin B_{12} and folate levels, serum methylmalonic acid and homocysteine levels are useful in distinguishing between vitamin B_{12} and folate deficiency. The serum methylmalonic acid concentration is high in patients with vitamin B_{12} deficiency ($>95\%$ sensitive) and normal in those with folate deficiency. In contrast, serum homocysteine concentrations are high with both vitamin B_{12} and folate deficiency. A therapeutic trial of intramuscular vitamin B_{12}, 1 μg per day for 10 days, may be useful. This dose produces reticulocytosis in patients with vitamin B_{12} deficiency but not in patients with folate deficiency. Once vitamin B_{12} deficiency is diagnosed, the cause must be determined. Useful ancillary tests include examination of parietal cell and intrinsic factor antibodies, a gastrin test and a Schilling test.

Folate Deficiency. Serum folate is low in patients with megaloblastic anemia due to folate deficiency but is usually normal or increased in patients with vitamin B_{12} deficiency. A low serum folate concentration precedes low RBC or tissue folate values. RBC folate is a better test of tissue stores than serum folate; however, the RBC folate concentration is also low in the majority of cases of vitamin B_{12} deficiency, so vitamin B_{12} deficiency must be excluded. A therapeutic trial of (oral folate) 100 μg per day for 10 days is useful. This dose produces reticulocytosis in patients with folate deficiency but not in patients with vitamin B_{12} deficiency. Once folate deficiency is diagnosed, the cause must be determined.

MACROCYTIC NONMEGALOBLASTIC ANEMIA

In patients with macrocytic nonmegaloblastic anemia macrocytic RBCs are in the peripheral blood, but no megaloblasts are in the marrow (i.e., the marrow shows normoblasts). Causes include reticulocytosis, alcoholism, liver disease, hypothyroidism, aplastic anemia, and sideroblastic anemia. Since a normal to low reticulocyte count excludes reticulocytosis as a cause, only the other causes are considered here.

Alcoholism and Liver Disease. In alcoholic individuals macrocytic RBCs (MCV usually 100 to 110 fL) that are not due to reticulocytosis or a vitamin deficiency are seen in the peripheral blood smear. It is unclear whether this represents a nonspecific effect of marrow damage or a direct effect of alcohol on RBCs or RBC precursors. Macrocytic RBCs may also occur in patients with liver disease.

Patients with alcoholism may have a variety of causes for anemia: toxic suppression of the marrow, folate deficiency, iron deficiency, decreased RBC survival, abnormal iron metabolism, and hemodilution.

Hypothyroidism. There is a tendency to develop macrocytic RBCs with hypothyroidism and microcytic RBCs with hyperthyroidism. Typically, however, the anemia of hypothyroidism or hyperthyroidism is normocytic. These changes can occur even in the presence of adequate amounts of vitamins and iron.

Aplastic Anemia. In patients with aplastic and hypoplastic anemia the peripheral blood count may show pancytopenia. Macrocytic RBCs may be seen.

Sideroblastic Anemia. In patients with sideroblastic anemia the peripheral blood shows a dimorphic picture: hypochromic microcytes and macrocytes. If macrocytes prevail, the MCV may be high. See additional information about sideroblastic anemia in the discussion of microcytic anemia without reticulocytosis.

4.   In patients with macrocytic anemia the following additional abnormal blood test results may occur:

↑ **Indirect bilirubin** in megaloblastic anemia due to hemolysis of some abnormal RBCs.

↑ **Lactate dehydrogenase** in megaloblastic anemia due to intramedullary destruction of red cells.

↑ **Gastrin** in pernicious anemia.

BIBLIOGRAPHY

Brown RG: Normocytic and macrocytic anemias. Postgrad Med 89:125, 1991.
   Good discussion of the differential diagnosis of normocytic and macrocytic anemias.
Kassirer JP, Kopelman RI: Case 19—Searching for a pony. In Learning Clinical Reasoning. Baltimore, Williams & Wilkins, 1991, p 124.
   Discusses clinical reasoning in a patient with vitamin B_{12} deficiency.
Rapoport AP, Rowe JM: Macrocytosis. In Panzer RJ, Black ER, Griner PF (eds): Diagnostic Strategies for Common Medical Problems. Philadelphia, American College of Physicians, 1991, p 458.
   Suggests strategies for the differential diagnosis of macrocytic anemias.
Scates S, Glaspy J: The macrocytic anemias. Laboratory Medicine 21:736, 1990.
   Good discussion of the differential diagnosis of the macrocytic anemias.
Spivak JL: Folic acid deficiency; Vitamin B_{12} deficiency. In Spivak JL, Barnes HV (eds):

Manual of Clinical Problems in Internal Medicine, 4th ed. Boston, Little, Brown & Co, 1990, pp 313, 389.
Discusses diagnosis and management with annotated key references.
Wymer A, Becker DM: Recognition and evaluation of red blood cell macrocytosis in the primary care setting. J Gen Intern Med 5:192, 1990.
Macrocytosis is common in outpatients. Treatable causes include alcohol abuse, vitamin B_{12} deficiency, folate deficiency, and hypothyroidism.

Normocytic Anemia Without Reticulocytosis

1. In patients with normocytic anemia and a normal to low reticulocyte count, causes include primary and secondary bone marrow failure and other miscellaneous disorders. Consider the following studies: examination of a peripheral blood smear and bone marrow aspirate; determinations of serum iron, total iron-binding capacity, percent saturation, and ferritin; creatinine determination; liver function tests; and tests of endocrine function—especially thyroid function tests.

Before considering bone marrow failure as a cause, remember that normocytic anemia with a normal to low reticulocyte count may have other miscellaneous causes: early stages of iron deficiency anemia, anemia of chronic disease, acquired sideroblastic anemia, and dilutional anemia due to hypervolemia. Moreover, mixed anemias (e.g., from folate and iron deficiency) may be normocytic.

The anemias of primary bone marrow failure include the aplastic and hypoplastic anemias and the bone marrow replacement disorders.

The anemias of secondary bone marrow failure include uremia, endocrinological causes, and HIV infection.

2. Interpret test results in the context of clinical findings.

MISCELLANEOUS CAUSES

Early Stages of Microcytic Anemia. Mild cases of iron deficiency anemia, anemia of chronic disease, and sideroblastic anemia may be seen as normocytic anemia without reticulocytosis.

Dilutional Anemia. Normocytic anemia can occur with an increased plasma volume. This happens in alcoholic patients who have splenomegaly and with the use of drugs such as α-adrenergic blockers.

PRIMARY BONE MARROW FAILURE

Aplastic and Hypoplastic Anemia. Aplastic and hypoplastic anemias are typically normocytic but may be macrocytic. Hereditary forms of these anemias can occur in children, and acquired forms can occur at any age. Acquired anemias include acquired aplastic anemia (from drugs, toxins, infections, miscellaneous conditions) and acquired pure RBC aplasia (from thymoma, drugs, toxins, neoplasms, autoimmune disorders, viral infections).

Bone Marrow Replacement Disorders. Bone marrow replacement patients have normocytic anemia because of failure of hematopoiesis secondary to replacement of the bone marrow by fibrosis, neoplastic cells, or nonneoplastic cells (e.g., Gaucher's cells). Pancytopenia may be present.

SECONDARY BONE MARROW FAILURE

Normocytic anemia can occur in patients with uremia, liver disease, endocrinological disease, and HIV infection. Normocytic anemia occurs with chronic renal insufficiency, and its severity is roughly proportional to the degree of renal failure. It is caused by erythropoietin deficiency and other metabolic abnormalities that accompany uremia. It is not dependent on the presence of inflammation. Normocytic anemia frequently occurs with diseases of the thyroid, adrenal glands, and gonads. With endocrinological disease, especially hypothyroidism, a decreased hemoglobin concentration is related to reduced oxygen consumption. Decreased erythropoietin production may also be a factor in endocrinological disorders. The prevalence of anemia in HIV-infected persons increases as the disease worsens. The anemia is typically normocytic.

BIBLIOGRAPHY

Björkholm M: Aplastic anemia: Pathogenetic mechanisms and treatment with special reference to immunomodulation. J Intern Med 231:575, 1992.
  Reviews the disease and emphasizes immune mechanisms.
Brown RG: Normocytic and macrocytic anemias. Postgrad Med 89:125, 1991.
  Good discussion of the differential diagnosis of normocytic and macrocytic anemias.
Schilling RF: Anemia of chronic disease: A misnomer. Ann Intern Med 115:572, 1991.
  Scholarly discussion of anemia due to inflammation, iron deficiency anemia, hypothyroidism, and malignancy.
Spivak JL: Anemia and renal disease; Aplastic anemia. In Spivak JL, Barnes HV (eds): Manual of Clinical Problems in Internal Medicine, 4th ed. Boston, Little, Brown & Co, 1990, pp 289, 293.
  Discusses diagnosis and management with annotated key references.

Anemia With Reticulocytosis

1.   In patients with anemia and a high reticulocyte count causes include acute blood loss and hemolytic anemia. First consider acute blood loss.

A high reticulocyte count may cause some of these patients to have a high MCV. Others will have a normal MCV.

ACUTE BLOOD LOSS

After acute blood loss, it may take a few days for the onset of reticulocytosis. In the bleeding patient reticulocytosis will continue until iron stores are depleted. Usually the source of bleeding is obvious (gastrointestinal or genitourinary), but it may be occult (into a fractured hip or into the retroperitoneum). Even though a bleeding source is obvious, it is still advisable to do an adequate workup (i.e., there may be other coexisting causes for anemia).

2.   If acute blood loss is not the cause, consider hemolytic anemia. Consider obtaining the following studies: examination of a peripheral blood smear and determinations of plasma haptoglobin, serum unconjugated bilirubin and lactate dehydrogenase, and urinary hemoglobin and hemosiderin.

A Wright-stained peripheral blood smear may show helpful RBC changes: spherocytes suggest hereditary spherocytosis; elliptocytes suggest hereditary elliptocytosis; abnormal RBC shapes and increased target cells suggest hemoglobinopathies; and fragmented cells suggest intravascular coagulation and a variety of other disorders that may cause mechanical fragmentation of RBCs.

Hemolytic anemias are less common than those caused by marrow failure or blood loss. Two questions should be addressed in the diagnosis:

1. Is hemolysis present?
2. What is its cause?

COMMONLY USED TESTS INDICATING PRESENCE OF HEMOLYSIS

TEST	RESULT
Plasma haptoglobin	Decreased
Serum unconjugated bilirubin	Increased
Serum lactate dehydrogenase	Increased
Urine hemoglobin	Present
Urine hemosiderin	Present

Source: Lindenbaum J: An approach to the anemias. In Wyngaarden JB, Smith LH Jr, and Bennett JC (eds): Cecil Textbook of Medicine, 19th ed. Philadelphia, WB Saunders Co, 1992, p 829.

The above tests detect hemolysis in an indirect manner. Although rarely needed, a direct estimate of RBC survival is available using radioactive chromium (^{51}Cr): reference range for the normal RBC half-life is 25 to 32 days (elution of ^{51}Cr from RBCs at 1% per day produces this reference range instead of 60 days).

SOME RELATIVELY COMMON CAUSES OF HEMOLYTIC ANEMIA

MECHANISM	EXAMPLES
Congenital	
Enzyme deficiency	Glucose-6-phosphate dehydrogenase, pyruvate kinase
Membrane skeletal protein abnormalities (e.g., spectrin)	Hereditary spherocytosis, hereditary elliptocytosis
Hemoglobinopathies	Hemoglobin SS, SC, CC, S-thalassemia
Acquired	
Antibody induced	Autoimmune hemolysis (warm antibodies), cold agglutinin disease, hemolytic transfusion reaction
Mechanical fragmentation	Intravascular coagulation, malignant hypertension, cancer chemotherapy, malfunctioning valve prosthesis, thrombotic thrombocytopenic purpura
Membrane protein anchoring abnormality	Paroxysmal nocturnal hemoglobinuria

Source: Lindenbaum J: An approach to the anemias. In Wyngaarden JB, Smith LH Jr, and Bennett JC (eds): Cecil Textbook of Medicine, 19th ed. Philadelphia, WB Saunders Co, 1992, p 829.

3. If there is evidence of hemolysis, perform appropriate studies as indicated by the clinical findings and peripheral blood smear.

The causes of hemolysis are many, and the list of available tests is long. Therefore testing should be based on clues discovered in the clinical findings and peripheral blood smear. Testing strategies for some common causes of hemolytic anemia follow.

CONGENITAL CAUSES

Enzyme Deficiency. Glucose-6-phosphate dehydrogenase (G6PD) deficiency is a prevalent X-linked genetic abnormality that can cause hemolytic anemia. The anemia can be induced by drugs, chemicals, infections, and fava beans. The fluorescent screening test for G6PD deficiency is reliable for detecting the disease. A quantitative G6PD assay is also available.

Pyruvate kinase deficiency is a less prevalent autosomal recessive abnormality that can cause hemolytic anemia. A fluorescent screening test for pyruvate kinase deficiency is available, and RBC enzyme levels can also be measured.

Membrane Skeletal Protein Abnormalities. Hereditary spherocytosis is the most prevalent hemolytic anemia among individuals of Northern European origin. It has an autosomal dominant inheritance, although some recessive forms may exist. The peripheral blood smear shows spherocytes. Laboratory tests include the osmotic fragility test and the autohemolysis test.

Hereditary elliptocytosis is another hemolytic anemia with an autosomal dominant inheritance. The peripheral blood smear shows at least 25% elliptocytes.

Hemoglobinopathies. Hemolytic anemias can occur with RBC Hb defects such as Hb SS, SC, CC, and S-thalassemia. These defects can be diagnosed using Hb electrophoresis and other tests: sickle cell test, solubility test for Hb S, alkali denaturation test for Hb F, quantitation of Hb A_2 by chromatography, acid elution test for hemoglobin in RBCs, test for Hb H inclusion bodies, and other ancillary tests (Heinz bodies, crystal cells of Hb C disease, and RBC inclusions in Hb H disease).

ACQUIRED CAUSES

Antibody-Induced Anemia. Antibody-induced anemia can be caused by autoimmune hemolysis (warm antibodies), cold agglutinin disease, or a hemolytic transfusion reaction. The direct antiglobulin test (Coombs' test) is useful for detecting antibodies attached to RBCs.

In patients with warm antibody–induced hemolysis the antibodies are usually IgG, react best at body temperature, usually do not activate complement, and never cause agglutination. The antibodies are usually nonspecific, panspecific for Rh antigens, or drug induced. Women are affected more than men; 55% of cases are idiopathic, 20% to 25% drug induced, 15% to 20% associated with lymphoproliferative disorders, and 5% to 10% other.

In patients with cold agglutinin–induced hemolysis the antibodies are usually IgM, are highly reactive at 0° C (32° F), activate complement, and cause agglutination. Specificity against I antigen is 95% and against i, 5%. Anti-I is associated with *Mycoplasma pneumoniae* and anti-i with infectious mononucleosis. These antibodies can occur with lymphoproliferative disorders or be idiopathic. Another rare hemolytic disorder is paroxysmal cold hemoglobinuria.

Membrane Protein Anchoring Abnormality. Paroxysmal nocturnal hemoglobinuria is a rare cause of chronic hemolytic anemia due to an abnormality of the RBC membrane. The sucrose hemolysis test and the test for urinary hemosiderin are useful for screening, and the acid hemolysis test is the definitive diagnostic test.

Mechanical Fragmentation. In mechanical fragmentation traumatic hemolysis occurs because of shear forces on RBCs in turbulent flow, producing schistocytes, triangular cells, and helmet cells. In addition to occurring with intravascular coagulation, malignant hypertension, cancer, cardiac valve prosthesis, and thrombotic thrombocytopenic purpura, traumatic hemolysis can occur in patients with the hemolytic uremic syndrome, vasculitis, and giant hemangioma.

Infections. Various infections can cause hemolysis, and different tests are necessary for diagnosis: blood cultures for *Clostridium perfringens,* wound cultures for *Escherichia coli* sepsis, stool cultures for cholera, and examination of RBCs in a peripheral blood smear for malaria.

Physiochemical Injuries. Burns, chemical toxins, and drugs can cause hemolytic anemia.

BIBLIOGRAPHY

Hoffman GC: The sickling disorders. Laboratory Medicine 21:797, 1990.
   Good discussion of not only sickle cell trait and sickle cell anemia, but also the combinations of sickle hemoglobin with thalassemia and other structurally abnormal hemoglobins.
Spivak JL: Hemolytic anemia; Paroxysmal nocturnal hemoglobinuria; Sickle cell anemia. In Spivak JL, Barnes HV (eds): Manual of Clinical Problems in Internal Medicine, 4th ed. Boston, Little, Brown & Co, 1990, pp 321, 345, 367.
   Good discussion of diagnosis and management with annotated key references.

Classifying Bleeding Disorders by Laboratory Tests

1.   For patients with clinical findings of a bleeding disorder or to screen for such a disorder, request appropriate tests: CBC, examination of a peripheral blood smear, and determinations of bleeding time, prothrombin time (PT), and activated partial thromboplastin time (APTT).

In patients with clinical findings of a bleeding disorder, these tests provide a useful initial workup. In patients without a personal or family history of bleeding who are to undergo surgery, these tests are adequate to exclude a bleeding tendency. Some experts believe that routine screening tests for a bleeding disorder in asymptomatic medical patients or healthy patients about to undergo surgery are unnecessary. Occasionally a patient with a history of bleeding will have normal screening test results (e.g., mild von Willebrand disease, factor XIII deficiency). In this situation additional special tests can demonstrate the abnormality.

Clinical findings, if present, should be scrutinized to determine any family history of bleeding, the age and circumstances of onset, and the presence or absence of any underlying disorder. Bleeding due to thrombocytopenia (petechiae and purpura) should be distinguished from bleeding due to defective fibrin clot formation. Platelet disorders are caused by either decreased platelets or functional platelet disorders, which may be acquired or hereditary. Defective fibrin clot disorders can also be hereditary or acquired.

Platelet-type bleeding is characterized by mucocutaneous and posttraumatic bleeding. Patients with petechiae and purpura usually lack a sex-linked hereditary history, and affected individuals may be males or females. Bleeding episodes may follow dental procedures and operations, but the bleeding starts immediately at the time of the operation and often can be controlled by pressure. Epistaxis and gastrointestinal bleeding are often major problems.

Defective fibrin clot bleeding is commonly associated with hemarthrosis and intramuscular hematoma formation. Defective fibrin clot disorders are often sex-linked recessive diseases of males (hemophilia A and B), and almost 50% of patients will have a sex-linked history of the disorder. The milder forms of hemophilia A and B resemble von Willebrand's disease. Bleeding frequently follows surgery or trauma such as venipuncture, dental procedures, surgical wounds, and bruises. Hematuria and hemarthroses may occur.

2.   Evaluate the tests.

The CBC is useful to determine any quantitative blood cell abnormalities such as anemia and thrombocytopenia, and the peripheral blood smear is valuable for detecting morphological changes such as RBC fragments, which may be a clue to disseminated intravascular coagulation, and large platelets, which may be a clue to immune thrombocytopenia. Any WBC abnormalities can be evaluated.

The bleeding time is useful to evaluate platelet function. A prolonged bleeding time may be due to either thrombocytopenia, a functional platelet disorder (e.g., aspirin ingestion), or a poorly done test. The combination of a long bleeding time and a platelet count $>100 \times 10^3/\mu L$ ($100 \times 10^9/L$) is indicative of abnormal platelet function. The combination of a long bleeding time and APTT with a normal PT and platelet count suggests von Willebrand's disease. The response of platelets to a variety of aggregating agents (adenosine diphosphate [ADP], collagen, epinephrine) is useful to diagnose functional platelet disorders.

The PT and APTT are useful to detect abnormalities of the extrinsic and intrinsic pathways, respectively. Both tests are sensitive to defects in the common pathway. When the PT and/or APTT are prolonged, mixing experiments of normal plasma and the abnormal plasma will determine whether the problem is a simple deficiency of a coagulation factor(s) (in which case the abnormal test result will be corrected) or an inhibitor of coagulation (in which case the abnormal test result will not be corrected). In a patient with a factor deficiency the diagnosis can be established by mixing studies, using a series of plasmas with specific factor deficiencies.

3.   In patients with clinical findings of platelet-type bleeding (i.e., mucocutaneous and posttraumatic bleeding) consider a platelet disorder. When the platelet count is less than $50 \times 10^3/\mu L$ ($50 \times 10^9/L$), determining a bleeding time is unnecessary because it will be greatly prolonged. In a patient with thrombocytopenia decreased platelet production can be distinguished from increased platelet destruction by a bone marrow aspirate, which also provides information about primary bone marrow disease such as leukemia. A normal PT and a normal APTT exclude an asso-

ciated coagulation abnormality such as a lupus anticoagulant. Occasionally purpura is caused by a vascular or connective tissue abnormality.

Clinical bleeding and purpura do not occur unless the platelet count is less than 50 to 70 $\times$ $10^3/\mu L$ (50 to 70 $\times$ $10^9/L$) or there is an associated qualitative platelet defect. When the count decreases to less than 10 to 20 $\times$ $10^3/\mu L$ (10 to 20 $\times$ $10^9/L$), major spontaneous bleeding may occur.

Causes of nonthrombocytopenic purpura include connective tissue disorders (Marfan syndrome, Ehlers-Danlos syndrome, osteogenesis imperfecta); vasculitis (drug hypersensitivity, Henoch-Schönlein syndrome); infections (bacterial, viral, rickettsial); and miscellaneous diseases (Cushing's syndrome, systemic lupus erythematosus).

QUANTITATIVE PLATELET DISORDERS

Quantitative platelet disorders may be due to either too few platelets (thrombocytopenia) or too many platelets (thrombocytosis). Thrombocytosis may be reactive (secondary) or primary. Interestingly, bleeding or thrombosis is usually seen only in patients with primary thrombocytosis (e.g., essential thrombocythemia, chronic myelocytic leukemia, polycythemia vera).

QUALITATIVE PLATELET DISORDERS

Qualitative platelet disorders may be either hereditary or acquired.

Hereditary Disorders. Hereditary disorders are due to problems with platelet adhesion, secretion or release, or aggregation. von Willebrand's disease, the most common hereditary bleeding disorder, is due to abnormal platelet adhesion caused by a quantitative or qualitative abnormality of von Willebrand factor. Because this factor also acts as a carrier for factor VIII, the APTT and the bleeding time are also prolonged. Other functional platelet disorders are rare and can be differentiated with special platelet aggregation studies.

Acquired Disorders. Acquired platelet disorders commonly cause abnormal platelet function. The most prevalent of them is drug therapy, but there are additional causes (e.g., platelet antibodies, renal disease, myeloproliferative disorders). A variety of different drugs can interfere with platelet function (e.g., anti-inflammatory agents [commonly aspirin], antibiotics, tricylic antidepressants, beta-blockers, calcium channel blockers, lipid-lowering drugs, antihistamines, and miscellaneous agents [ethanol, hydrocortisone]). Diagnosis can be made using the clinical history and the demonstration of a prolonged bleeding time. Platelet aggregation studies are not usually necessary.

4.   In patients with clinical findings of defective fibrin clot bleeding (i.e., hemarthrosis, intramuscular bleeding) consider a disorder of fibrin clot formation. Any or all of the initial bleeding disorder tests may be abnormal:

the CBC, the peripheral blood smear, the bleeding time, the PT, and the APTT.

The differential for abnormal screening tests of fibrin clot formation follows:

PROLONGED APTT	PROLONGED PT	PROLONGED PT AND APTT
Common		
Heparin	Vitamin K deficiency	Vitamin K deficiency
Lupus anticoagulants	Oral anticoagulants	Oral anticoagulants
Hemophilia A	Liver disease	Liver disease
Hemophilia B		Consumptive coagu-
VWD (plus long BT)		lopathies
Uncommon		
Specific factor inhibi-	Factor VII deficiency	Factor II, V, or X
tors		deficiency
Factor XI or XII de-		Hereditary dysfibrin-
ficiency		ogenemia
Prekallikrein defi-		Afibrinogenemia
ciency		Specific factor inhib-
High-molecular-		itors
weight kininogen		Amyloidosis
deficiency		

Source: Brandt JT: Hemostasis. In Howanitz JH, Howanitz PJ (eds): Laboratory Medicine: Test Selection and Interpretation. New York, Churchill Livingstone, 1991, p 518.
APTT = activated partial thromboplastin time; PT = prothrombin time; VWD = von Willebrand disease; BT = bleeding time.

Disorders of fibrin clot formation may be hereditary or acquired.

Hereditary Disorders. Hereditary disorders usually are seen initially as soft tissue bleeding in childhood. Hemophilia A (factor VIII deficiency) and hemophilia B (factor IX deficiency), together with von Willebrand's disease, constitute the vast majority of these conditions. The diagnosis is established by demonstrating the specific defect by factor assays.

Acquired Disorders. A number of acquired disorders can affect fibrin clot formation.

ACQUIRED DEFICIENCY STATES	INHIBITION OF CLOT FORMATION
Liver disease	Heparin
Vitamin K deficiency	Lupus anticoagulants*
Oral anticoagulants	Neutralizing factor inhibitors
Amyloidosis	Non-neutralizing factor inhibitors

Acquired Deficiency States	Inhibition of Clot Formation
Consumptive coagulopathies	Macromolecules (e.g., dextran)
Hematin	Dysfibrinogenemia
Snake venoms	

Source: Brandt JT: Hemostasis. In Howanitz JH, Howanitz PJ (eds): Laboratory Medicine: Test Selection and Interpretation. New York, Churchill Livingstone, 1991, p 517.
*Generally not associated with bleeding.

These disorders can be differentiated with special studies.

Some acquired disorders are complex and may be seen initially with simultaneous bleeding and microvascular thrombosis.

Disorder	Laboratory Manifestations
Disseminated intravascular co-agulation	Thrombocytopenia, low fibrinogen, long PT, long APTT, increased FDPs, low AT III
Thrombotic thrombocytopenic purpura; hemolytic uremic syndrome	Thrombocytopenia, microangiopathic peripheral blood film, normal fibrinogen, normal AT III
Liver disease	Long PT, normal to low fibrinogen, low AT III

Source: Brandt JT: Hemostasis. In Howanitz JH, Howanitz PJ (eds): Laboratory Medicine: Test Selection and Interpretation. New York, Churchill Livingstone, 1991, p 522.
PT = prothrombin time; APTT = activated partial thromboplastin time; FDPs = fibrin degradation products; AT III = antithrombin III.

BIBLIOGRAPHY

AbuRahma AF, Boland JP, Witsberger T: Diagnostic and therapeutic strategies of white clot syndrome. Am J Surg 162:175, 1991.
  Describes two kinds of heparin-induced thrombocytopenia and makes management recommendations.
Burns ER, Lawrence C: Bleeding time: A guide to its diagnostic and clinical utility. Arch Pathol Lab Med 113:1219, 1989.
  Concludes that determining a preoperative bleeding time is only necessary in the presence of a positive history of bleeding.
Colon-Otero G, Cockerill KJ, Bowie EJ: How to diagnose bleeding disorders. Postgrad Med 90:145, 1991.
  Recommends practical strategies.
Erban SB, Kinman JL, Schwartz JS: Routine use of the prothrombin and partial thromboplastin times. JAMA 262:2428, 1989.
  Believe that routine screening using the PT and APTT is inappropriate.
Remaley AT, Kennedy JM, Laposata M: Evaluation of the clinical utility of platelet aggregation studies. Am J Hematol 31:188, 1989.
  Concludes that platelet aggregation studies are rarely useful in the diagnosis of specific bleeding disorders.

Santhosh-Kumar CR, Yohannan MD, Higgy KE, et al: Thrombocytosis in adults: Analysis of 777 patients. J Intern Med 229:493, 1991.
Studied the causes of thrombocytosis found on routine blood counts.

Spivak JL: Disseminated intravascular coagulation; Nonthrombocytopenic purpura; Thrombocytopenia; Thrombocytosis; Thrombotic thrombocytopenic purpura. In Spivak JL, Barnes HV (eds): Manual of Clinical Problems in Internal Medicine, 4th ed. Boston, Little, Brown & Co, 1990, pp 306, 342, 377, 382, 385.
Good discussion of diagnosis and management with annotated key references.

Suchman AL, Griner PF: Coagulation disorders. In Panzer RJ, Black ER, Griner PF (eds): Diagnostic Strategies for Common Medical Problems. Philadelphia, American College of Physicians, 1991, p 478.
Believe that no coagulation tests are indicated before surgery in asymptomatic individuals without risk factors.

Suchman AL, Griner PF: Common uses of the activated partial thromboplastin time and prothrombin time. In Sox HC Jr (ed): Common Diagnostic Tests: Use and Interpretation, 2nd ed. Philadelphia, American College of Physicians, 1990, p 227.
Recommends against routine screening of medical or surgical patients who have no clinical findings of a bleeding disorder.

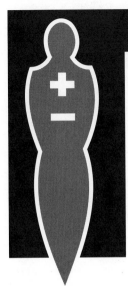

CHAPTER 10

ACID-BASE DISTURBANCES AND ELECTROLYTE DISEASES

Classifying Fluid Volume, Acid-Base, Electrolyte, and Osmolality Disorders by Laboratory Tests

1.   In patients with clinical findings of a fluid volume, acid-base, and/or electrolyte disorder, assess the patient's hydration (hypovolemia, normovolemia, hypervolemia) using clinical findings and request appropriate laboratory tests: arterial blood gas analysis and determinations of serum electrolytes and serum osmolality.

The American College of Physicians does not recommend arterial blood gas analysis and determinations of serum electrolytes and serum osmolality for screening but does recommend these tests to diagnose and manage patients with a serious illness in which these analytes are affected. In intensive care units Canadian researchers developed guidelines for measuring blood gases in stable patients every 12 hours with greater reliance on pulse oximetry—special indications were outlined for unstable patients and those being weaned from a ventilator. In the emergency department 10 clinical criteria are helpful in deciding which patients need serum electrolyte determinations: poor oral intake, vomiting, chronic hypertension, taking a diuretic, recent seizure, muscle weakness, age 65 years or older, alcoholism, abnormal mental status, and recent history of an electrolyte abnormality.

Acid-base and electrolyte disorders occur in the context of fluid volumes that are decreased (hypovolemic disorders), normal (normovolemic disorders), or increased (hypervolemic disorders). The history and physical examination are the mainstays of evaluating the existence and causes of volume disorders.

Clinical findings of hypovolemia include increased thirst, decreased sweating and skin turgor, decreased mucous membrane secretions, oliguria with increased urine concentration, central nervous system (CNS) depression, weakness and muscle cramps, decreased blood pressure, increased pulse rate, and decreased central venous pressure. Clinical findings of normovolemia include well-being and alertness and normal vital signs, skin turgor, thirst, sweating, and urination. Clinical findings of hypervolemia include edema, shortness of breath, paroxysmal nocturnal dyspnea, orthopnea, and hypertension.

2.   Evaluate the tests.

Arterial blood gas and serum electrolyte and osmolality tests should be evaluated with an understanding of the body fluid compartments. Body water comprises approximately 60% of body weight and is divided into two compartments: the intracellular fluid (ICF) compartment and the extracellular fluid (ECF) compartment. The ICF compartment contains two thirds of the body water and the ECF compartment one third. The ECF, in turn, is divided into two parts: the intravascular part (blood) and the extravascular part. Thus in a healthy 70-kg man total body water is approximately 40 L, of which 25 L are intracellular and 15 L extracellular, of which 5 L are blood. Since the normal hematocrit value is 40% to 45%, total plasma (serum) volume is 2.75 to 3 L. Arterial blood gas and serum electrolyte analyses are determined using whole blood and serum, respectively, and the test results represent concentrations in blood and serum, respectively. Assumptions about changes in the ICF are based on blood and serum gas and electrolyte concentrations interpreted in the context of a clinical assessment of body fluid volume. In addition to acid-base and electrolyte balance, serum osmolality must be considered. Besides the maintenance of normal pH and electrolyte concentrations, the serum osmolality is maintained in a narrow range of 275 to 295 mOsmol/kg. Serum osmolality is either measured directly or calculated using the following formula:

Calculated osmolality (mOsm/kg) =

$$2X \text{ Sodium (mEq/L)} + \frac{\text{Glucose (mg/dL)}}{18} + \frac{\text{Urea nitrogen (mg/dL)}}{2.8}$$

or

Calculated osmolality (mOsm/kg) =

$$2X \text{ Sodium (mmol/L)} + \text{Glucose (mmol/L)} + \text{Urea nitrogen (mmol/L)}$$

3.   Interpret arterial blood gas, serum electrolyte, and serum osmolality test results in the context of body fluid status.

Arterial blood gas, electrolyte, and serum osmolality test results should be interpreted in the context of a clinical assessment of fluid volume status. This is especially true of serum sodium, which is the principal cation of the ECF, in which 95% of total body sodium is located. For example, hyponatremic disorders can occur with decreased extracellular volume, normal extracellular volume (adrenal or thyroid insufficiency, redistribution of sodium), or increased extracellular volume (congestive heart failure, cirrhosis, nephrotic syndrome). Potassium is the principal cation of the ICF, which contains nearly 90% of total body potassium.

BIBLIOGRAPHY

Beck LH, Kassirer JP: Serum electrolytes, serum osmolality, blood urea nitrogen, and serum creatinine; and Raffin TA: Indications for arterial blood gas analysis. In Sox HC Jr (ed): Common Diagnostic Tests: Use and Interpretation, 2nd ed. Philadelphia, American College of Physicians, 1990, pp 367, 100.
  Review of arterial blood gas analysis, serum electrolytes, serum osmolality, blood urea nitrogen, and serum creatine with American College of Physicians guidelines for appropriate use.
Kapsner CO, Tzamaloukas AH: Understanding serum electrolytes: How to avoid mistakes. Postgrad Med 90:151, 1991.
  Discusses pitfalls in the interpretation of serum electrolytes.
Lowe RA, Arst HF, Ellis BK: Rational ordering of electrolytes in the emergency department. Ann Emerg Med 20:16, 1991.
  Summarizes 10 clinical criteria that should trigger a request for serum electrolytes.
Roberts D, Ostryzniuk P, Loewen E, et al: Control of blood gas measurements in intensive-care units. Lancet 337:1580, 1991.
  Canadian guidelines for blood gas analysis in intensive care units that produced favorable outcomes and decreased costs.

Acid-Base Disorders

1.   For patients with clinical findings of an acid-base disorder, request arterial blood gas analysis and serum electrolyte determinations.

2.   Evaluate the test results.

a.   Determine pH status.

A pH >7.45 indicates alkalosis, and a pH <7.35 indicates acidosis.

b.   Determine whether the primary process is respiratory or metabolic (or both).

Consider whether the pH is above or below 7.4. The process or processes that caused it to shift to that side are the primary abnormalities.

PRIMARY UNCOMPENSATED ALKALOSIS

- Respiratory alkalosis: pH >7.45 and partial pressure of carbon dioxide (Pco_2) <35 mmHg
- Metabolic alkalosis: pH >7.45 and bicarbonate >23 mEq/L (23 mmol/L)

PRIMARY UNCOMPENSATED ACIDOSIS

- Respiratory acidosis: pH <7.35 and Pco_2 >45 mmHg
- Metabolic acidosis: pH <7.35 and bicarbonate <18 mEq/L (18 mmol/L)

   c.   **Calculate the serum anion gap. Use the anion gap reference range established by your laboratory.**

$$\text{Anion gap} = \text{Sodium} - (\text{Chloride} + \text{Bicarbonate})$$

An anion gap that is increased more than 15 mEq/L (15 mmol/L) may indicate metabolic acidosis. An anion gap increased more than 25 mEq/L (25 mmol/L) always indicates metabolic acidosis.

   d.   **Check the degree of compensation.**

In a patient with metabolic acidosis compensation is evidenced by a decreasing arterial Pco_2 and an increasing arterial pH, whereas in a patient with metabolic alkalosis compensation is shown by an increasing arterial Pco_2 and a decreasing arterial pH.

In a patient with respiratory acidosis compensation occurs secondary to an increasing serum bicarbonate concentration and an increasing arterial pH, whereas in a patient with respiratory alkalosis compensation occurs because of a decreasing serum bicarbonate concentration and a decreasing arterial pH.

   e.   **Determine whether there is a 1:1 relationship between anions in blood.**

PURE INCREASED ANION GAP METABOLIC ACIDOSIS

Every one-point increase in anion gap should be accompanied by a 1 mEq/L (1 mmol/L) decrease in bicarbonate.

PURE NORMAL ANION GAP METABOLIC ACIDOSIS

Every 1 mEq/L (1 mmol/L) increase in chloride should be accompanied by a 1 mEq/L (1 mmol/L) decrease in bicarbonate.

3.   Interpret test results in the context of clinical findings.

SIMPLE ACID-BASE DISORDERS

Respiratory Alkalosis. With respiratory alkalosis the pH is greater than 7.45, and the Pco_2 is less than 35 mmHg. A normal bicarbonate concentration means lack of metabolic compensation, which indicates an acute respiratory alkalosis, whereas a low bicarbonate concentration with a normal pH value means metabolic compensation, which indicates a chronic respiratory alkalosis.

The causes of acute respiratory alkalosis include anxiety; lung disease, with or without hypoxia; drug use (salicylates, catecholamines, progesterone); mechanical ventilation; CNS disease; pregnancy; sepsis; and hepatic encephalopathy.

Metabolic Alkalosis. With metabolic alkalosis the pH is greater than 7.45, and the serum bicarbonate concentration is greater than 23 mEq/L (23 mmol/L). The Pco_2 can rise modestly in compensation for metabolic alkalosis, with a concomitant decrease in pH, but Pco_2 >55 mmHg probably is not just compensatory, and an additional primary respiratory abnormality should be excluded.

The causes of metabolic alkalosis with respiratory compensation include disorders in which the urinary chloride level is low and disorders in which the urinary chloride concentration is normal or high. Conditions in which the urinary chloride concentration is low include vomiting; nasogastric suction; diuretic use in the past; and posthypercapnia. Conditions in which the urinary chloride level is normal or high include excess mineralocorticoid activity (Cushing's syndrome, Conn's syndrome, exogenous steroids, licorice ingestion, increased renin states, Bartter's syndrome); current or recent diuretic use; and excess alkali administration.

Respiratory Acidosis. With respiratory acidosis the pH is less than 7.35 and the Pco_2 greater than 45 mmHg. A normal bicarbonate concentration means lack of metabolic compensation, which indicates acute respiratory acidosis, whereas a high bicarbonate concentration with a normal pH level means metabolic compensation, which indicates chronic respiratory acidosis.

The causes of acute respiratory acidosis include CNS depression (drugs, CNS event); acute airway obstruction (in upper airway, laryngospasm, bronchospasm, severe pneumonia, pulmonary edema); thoracic cage injury (flail chest, ventilator dysfunction); neuromuscular disorders (myopathies, neuropathies); and impaired lung motion (hemothorax, pneumothorax).

The causes of chronic respiratory acidosis with metabolic compensation include chronic lung disease (obstructive or restrictive); chronic respiratory center depression (central hypoventilation); and chronic neuromuscular disorders.

Metabolic Acidosis. With metabolic acidosis the pH is less than 7.35 and the serum bicarbonate concentration less than 18 mEq/L (18 mmol/L). Low Pco_2 with a normal pH level indicates respiratory compensation.

The causes of metabolic acidosis are divided into those with an increased anion gap and those without an increased anion gap. Those with an increased anion gap include ketoacidosis (diabetic, alcoholic); renal failure; lactic acidosis (anion gap not always increased); rhabdomyolysis; and toxins (methanol, ethylene glycol, paraldehyde, salicylates). Those without an increased anion gap include gastrointestinal bicarbonate loss (diarrhea, ureteral diversions); renal bicarbonate loss (renal tubular acidosis, early renal failure, carbonic anhydrase inhibitors, aldosterone inhibitors); hydrochloric acid administration; and posthypocapnia.

MIXED ACID-BASE DISORDERS

See the article by Haber listed in the references for a discussion of the following mixed acid-base disorders:

- Respiratory alkalosis and metabolic acidosis
- Metabolic acidosis and metabolic alkalosis
- Respiratory alkalosis, metabolic acidosis, and metabolic alkalosis
- Respiratory acidosis, metabolic acidosis, and metabolic alkalosis
- Anion gap and nonanion gap metabolic acidoses

BIBLIOGRAPHY

Blanke RV: High anion-gap acidosis with high osmolal gap. In Tietz NW, Conn RB, Pruden EL (eds): Applied Laboratory Medicine. Philadelphia, WB Saunders Co, 1992, p 335.
   Case discussion of the use of anion and osmolar gaps in a patient with ethylene glycol poisoning.
Haber RJ: A practical approach to acid-base disorders. West J Med 155:146, 1991.
   Excellent discussion of how to diagnose simple and complex acid-base disorders.
Iberti TJ, Leibowitz AB, Papadakos PJ, et al: Low sensitivity of the anion gap as a screen to detect hyperlactatemia in critically ill patients. Crit Care Med 18:275, 1990.
   Increased anion gap is not always present in patients with lactic acidosis.
Rutecki GW, Whittier FC: Acid-base interpretation: Five rules, and how they help in everyday cases. Consultant 31:44, 1991; and Rutecki GW, Whittier FC: Acid-base interpretation: Five rules, and how they simplify complex cases. Consultant 31:19, 1991.
   Two short practical articles on acid-base interpretation.
Winter SD, Pearson JR, Gabow PA, et al: The fall of the serum anion gap. Arch Intern Med 150:311, 1990.
   Found that modern analyzers often generate anion gaps that are significantly lower than in the past (e.g., 3 to 11 mEq/L (3 to 11 mmol/L) compared with 8 to 16 mEq/L (8 to 16 mmol/L).

Hyponatremia

1.   In patients with hyponatremia or clinical findings of hyponatremia exclude pseudohyponatremia before proceeding with the workup. Request measurements of serum sodium and osmolality and urinary sodium.

Hyponatremia is a hypotonic disorder caused by a depressed serum sodium concentration, below 136 mEq/L (136 mmol/L). The clinical features are produced by brain swelling secondary to a decreased extracellular fluid osmolality. Causes include excessive total body water and sodium depletion. When evaluating hyponatremia, it is important to assess whether the patient is hypervolemic, hypovolemic, or euvolemic. Usually, hyponatremia is modest, the patient is asymptomatic, and if the cause is removed (e.g., diuretic therapy), the condition improves. On the other hand, severe symptomatic hyponatremia (serum sodium <120 mEq/L [120 mmol/L]) is rare but constitutes a medical emergency. The findings progress from lethargy, weakness, and somnolence to seizures, coma, and death as the hyponatremia worsens.

Hyponatremia is the most common serum electrolyte abnormality in hospitalized patients. It often occurs in patients in the intensive care unit. A serum sodium determination can be used to detect or verify hyponatremia, and serum osmolality and urinary sodium measurements are useful to determine the cause of hyponatremia. Dietary sodium, excessive water intake, and drugs may be contributing factors.

Using serum or heparinized plasma for the test is satisfactory, but avoid the use of sodium salts of heparin. When obtaining the blood specimen, avoid significant hemolysis, which can decrease the serum sodium concentration because of a dilutional effect from the erythrocyte fluid. Lipemia or hyperproteinemia can artifactually decrease the serum sodium concentration, causing a normal serum sodium value to appear decreased.

2. Evaluate the test results.

Exclude pseudohyponatremia (euosmolar hyponatremia) caused by severe hyperlipidemia or hyperproteinemia. If the serum is lipemic or the proteins are high (>10 g/dL [>100 g/L]), determine whether there is a significant osmolar gap, according to the following formula*:

$$\text{Osmolar gap} = \text{Measured osmolality} - \text{Calculated osmolality}$$

(See the first problem in this chapter for formula for calculated osmolality.)

If the measured osmolality is normal and there is a significant osmolar gap, the low serum sodium concentration is probably an artifact caused by lipemia or hyperproteinemia. This is true only if there are no unusual osmotically active substances (ethanol, methanol, mannitol) in the serum because these substances can also cause an increased osmolar gap (see the discussion of alcoholism in Chapter 1).

---

*All units in milliosmoles per kilogram (mOsm/kg).

The occurrence of pseudohyponatremia is method dependent; that is, it is observed when the serum sodium concentration is measured by flame photometry but not when sodium is measured in undiluted serum using an ion-specific electrode. It is important to recognize pseudohyponatremia because it requires no therapy.

A high serum glucose concentration (an osmotically active, low-molecular solute) can also contribute to a low serum sodium value because every 100 mg/dL (5.55 mmol/L) rise in the serum glucose concentration produces a decrease of approximately 1.6 mEq/L (1.6 mmol/L) in the serum sodium value. This phenomenon can also occur with mannitol. Increased serum immunoglobulins, particularly IgG (but also IgA), can behave as cations and cause a decreased serum sodium value and a low anion gap (anion gap =

$Na - [Cl + HCO_3])$. Normally the gap is 8 to 16 mEq/L (8 to 16 mmol/L) and is composed of phosphate, sulfate, organic acids, and proteinate. Myeloma patients have a mean anion gap of 6.8, whereas the mean gap of controls is 9.4. Patients with monoclonal gammopathy of undetermined significance have a mean anion gap of 9.1.

In a patient with true hyponatremia the severity of the clinical findings correlates with the degree of hyponatremia and the rate at which it develops. With acute hyponatremia the clinical features generally appear when the serum sodium concentration falls to 120 mEq/L (120 mmol/L) or less. With chronic hyponatremia clinical manifestations are far less common, even when the serum sodium concentration is below 120 mEq/L (120 mmol/L).

According to a recent study, neither hyponatremic encephalopathy nor its therapy is commonly associated with central pontine myelinolysis.

3. Interpret test results in the context of clinical findings.

HYPOVOLEMIC HYPONATREMIA

Gastrointestinal and renal loss of fluid and electrolytes can lead to hypovolemic hyponatremia. Gastrointestinal disorders include external loss (diarrhea, vomiting, external fistula) or internal loss (pancreatitis, peritonitis, internal fistula). Renal disorders include excessive diuretic use, osmotic diuresis, postobstructive diuresis, bicarbonaturia, renal salt wasting, ketonuria, and adrenocortical hormone deficiency.

The skin can be a site of substantial loss of fluid and electrolytes in long distance runners and patients with severe burns or widespread skin disorders.

A urinary sodium concentration >20 mEq/L (20 mmol/L) is characteristic of renal causes of hypovolemic hyponatremia, and a urinary sodium concentration <10 mEq/L (10 mmol/L) occurs with extrarenal disorders (gastrointestinal or skin disorders).

NORMOVOLEMIC HYPONATREMIA

Certain drugs can cause normovolemic hyponatremia, and severe emotional stress (acute psychosis) and physical stress (trauma, surgery) are additional causes. Two endocrine disorders, hypothyroidism and hypopituitarism, may be seen initially as normovolemic hyponatremia. The syndrome of inappropriate antidiuretic hormone (SIADH) secretion can also cause normovolemic hyponatremia. This syndrome has been described with a variety of cancers, pulmonary disorders, and brain disorders.

In a patient with normovolemic hyponatremia the urinary sodium concentration is typically greater than 20 mEq/L (20 mmol/L).

HYPERVOLEMIC HYPONATREMIA

Edematous patients often have hypervolemic hyponatremia (congestive heart failure, cirrhosis, nephrotic syndrome, renal failure).

In patients with cardiac failure, cirrhosis, and the nephrotic syndrome the urinary sodium concentration is less than 10 mEq/L (10 mmol/L), and in patients with acute or chronic renal failure the urinary sodium concentration is greater than 20 mEq/L (20 mmol/L).

An additional cause of hypervolemic hyponatremia is transurethral resection of the prostate: 5% to 10% of patients develop hypervolemic hyponatremia because of absorption of the irrigate solution used to clear the operative field.

BIBLIOGRAPHY

DeVita MV, Gardenswartz MH, Konecky A, et al: Incidence and etiology of hyponatremia in an intensive care unit. Clin Nephrol 34:163, 1990.
   Patients in the intensive care unit often develop hyponatremia.
Ellis RE, Carmichael JK: Hyponatremia and volume overload as a complication of transurethral resection of the prostate. J Fam Pract 33:89, 1991.
   Awareness of this complication of prostate surgery is important.
Flanagan NG, Ridway JC, Irving AG: The anion gap as a screening procedure for occult myeloma in the elderly. J R Soc Med 81:27, 1988.
   Anion gap can be used to detect myeloma.
Kassirer JP, Kopelman RI: Case 36—Leaving no stone unturned. In Kassirer JP, Kopelman RI: Learning Clinical Reasoning. Baltimore, Williams & Wilkins, 1991, p 192.
   Discusses clinical reasoning in a patient with confusion and disorientation secondary to hyponatremia.
Moran SM, Jamison RL: The variable hyponatremic response to hyperglycemia. West J Med 142:49, 1985.
   High serum glucose concentration can cause hyponatremia.
Schrier RW, Briner VA: The differential diagnosis of hyponatremia. Hosp Pract 25:29, 1990.
   Review of the differential diagnosis and management of patients with hyponatremia.
Tien R, Arieff AI, Kucharczyk W, et al: Hyponatremic encephalopathy: Is central pontine myelinolysis a component? Am J Med 92:513, 1992.
   Disproves the association between hyponatremia and central pontine myelinolysis.

Hypernatremia

1. For patients with hypernatremia or clinical findings of hypernatremia, request measurements of serum sodium and serum and urinary osmolality.

Hypernatremia is a hypertonic disorder caused by an elevated serum sodium concentration, above 146 mEq/L (146 mmol/L). The clinical features are produced by brain shrinkage secondary to an increased extracellular fluid osmolality. Causes include too much dietary salt, too little dietary water, or excessive water loss from the body. Clinical findings of hypernatremia progress from somnolence, confusion, and coma to respiratory paralysis and death as the hypernatremia worsens.

A serum sodium determination can be used to verify the presence of hypernatremia, and serum and urinary osmolality measurements are helpful to determine the cause of the hypernatremia. The specimen collection and handling considerations are the same as for hyponatremia.

2.   Evaluate the test results.

The severity of the clinical findings correlates with the degree of hypernatremia and the rate at which it develops. In a patient with acute hypernatremia symptoms may appear when serum osmolality exceeds 320 to 330 mOsm/kg, and respiratory arrest may occur when osmolality exceeds 360 to 380 mOsm/kg.

In diabetics nonketotic hyperglycemic hyperosmolality can produce clinical findings similar to hypernatremia. In patients with this syndrome the serum sodium concentration is initially low, but as hyperglycemia rapidly depletes extracellular water, the serum sodium concentration becomes normal or increases. Depressed consciousness is uncommon when serum osmolality is less than 350 mOsm/kg, whereas virtually all patients with serum osmolalities exceeding 400 mOsm/kg are comatose.

3.   Interpret test results in the context of clinical findings. Antidiuretic hormone (ADH) levels may be normal or low.

HYPERNATREMIC STATES WITH NORMAL ADH LEVELS

Hypovolemia With Excessive Water Loss

• Impaired water intake: if water intake is impaired and falls behind normal insensitive loss through the skin, lungs, and gastrointestinal tract, the ECF volume contracts, and the serum sodium concentration increases. The individual is appropriately thirsty, and the urine is highly concentrated.
• Excessive water loss: excessive water loss can occur through the skin (excessive sweating, burns), the lungs (hyperventilation), and the gastrointestinal tract (vomiting, diarrhea). The ECF volume contracts, the serum sodium concentration increases, and the urine is highly concentrated.
• Osmotic diuresis: osmotic diuresis secondary to glucose, urea, mannitol, or radiocontrast dye excretion can result in a contracted ECF volume and a high serum sodium concentration.

Normovolemia With Altered Regulation of Osmolality. Diseases of the hypothalamus and pituitary can alter the regulation of thirst and ADH secretion, causing a high serum sodium concentration. The ECF volume is normal.

Hypervolemia With Excessive Sodium Loads. A high serum sodium concentration and an expanded extracellular volume can occur with excessive salt intake either by ingestion or parenteral administration. Also, in patients with primary hyperaldosteronism and Cushing's syndrome, the serum sodium concentration may be high with an expansion of the ECF volume.

HYPERNATREMIC STATES WITH LOW ADH LEVELS

Central Diabetes Insipidus. A variety of diseases (traumatic, neoplastic, infiltrative, infectious, vascular) and drugs (ethanol, opiate antagonists, α-adrenergic agents, phenytoin) can affect the hypothalamus and cause an ADH deficiency, which results in polyuria with dilute urine. If the ADH deficiency is severe enough, the serum sodium concentration can increase.

Nephrogenic Diabetes Insipidus. Unresponsiveness of the kidneys to ADH can be either congenital or acquired. The congenital form is X linked and rare. The acquired forms (electrolyte disorders, drugs, tubulointerstitial nephropathies) are common.

BIBLIOGRAPHY

Felig P, Johnson C, Levitt M, et al: Hypernatremia induced by maximal exercise. JAMA 248:1209, 1982.
Intense exercise can cause hypernatremia.
Snyder NA, Feigal DW, Arieff AI: Hypernatremia in elderly patients: A heterogeneous, morbid, and iatrogenic entity. Ann Intern Med 107:309, 1987; and Beck LH, Lavizzo-Mourey R: Geriatric hyponatremia. Ann Intern Med 107:768, 1987.
Discusses the increased susceptibility to hypernatremia in the elderly.

Hypokalemia

1. For patients with hypokalemia or clinical findings of hypokalemia, request measurement of serum potassium. Consider measuring serum magnesium and the 24-hour urinary excretion of potassium to document potassium depletion of renal origin.

Hypokalemia is a depressed serum potassium concentration, below 3.5 mEq/L (3.5 mmol/L). The normal serum potassium concentration is greater than the plasma concentration because of the release of platelet potassium during clotting. The most significant effects of hypokalemia relate to neuromuscular and electrocardiographic disturbances. The causes of hypokalemia include diuretic therapy, inadequate potassium intake, excessive renal loss, excessive gastrointestinal loss, and shifts from the extracellular fluid to the intracellular fluid. Clinical features include skeletal muscle weakness and paralysis and derangements in cardiac conduction.

A serum potassium determination can be used to verify the presence of hypokalemia, and measurement of urinary potassium excretion is useful to determine the cause of hypokalemia. Hypomagnesemia is common in patients with hypokalemia and, unless corrected, impairs repletion of intracellular potassium.

Serum or heparinized plasma can be used for potassium measurements, but avoid the use of potassium salts of heparin and promptly separate the serum or plasma from the cells. Opening and closing of the patient's fist before venipuncture should be avoided since muscle action can increase the potassium concentration by 10% to 20%.

2.   Evaluate the test results.

At serum potassium concentrations of 2 to 2.5 mEq/L (2 to 2.5 mmol/ L), muscular weakness can occur. At lower values, areflexic paralysis can occur, with associated respiratory insufficiency and death. Electrocardiographic manifestations of hypokalemia include sagging of the ST segment, depression of the T wave, and elevation of the U wave. With marked hypokalemia, the T wave becomes progressively smaller, and the U wave shows increasing amplitude. In patients treated with digitalis, hypokalemia can precipitate serious arrhythmias. Recently hypokalemia has been reported to cause tetany.

3.   Interpret test results in the context of clinical findings.

Certain drugs such as the thiazides or loop diuretics and theophylline can cause a decreased serum potassium concentration. Other causes of hypokalemia include **inadequate intake and excessive renal loss,** for example, from mineralocorticoid excess (primary or exogenous and licorice ingestion), Bartter's syndrome, osmotic diuresis, chronic metabolic alkalosis, certain antibiotics (penicillin-like antibiotics, amphotericin B, gentamicin), renal tubular acidosis, leukemia, Liddle's syndrome, and magnesium depletion; **excessive gastrointestinal loss,** for example, from vomiting, diarrhea, secretory diarrhea, chronic laxative abuse, villous adenoma, fistulas, ureterosigmoidostomy, and inflammatory bowel disease; and **shifts from the extracellular fluid to the intracellular fluid,** for example, from hypokalemic periodic paralysis, ingestion of barium salts, insulin therapy, vitamin B_{12} therapy, epinephrine administration, and metabolic alkalosis.

BIBLIOGRAPHY

Ault MJ, Geiderman J: Hypokalemia as a cause of tetany. West J Med 157:65, 1992.
  Hypokalemia—A cause of tetany that has not previously been reported.
Kaplan NM: How bad are diuretic-induced hypokalemia and hypercholesterolemia? Arch Intern Med 149:2649, 1989.
  Believes that diuretic-induced hypokalemia may be harmful.
Kassirer JP, Kopelman RI: Case 2—Hypothesis triggering by an expert. In Learning Clinical Reasoning. Baltimore, Williams & Wilkins, 1991, p 53.
  Discusses clinical reasoning in a patient with weakness secondary to hypokalemia.
Schnaper HW, Freis ED, Friedman RG, et al: Potassium restoration in hypertensive patients made hypokalemic by hydrochlorothiazide. Arch Intern Med 149:2677, 1989.
  Many patients taking 50 mg per day of hydrochlorothiazide require triamterene or supplementary potassium to maintain their serum potassium in the normal range.
Shannon M, Lovejoy FH Jr: Hypokalemia after theophylline intoxication. Arch Intern Med 149:2725, 1989.
  Hypokalemia is common after theophylline intoxication.
Siegel D, Hulley SB, Black DM, et al: Diuretics, serum and intracellular electrolyte levels, and ventricular arrhythmias in hypertensive men. JAMA 267:1083, 1992.
  Potassium concentrations should be carefully monitored during initiation of diuretic therapy.

Stein JH: Hypokalemia: Common and uncommon causes. Hosp Pract 23:55, 1988.
  Reviews the differential diagnosis of hypokalemia.
Whang R, Whang DD, Ryan MP: Refractory potassium repletion: A consequence of magnesium deficiency. Arch Intern Med 152:40, 1992.
  Serum magnesium should be measured routinely in patients with hypokalemia.

Hyperkalemia

1. In patients with hyperkalemia or clinical findings of hyperkalemia measure serum potassium. Exclude artifactual hyperkalemia before proceeding with the workup.

Hyperkalemia is an increased serum potassium concentration, above 5.1 mEq/L (5.1 mmol/L). Normally, the serum potassium concentration is higher than the plasma concentration because of release of platelet potassium during clotting. The most important clinical features of hyperkalemia relate to alterations of cardiac excitability as manifested in the electrocardiogram and depression of neuromuscular activity. Causes of hyperkalemia include excessive intake of potassium, decreased excretion, and shifts of potassium from cells to extracellular fluid. Clinical features include cardiotoxic effects and depressive effects on skeletal muscle.

A serum potassium determination can be used to verify the presence of hyperkalemia. Artifactually high serum potassium concentrations can result from thrombocytosis, leukocytosis, hemolysis, fist clenching during phlebotomy, and allowing the serum to remain in contact with the clot for prolonged periods of time at room temperature. The specimen collection and handling issues are the same as for hypokalemia.

2. Evaluate the test results.

The earliest electrocardiographic manifestation of hyperkalemia consists of peaked T waves and occurs when the serum level exceeds 6.5 mEq/L (6.5 mmol/L). Between 7 and 8 mEq/L (7 to 8 mmol/L) the PR interval is prolonged, followed by a loss of P waves and widening of the QRS complex. When the serum potassium concentration exceeds 8 to 10 mEq/L (8 to 10 mmol/L), a sine wave pattern can develop, and cardiac asystole fibrillation can occur. Rarely skeletal muscle weakness and flaccid paralysis occur. Hyponatremia and acidosis can potentiate the adverse effects of hyperkalemia on the heart.

3. Interpret test results in the context of clinical findings.

Certain drugs such as antineoplastic agents, heparin, and potassium-sparing diuretics (triamterene, spironolactone) can cause an increased serum potassium concentration. Other causes of hyperkalemia include **excessive intake,** especially in patients with renal insufficiency; **increased cellular release of potassium** such as with metabolic acidosis, trauma, burns, rhabdomyolysis, hemolysis, lysis of tumor tissue, drug usage (succinylcholine, digitalis, beta-blocking agents), hyperosmolality, insulin deficiency, hyperkalemic periodic paralysis, severe muscle disease, and hypothermia; and **decreased renal excretion of potassium** such as in acute oliguric renal failure, chronic renal failure, renal tubular disorders, Addison's disease, and hypoaldosteronism.

BIBLIOGRAPHY

Alvo M, Warnock DG: Hyperkalemia. West J Med 141:666, 1984.
 Discussion of the diagnosis and management of hyperkalemia.
Don BR, Sebastian A, Cheitlin M, et al: Pseudohyperkalemia caused by fist clenching during phlebotomy. N Engl J Med 322:1290, 1990.
 Another cause of pseudohyperkalemia.
Schaller M-D, Fischer AP, Perret CH: Hyperkalemia: A prognostic factor during acute severe hypothermia. JAMA 264:1842, 1990.
 In patients with serum hypothermia, marked hyperkalemia >10 mEq/L (10 mmol/L) is considered an index of irreversibility.

Hypophosphatemia

1.   For patients with hypophosphatemia or clinical findings of hypophosphatemia, request a serum phosphorous measurement. Consider obtaining a complete blood count (CBC), serum glucose, urea nitrogen, creatinine, calcium, and creatine kinase determinations, liver function tests, and a urinalysis.

Hypophosphatemia is a decreased serum phosphorus concentration, below 2.7 mg/dL (0.87 mmol/L). The clinical features are produced by a deficiency of phosphorus for key metabolic functions, including the integrity of all cell membranes, the structure of nucleic acids, a second messenger in endocrinology (cAMP, cGMP), the release of oxygen by hemoglobin (2,3-DPG), and the buffering of urine. Causes include decreased intake of phosphate, impaired absorption of phosphate, excessive renal loss of phosphate, and a shift of phosphate into cells and bone. The diagnosis of hypophosphatemia and its cause depends on obtaining appropriate tests in the context of the clinical findings. These findings include red cell dysfunction and hemolysis, leukocyte dysfunction, platelet dysfunction, weakness, congestive cardiomyopathy, rhabdomyolysis, central nervous system dysfunction, and possible hepatic dysfunction.

A serum phosphorus determination can be used to verify the presence of hypophosphatemia, and a CBC is useful to detect hemolytic anemia and thrombocytopenia. The serum glucose value can be used to assess carbohydrate homeostasis; and serum urea nitrogen and creatinine determinations and a urinalysis are useful to determine renal function. Cardiac or skeletal muscle damage can be detected by a serum creatine kinase assay, and hepatic function can be assessed with liver function tests.

Use of serum or heparinized plasma is satisfactory for testing. The patient should be fasting since postprandial phosphorylation of glucose decreases serum phosphorus. Collection of the specimen after an overnight fast is ideal. Hemolysis and prolonged contact with the clot should be avoided because they will increase serum phosphorus.

2. Evaluate the test results.

It is unusual for hypophosphatemia to cause metabolic disturbances at concentrations >1.5 mg/dL (0.48 mmol/L). If you decide to treat with parenteral phosphate, be careful because hyperphosphatemia can result and ionized calcium can fall, producing tetany or convulsions. In addition, metastatic calcification of soft tissues can occur.

3. Interpret test results in the context of clinical findings.

Certain drugs such as steroids, diuretics, and insulin can decrease serum phosphorus. Vomiting and prolonged nasogastric suction can limit phosphorus intake. Other causes include **decreased phosphate intake; impaired phosphate absorption** with drugs (aluminum- and magnesium-containing antacids) and in alcoholism; **excessive renal loss of phosphate** such as in patient's with hyperparathyroidism, renal tubular disorders, acidosis, and severe trauma; and **intracellular shifts of phosphate** such as in patients with carbohydrate loading, hyperalimentation, respiratory alkalosis, rapid tumor growth, the nutritional recovery syndrome, burns, treatment of respiratory failure (severe asthma and obstructive pulmonary disease), and the hungry bone syndrome (hypocalcemia and hypophosphatemia caused by bone remineralization after parathyroid surgery).

BIBLIOGRAPHY

Brasier AR, Nussbaum SR: Hungry bone syndrome: Clinical and biochemical predictors of its occurrence after parathyroid surgery. Am J Med 84:654, 1988.
  Hypophosphatemia can occur after parathyroid surgery.
Daily WH, Tonnesen AS, Allen SJ: Hypophosphatemia: Incidence, etiology, and prevention in the trauma patient. Crit Care Med 18:1210, 1990.
  Severe hypophosphatemia occurs frequently after severe trauma, probably because of urinary loss.
Laaban J-P, Grateau G, Psychoyos I, et al: Hypophosphatemia induced by mechanical ventilation in patients with chronic obstructive pulmonary disease. Crit Care Med 17:1115, 1989.
  After starting mechanical ventilation, patients with acute respiratory failure should be monitored to detect hypophosphatemia.
Laaban J-P, Waked M, Laromiguiere M, et al: Hypophosphatemia complicating management of acute severe asthma. Ann Intern Med 112:68, 1990.
  After starting therapy, patients with acute severe asthma should be monitored to detect hypophosphatemia.

Scott MG: Inorganic phosphorus: Review of methods. Chicago, American Society of Clinical Pathologists, Core Analyte PTS 92-5 (PTS-63), 1992.
Discusses causes of hypophosphatemia.

Singhal PC, Kumar A, Desroches L, et al: Prevalence and predictors of rhabdomyolysis in patients with hypophosphatemia. Am J Med 92:458, 1992; and Knochel JP: Hypophosphatemia and rhabdomyolysis. Am J Med 92:455, 1992.
Clinical study and editorial that describe the common occurrence of rhabdomyolysis in hypophosphatemia patients.

Yu GC, Lee DBN: Clinical disorders of phosphorus metabolism. West J Med 147:569, 1987.
Discusses the diagnosis and management of hypophosphatemia.

Zaloga GP: Hypophosphatemia in COPD: How serious—And what to do? J Crit Illness 7:364, 1992.
Patients with COPD are vulnerable to hypophosphatemia.

Hyperphosphatemia

1.   For patients with hyperphosphatemia, request a determination of serum phosphorus. Consider obtaining measurements of serum calcium, glucose, urea nitrogen, and creatinine and a urinalysis.

Hyperphosphatemia is an elevated serum phosphorus concentration, above 4.5 mg/dL (1.45 mmol/L). When severe, hyperphosphatemia can contribute to the acidosis of uremia, further reduce the concentration of ionized calcium in the extracellular fluid, and cause metastic calcification in soft tissues. The most common cause is renal insufficiency. Hyperphosphatemia produces no direct clinical symptoms.

A serum phosphorous determination can be used to verify the presence of hyperphosphatemia. Hypocalcemia may be a clue to hypoparathyroidism; hyperglycemia a clue to acromegaly; and urea nitrogen and creatinine values and urinalysis indications of renal insufficiency.

Specimen collection and handling are the same as for hypophosphatemia.

2.   Evaluate the test results.

Hyperphosphatemia can indirectly produce tetany by lowering serum calcium levels. With rapid elevations of serum phosphorus, hypocalcemia and tetany can occur with a serum phosphorous concentration as low as 6 mg/dL (1.94 mmol/L), a concentration that, if reached more slowly, has no detectable effect on serum calcium levels.

3.   Interpret test results in the context of clinical findings.

Certain drugs such as steroids and thiazides can increase the serum phosphate concentration. If truly large amounts of phosphate are administered orally, parenterally, or rectally, hyperphosphatemia can occur, even in the presence of normal renal function. **Other causes of hyperphosphatemia** include increased tubular reabsorption (hypoparathyroidism, pseudohypoparathyroidism, acromegaly, hyperthyroidism, tumoral calcinosis), transcellular shifts (acidosis), cell lysis (rhabdomyolysis, hemolysis, chemotherapy, malignant pyrexia), and miscellaneous factors (e.g., familial intermittent hyperphosphatemia).

BIBLIOGRAPHY

Scott MG: Inorganic Phosphorus: Review of methods. Chicago, American Society of Clinical Pathologists, Core Analyte PTS 92-5 (PTS-63), 1992.
  Discusses causes of hyperphosphatemia.
Yu GC, Lee DBN: Clinical disorders of phosphorus metabolism. West J Med 147:569, 1987.
  Discusses the diagnosis and management of hyperphosphatemia.

Hypomagnesemia

1. For patients with hypomagnesemia or clinical findings of hypomagnesemia, request measurements of serum magnesium, calcium, and potassium.

Hypomagnesemia is a depression of the serum magnesium concentration to below 1.3 mEq/L (0.65 mmol/L). It is more common than hypermagnesemia and usually occurs as a component of a more complex deficiency state. Low levels of magnesium ions cause hyperirritability of nerves and muscles with manifestations in the neuromuscular, cardiovascular, and gastrointestinal systems. Causes of hypomagnesemia include decreased absorption from dietary sources, increased loss from the body, and internal redistributions. Clinical manifestations include lethargy, weakness, irritability, short attention span, fainting, convulsions, and Chvostek's and Trousseau's signs. There may be anorexia, nausea, vomiting, paralytic ileus, and cardiac arrhythmias.

In the context of other electrolyte disorders, physicians should consider hypomagnesemia, which can be detected or verified by a serum magnesium determination. Measurements of calcium and potassium can be helpful because hypocalcemia and hypokalemia frequently accompany hypomagnesemia. The hypocalcemia and hypokalemia are resistant to treatment unless the hypomagnesemia is corrected first. Routine determinations of serum magnesium are unnecessary in patients with uncomplicated hypertension who are receiving triamterene-containing diuretics or low-dose (50 mg/day or less) hydrochlorothiazide.

2. Evaluate the test results.

Clinical findings increase in number and severity as the serum magnesium level becomes progressively decreased. Values of 1.2 mEq/L (0.60 mmol/L) or lower are associated with weakness, irritability, tetany, and convulsions.

3. Interpret test results in the context of clinical findings.

Certain drugs such as diuretics and digoxin can cause hypomagnesemia. Other causes include **decreased absorption from dietary sources** such as with a low magnesium diet, inhibition of absorption by ethanol, malabsorption, uremia, and a selective defect in magnesium absorption (rare); **increased magnesium loss** such as with gastrointestinal disorders (diarrhea) and renal disorders (tubular defects); and **internal redistribution of magnesium** such as with acute pancreatitis and increased loss into bone.

BIBLIOGRAPHY

Kroenke K, Wood DR, Hanley JF: The value of serum magnesium determination in hypertensive patients receiving diuretics. Arch Intern Med 147:1553, 1987.
It is not necessary to measure serum magnesium routinely in patients receiving low-dose hydrochlorothiazide.
Reinhart RA: Magnesium metabolism: A review with special reference to the relationship between intracellular content and serum levels. Arch Intern Med 148:2415, 1988.
Discusses the diagnosis and management of hypomagnesemia.
Shechter M, Hod H, Marks N, et al: Beneficial effect of magnesium sulfate in acute myocardial infarction. Am J Cardiol 66:271, 1990.
Cardioprotective effect of adequate magnesium deserves additional study.
Varsou A, Papadimitiou JC, Koch TR, et al: Occurrence of abnormal serum magnesium concentrations in uremic and nonuremic patients treated with digoxin. Laboratory Medicine 21:226, 1990.
Patients receiving digoxin therapy frequently develop hypomagnesemia.
Whang R, Ryder KW: Frequency of hypomagnesemia and hypermagnesemia: Requested vs routine. JAMA 263:3063, 1990.
Hypomagnesemia frequently is not suspected by physicians.

Hypermagnesemia

1. In patients with hypermagnesemia or clinical findings of hypermagnesemia measure serum magnesium, urea nitrogen, creatinine, calcium, and potassium.

Hypermagnesemia is an elevation of the serum magnesium concentration above 2.1 mEq/L (1.05 mmol/L). The magnesium ion exerts a depressive effect on the neuromuscular junction, and the clinical manifestations of hypermagnesemia are related to toxic effects on the central nervous and cardiovascular systems. Hypermagnesemia occurs in patients with renal insufficiency who ingest excessive amounts of magnesium, such as in magnesium-containing antacids. It can result from parenteral administration of magnesium, such as in the treatment of acute hypertension. Clinical manifestations include hypotension and cardiac arrhythmias. The cardiotoxicity of magnesium is aggravated by hypocalcemia, hyperkalemia, acidosis, digitalis therapy, and renal insufficiency (beyond its effect on the magnesium level).

In the context of other electrolyte disorders, physicians should consider hypermagnesemia, which can be detected or verified by a serum magnesium determination. Measurements of calcium and potassium can be helpful because of the synergistic effects of hypocalcemia and hyperkalemia. Serum urea nitrogen and creatinine determinations are useful to assess renal function.

2.   Evaluate the test results.

The cardiac effects of magnesium usually begin at values >10 mEq/L (5 mmol/L) and consist of peripheral vasodilation with hypotension, depression of the cardiac conduction system, bradyrhythmias, and cardiac arrest in asystole, with more serious effects at higher levels (e.g., asystole at levels >25 mEq/L [12.50 mmol/L]). Occasionally patients develop cardiotoxicity at 4.5 to 5.5 mEq/L (2.25 to 2.75 mmol/L).

3.   Interpret test results in the context of clinical findings.

Certain drugs such as magnesium-containing medications can increase the serum magnesium concentration. **Another common cause of hypermagnesemia** is renal insufficiency. Miscellaneous causes of mild hypermagnesemia include Addison's disease, diabetic ketoacidosis, hypothyroidism, pituitary dwarfism, lithium therapy, viral hepatitis, and the milk-alkali syndrome.

BIBLIOGRAPHY

Kassirer JP, Kopelman RI: Case 33—Post hoc, ergo propter hoc. In Learning Clinical Reasoning. Baltimore, Williams & Wilkins, 1991, p 180.
  Discusses clinical reasoning in a patient with flaccid quadraplegia secondary to hypermagnesemia.
Reinhart RA: Magnesium metabolism: A review with special reference to the relationship between intracellular content and serum levels. Arch Intern Med 148:2415, 1988.
  Discusses the diagnosis and management of hypermagnesemia.
Varsou A, Papadimitiou JC, Koch TR, et al: Occurrence of abnormal serum magnesium concentrations in uremic acid and nonuremic patients treated with digoxin. Laboratory Medicine 21:226, 1990.
  Patients taking digoxin may develop abnormal serum magnesium values.
Whang R, Ryder KW: Frequency of hypomagnesemia and hypermagnesemia: Requested vs routine. JAMA 263:3063, 1990.
  Hypermagnesemia frequently is not suspected by physicians.

GENERAL BIBLIOGRAPHY

Bakerman S: ABC's of Interpretive Laboratory Data, 2nd ed. Greenville, NC, Interpretive Laboratory Data, Inc, 1984.

Branch WT Jr (ed): Office Practice of Medicine, 2nd ed. Philadelphia, WB Saunders Co, 1987.

Cogan MG: Fluid and Electrolytes: Physiology and Pathophysiology. Norwalk, Conn, Appleton & Lange, 1991.

Cotran RS, Kumar V, Robbins SL: Robbins Pathologic Basis of Disease, 4th ed. Philadelphia, WB Saunders Co, 1989.

Friedman RB, Young DS: Effects of Disease on Clinical Laboratory Tests, 2nd ed. Washington, DC, American Association for Clinical Chemistry Press, 1989.

Henry JB (ed): Clinical Diagnosis and Management by Laboratory Methods, 18th ed. Philadelphia, WB Saunders Co, 1991.

Hoffman R, Benz EJ Jr, Shattil SJ, et al (eds): Hematology: Basic Principles and Practice. New York, Churchill Livingstone, 1991.

Howanitz JH, Howanitz PJ (eds): Laboratory Medicine: Test Selection and Interpretation. New York, Churchill Livingstone, 1991.

Kjeldsberg CR (ed): Practical Diagnosis of Hematologic Disorders. Chicago, American Society of Clinical Pathologists Press, 1989.

Lippert H, Lehmann HP: SI Units in Medicine. Baltimore, Urban & Schwarzenberg, 1978.

Lott JA, Wolf PL: Clinical Enzymology: A Case-Oriented Approach. New York, Field, Rich & Associates, 1986.

Ravel R: Clinical Laboratory Medicine: Clinical Application of Laboratory Data, 5th ed. Chicago, Year Book Medical Publishers, 1989.

Rubenstein E, Federman DD (eds): Scientific American Medicine. New York, Scientific American, Inc, 1978-1992.

Speicher CE: The Right Test: A Physician's Guide to Laboratory Medicine, 1st ed. Philadelphia, WB Saunders Co, 1990.

Speicher CE, Smith JW: Choosing Effective Laboratory Tests. Philadelphia, WB Saunders Co, 1983.

Statland BE: Clinical Decision Levels for Lab Tests. Oradell, NJ, Medical Economics Books, 1983.

Tietz NW (ed): Clinical Guide to Laboratory Tests, 2nd ed. Philadelphia, WB Saunders Co, 1990.

Tietz NW, Conn RB, Pruden RL (eds): Applied Laboratory Medicine. Philadelphia, WB Saunders Co, 1992.

Wallach J: Interpretation of Diagnostic Tests: A Synopsis of Laboratory Medicine, 5th ed. Boston, Little, Brown & Co, 1992.

Watts NB, Keffer JH: Practical Endocrinology, 4th ed. Philadelphia, Lea & Febiger, 1989.

Wilson JD, Braunwald E, Isselbacher KJ, et al (eds): Harrison's Principles of Internal Medicine, 12th ed. New York, McGraw-Hill, 1991.

Wyngaarden JB, Smith LH Jr, Bennett JC: Cecil Textbook of Medicine, 19th ed. Philadelphia, WB Saunders Co, 1992.

Young DS: Effects of Drugs on Clinical Laboratory Tests, 3rd ed. Washington, DC, American Association for Clinical Chemistry Press, 1990.

Young DS: Effects of Drugs on Clinical Laboratory Tests (1991 Supplement to the 3rd ed). Washington, DC, American Association for Clinical Chemistry Press, 1991.

INDEX

Page numbers in *italics* refer to illustrations; page numbers followed by t refer to tables.

241

Borrelia burgdorfii infection (Lyme disease), 61-64
Botulism, 69t
Brief Michigan Alcoholism Screening Questionnaire, 46-48
Budd-Chiari syndrome (hepatic vein occlusion), 145
BUN (blood urea nitrogen/serum urea nitrogen). *See* Urinalysis; Urinary tract disease.

CAGE questionnaire for alcohol abuse, 47t, 48
Calcium disorder(s), 174-180. *See also* Endocrine disease(s).
 in coronary heart disease, 33
 in pregnancy, 26
Cancer, American Cancer Society screening recommendations for, 16t-17t
 hypercalcemia/hyperparathyroidism and, 176-180, 177t, 178t
 of cervix, 27-29
 of colon and rectum, 37-39
Candidiasis, 67t, 163
Carcinoembryonic antigen, in cervical cancer, 29
 in colorectal cancer, 39
Cardiovascular diseases, 30-36, 81-95
 acute myocardial infarction as, 81-85
 congestive heart failure as, 87-89
 coronary heart disease as, 30-36, 31t, 33t, 34t-35t
 digoxin monitoring in, 93-95
 hypertension as, 90-92
Case finding, 14t, 14-15. *See also* Screening.
CBC (complete blood count) with differential, as case-finding tool, 17
 automated methods for, 15
 in hematological diseases, 196-198, *197*
 red cell disorders and, 198t, 198-200, 199t
 white cell disorders and, 200-201, 201t
CD4 lymphocyte count, in AIDS/HIV, 56-58
CEA. *See* carcinoembryonic antigen.
Cerebrospinal fluid. *See* CSF assays.
Chancroid, 65t
Chemical food poisoning, 70t
Chinese restaurant syndrome, 70t
Chlamydia, 66t
 in respiratory infection, 97

Chlamydia (Continued)
 in urinary tract infection, 163, 164
Chloride disorders, in pregnancy, 26
Cholecystokinin. *See* CKK.
Cholescystitis, 116
Cholestasis, 131-132, 151-152
Cholesterol, in coronary heart disease screening, 30-36, 33t, 35t
 HDL cholesterol and, 32-33
 LDL cholesterol and, 33-36
 selected drug effects and, 33-34t
 total cholesterol measurement and, 30-32
 in pregnancy, 27
Chronic disease, anemia of, 204t, 205-206
Chronic obstructive pulmonary disease (COPD), 108-110
Cigarette smoking, 109
CK (creatine kinase), in acute myocardial infarction, 81-84
 in colorectal cancer, 39
 in pregnancy, 27
CKK (cholecystokinin) test, 125
Clinical decision making and problem solving, 4t, 4-6
Clostridium difficile, 121
Coagulopathies. *See* Bleeding disorders.
Coarctation of aorta, 91
Cocaine. *See* Drug abuse.
Complete blood count. *See* CBC and differential.
Congestive heart failure, 87-89
 digoxin monitoring in, 93t, 93-95
 hepatitis in, 145
Coombs' test, 214
COPD (chronic obstructive pulmonary disease), 108-110
Coronary heart disease, screening for hypercholesterolemia in, 30-36, 31t, 33t, 34t-35t. *See also* Cardiovascular disease.
Cortisol, in adrenal insufficiency, 193-194, 194t
Cosyntropin (rapid ACTH) test, 193, 194t
Creatine kinase. *See* CK.
Creatinine (serum), in pregnancy, 27
 in renal failure, 167
CSF (cerebrospinal fluid) analysis, 73-76
 contraindications to, 74
 in AIDS and HIV, 60
 indications for, 73
 in meningitis, 75
 in neurologic disorders, 75-76